Occupational Health

Department of Occupational Health and Safety
Central Manchester Healthcare NHS Trust
Cobbett House
Oxford Road
Manchester M13 9WL
Tel: 0161 276 4289

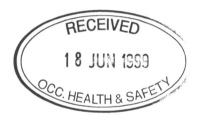

Occupational Health

J.M. Harrington CBE
BSc, MSc, FRCP, FFOM, FFOM(I), FACE, MFPHM
Professor of Occupational Health,
Institute of Occupational Health, University of Birmingham

F.S. Gill BSc, MSc, CEng, MIMinE, FIOH, Dip Occ Hyg, FFOM(Hon)
Consultant in Occupational Health

T.C. Aw MBBS, MSc, PhD, FFOM, FRCP(Canada), FRCP(Lond), FFOM
Senior Lecturer in Occupational Medicine,
Institute of Occupational Health, University of Birmingham

K. Gardiner BSc, PhD, Dip Occ Hyg, MIOH, MIOSH
Senior Lecturer in Occupational Hygiene,
Institute of Occupational Health, University of Birmingham

In collaboration with
Gillian Howard LLB, Dip Comp Lab Cantab
Employment Lawyer

Anne Spurgeon BSc, PhD, C Psychol
Senior Lecturer in Occupational Psychology,
Institute of Occupational Health, University of Birmingham

Stuart Whitaker MMedSc, PhD, RGN, RMN, OHNC MIOSH
Research Fellow, Institute of Occupational Health, University of Birmingham

Christine McRoy BA, ALA
Librarian and Information Officer,
Institute of Occupational Health, University of Birmingham

Fourth edition

**Blackwell
Science**

© 1983, 1987, 1992, 1998 by
Blackwell Science Ltd
Editorial Offices:
Osney Mead, Oxford OX2 0EL
25 John Street, London WC1N 2BL
23 Ainslie Place, Edinburgh EH3 6AJ
350 Main Street, Malden
  MA 02148 5018, USA
54 University Street, Carlton
  Victoria 3053, Australia
10, rue Casimir Delavigne
  75006 Paris, France

Other Editorial Offices:
Blackwell Wissenschafts-Verlag GmbH
Kurfürstendamm 57
10707 Berlin, Germany

Blackwell Science KK
MG Kodenmacho Building
7–10 Kodenmacho Nihombashi
Chuo-ku, Tokyo 104, Japan

First published 1983
Second edition 1987
Third edition 1992
Fourth edition 1998

Set by Semantic Graphics, Singapore
Printed and bound in Great Britain
at the University Press, Cambridge

DISTRIBUTORS

  Marston Book Services Ltd
  PO Box 269
  Abingdon, Oxon OX14 4YN
  (Orders: Tel: 01235 465500
          Fax: 01235 465555)

USA
  Blackwell Science, Inc.
  Commerce Place
  350 Main Street
  Malden, MA 02148 5018
  (Orders: Tel: 800 759 6102
          781 388 8250
          Fax: 781 388 8255)

Canada
  Login Brothers Book Company
  324 Saulteaux Crescent
  Winnipeg, Manitoba R3J 3T2
  (Orders: Tel: 204 837-2987)

Australia
  Blackwell Science Pty Ltd
  54 University Street
  Carlton, Victoria 3053
  (Orders: Tel: 3 9347 0300
          Fax: 3 9347 5001)

A catalogue record for this title
is available from the British Library
and the Library of Congress

ISBN 0-632-04832-8

For further information on
Blackwell Science, visit our website:
www.blackwell-science.com

Contents

Preface

A new edition of this little book has appeared at intervals of about 5 years — a sign from the publishers, we presume, of steady sales and therefore of continuing use. Nevertheless, the request for this fourth edition resulted in my canvassing a score of colleagues around the world for their views on content, as I feared that after a decade I risked mistaking the wood for the trees. I am most grateful to them for their unselfish and honest advice.

The result is a book of similar size and scope but with a complete overhaul of content and emphasis. To undertake this much larger task I have recruited two additional colleagues as major contributors. Ching Aw and Kerry Gardiner have taken to their task with enthusiasm and have added immeasurably to the quality of the final product.

The book now has much greater emphasis on prevention. In particular, the occupational hygiene component has been revamped as risk assessment and as hazard control, in an attempt to emphasise the multidisciplinary nature of modern occcupational health. Special sections have benefited from special authorship. Gillian Howard kindly agreed to write the chapter on law which is becoming such an important aspect of day-to-day practice. Stuart Whitaker has provided the section on audit, and Christine McRoy has undertaken the task of providing guidance on access of information. Finally, psychosocial aspects of the workplace have grown in importance in the past decade and now warrant a chapter on their own. Anne Spurgeon has succinctly summarised the issues.

In short, I hope this text helps the occupational health practitioner tackle the increasingly complex world of work and health, and that it will serve a useful purpose as we enter the next millennium.

Malcolm Harrington
Birmingham, 1998

Acknowledgements

Tackling a major overhaul of the book, recruiting two new contributors and adding three specialist sections has greatly increased the chore of secretarial support. This is particularly so as most of the main chapters were the result of contributions from more than one author. We then made matters worse for Caroline Baxter by putting the whole task in her hands. It is bad enough being my personal assistant, but she has undertaken a complex and difficult task with skill, fortitude and good humour. The fact that this edition appeared at all is largely due to her determination to keep us to deadlines and to insist on our continued coordination of effort. She has had meagre reward for a priceless contribution.

We are also grateful to Stuart Taylor of Blackwell Science for his support and advice as we planned this more complex fourth edition. He, too, has gently but firmly kept us on track for the delivery of the manuscript.

We are grateful to the Controller of The Stationery Office for permission to reproduce material on noise and hood design as well as the agreement to use the full list of UK Prescribed Diseases as published by the Department of Social Security. Finally, we would like to thank the Health and Safety Executive for permission to reproduce material from EH40/98 in section 4.1 (Crown copyright is reproduced with the permission of the Controller of Her Majesty's Stationery Office); Mike Griffin for permission to reproduce part of his chapter on noise in *Occupational Hygiene* (Blackwell Science, 1995) in section 5.4 and Richard Booth and Oxford University Press for permission to reproduce material from the *Oxford Textbook of Medicine* in section 10.3.

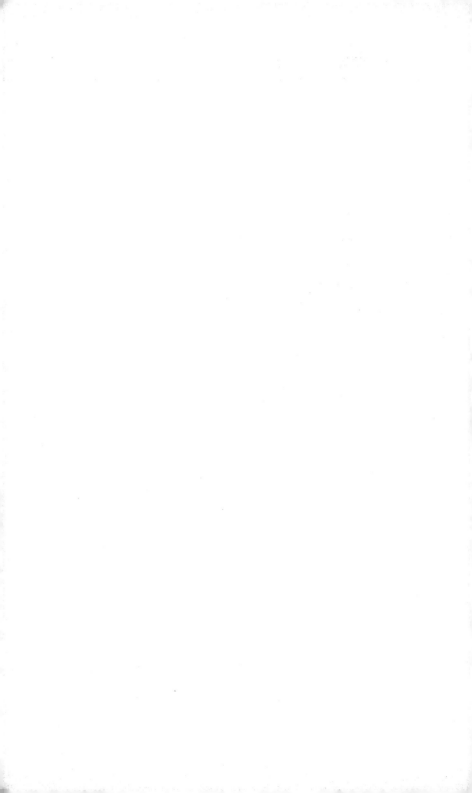

1 Introduction

1.1 What is occupational health?

Occupational health is a multifaceted activity concerned with the prevention of ill health in employed populations. This involves a consideration of the two-way relationship between work and health. It is as much related to the effects of the working environment on the health of workers as to the influence of the workers' state of health on their ability to perform the tasks for which they were employed. Its main aim is to prevent, rather than cure, ill health from wherever it arises in the workplace.

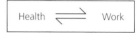

A joint International Labour Organization/World Health Organization (ILO/WHO) Committee defined the subject back in 1950 as: 'the promotion and maintenance of the highest degree of physical, mental and social well being of workers in all occupations'.

The relationship between the worker and the world of work is, necessarily, complex (Fig. 1.1). The worker brings to the place of work a pre-existent health status influenced by many factors — only some of which are under the workers' direct control. Any illness that occurs in the employed worker has to be viewed in this context. The health outcome could be caused by work, modulated by work or unrelated to it. Such a view of occupational health is, however, predominantly a medical model. Things are much more complex nowadays.

1.2 Who is involved in occupational health?

Traditionally, occupational health has been viewed as a clinical subject, implying that the dominant roles in prevention should be played by the physician and the nurse. The ILO/WHO definition from nearly half a century ago suggests that a broader view is necessary.

Thus the list of relevant professionals is extensive and includes:
- physicians;
- nurses;
- occupational hygienists;
- sociologists;
- toxicologists;
- psychologists;
- health physicists;

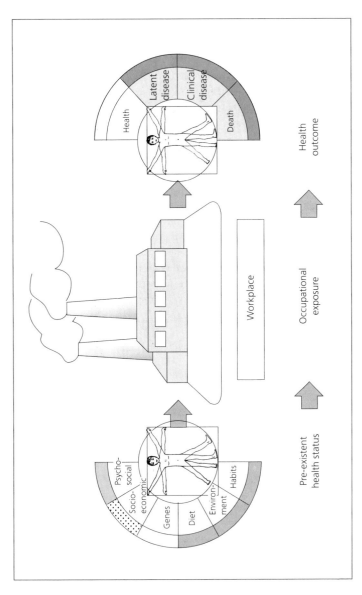

Fig. 1.1 The problems facing the practitioner attempting to establish a link between work and health. The new employee brings a legacy of genetic, social, dietary and environmental factors affecting health to the new workplace, which may influence his or her response to workplace hazards.

- microbiologists;
- epidemiologists;
- ergonomists;
- safety engineers;
- lawyers.

Yet, the ultimate responsibility for maintaining the health of the workforce rests with the employer, and, to a lesser extent, with the employee. This is the way most health and safety law is formulated. On the basis of this model, one can begin to view those involved as an even broader group. The 'stakeholders' would thus include a number of groups who, although they may not be professionally responsible for ensuring the well being of the workers, do have a crucial interest in the outcome (Fig. 1.2).

1.3 The world of work

The changing patterns of employment in world industry will have important implications for the future style and thrust of occupational health, as well as for the competence needed to deliver the goods. Across the world, the days of full-time, long-term employment in one industry for a worker with one set of skills are rapidly disappearing. The main features for the future seem to be:

- fragmented industry;
- smaller workforces;
- more mobile employees;
- multiskilled workers;
- greater use of subcontracted tasks;
- less job stability;
- less job security;
- more part-time work;
- more mechanised (? more dehumanised) workplaces.

1.4 The roles of the occupational health professional

In developed countries, many of the older occupational diseases have been controlled — or, at least, the means for controlling them are known. In such settings, the delivery of an effective occupational health service to employed people will become more complex and more difficult in the future — although with greater emphasis on control, there should be less to do in dealing with the injured or sick. These, after all, represent the 'failings' of an effective preventive programme.

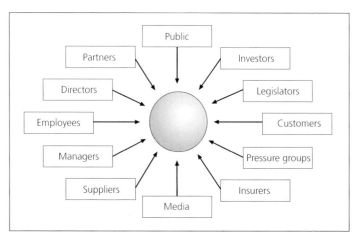

Fig. 1.2 The occupational health stakeholders.

Moreover, the influences of the stakeholder and the complexities of the employment scene have shifted the traditional emphasis away from the structure of 'see the health effect, diagnose the illness, find the cause' to the more proactive stance of 'control the exposure and monitor the effects'. In this model, the roles of the safety engineer and the occupational hygienist become more central, and now sit alongside the clinical aspects rather than being secondary to them. One further aspect of occupational health services is worth mentioning: in the market economies, there has been a shift towards demonstrating to employers the economic value to them of such a service. A recent UK Faculty of Occupational Medicine brochure listed the ways in which occupational physicians can help the employer to 'meet their obligations' under European health and safety legislation. These included:
• helping with company compliance with the law;
• advising on health and safety policy;
• assisting in the control of sickness absence;
• reviewing the fitness of employees' post sickness absence;
• managing rehabilitation;
• advising on fitness to work;
• managing access to first aid services;
• organising health promotion initiatives;
• designing and managing substance abuse programmes at work;
• advising on the management and alleviation of stress;

- advising employees for overseas travel on company business;
- assessing employees' eligibility for long-term disability benefits or retirement on health grounds.

The order of these functions is probably not random, and many might dispute the contents of this list and certainly the order. Nevertheless, it demonstrates the move towards delivering an economically attractive package to the employer. Whether this is what the employee needs is another matter. Indeed, one can dispute whether this medical model has real validity for the twenty-first century.

In developing countries, an occupational health service often starts with the provision of medical care for the workforce (akin to a general practice at the worksite, and often with provision for the workers' dependants) (see Chapter 2). In the newly emergent countries of Eastern Europe, the 'prophylactic' medical examination remains at the heart of the health care system in the workplace. Even in Poland — arguably the most advanced of this group of countries — the new Occupational Health Services Act of 1997 continues to place medical examinations at the core of the service activities.

Many of these functions will be performed by the occupational health nurse, who frequently works in isolation from any form of medical advice. Both physicians and nurses, however, have to be aware of their clinical limitations (either by training or by the fact that the employee is another physician's patient), and both also must see the workplace in the context of what goes on at the worksite (see Section 1.5).

Such a knowledge of the workplace activity and process is a central feature of the work of the occupational hygienist and (probably) the ergonomist. These professionals are in short supply, and few businesses employ their own. Yet, their role is to recognise and understand the complexities of the work process, the nature of the materials used, produced and disposed of and the methods of production. In addition, the hygienist is an expert in identifying the sources and measuring the concentrations and emissions of workplace contaminants to ensure that appropriate controls can be put in place.

The investigation of a putative link between a hazard and health effect requires a study of the populations exposed (a task for the epidemiologist), as well as a knowledge of the toxicological effects with the necessary accompaniment of a risk assessment (a task for the toxicologist).

Safety is often considered separately from health. This is inappropriate and counter-productive to the development and execution of an

integrated health and safety strategy to protect health in the workplace. The key functions of safety management are:
- policy and planning — determining safety goals and a plan of work to achieve these goals;
- the provision of a clear basis of responsibility and communication to achieve control;
- the identification and assessment of risks and the control measures necessary to counter such risks;
- the monitoring and review of these policies and practices.

Whilst safety engineers tend to concentrate on the mechanical aspects of the workplace process, a similar structure of activity and function could be established for all occupational health professionals.

Who does what then comes down to the resources available to the employer, as well as the hazards and risks inherent in the process. As industry becomes more fragmented, the large, company-financed, multidisciplinary teams will disappear as well. The role of independent consultant advisers will then come to the fore, but the integrated activity of several professional groups working together to achieve long-term goals could be lost.

Every professional providing occupational health advice and service must ensure that they have had the relevant training by professional bodies in their speciality which oversee competence. Training and education schemes are available for the main groups listed in Section 1.2. Furthermore, many of these bodies now insist upon programmes of continuing professional development for the career lifetime after successful completion of the examinations for competence.

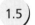

1.5 Industrial processes and health outcomes

Although there has been a dramatic rise in service industries in most developed countries, manufacturing industries remain a vital part of the economy. These industries, together with the extractive process and power generation enterprises, remain the main source of concern regarding workplace exposures leading to ill health and injury.

The main industries and their health effects are summarised in Table 1.1.

Whatever the workplace activity and whoever is responsible for managing health and safety, the means of protecting the workforce can be summarised as:
- hazard identification;
- risk assessment;

Table 1.1 *Industrial processes and potential occupational health exposures.* Industrial processes release hazardous substances and physical agents which can cause ill health to the operators if encountered in sufficiently large doses. Substances which can be inhaled will appear in the form of dusts, fibres, fumes, mists, micro-organisms, gases and vapours. Those which come into contact with the skin will be liquid or particulate. Substances can also be ingested or inoculated. Hazardous agents take the form of emissions of noise, heat, barometric pressure, electromagnetic waves and ionising particles which target one or more organs. The table lists some of these in relation to industry or occupation.

Industry	Substance	Main agents
Extractive		
Mining and quarrying of basic raw materials	Siliceous rock — fine crystalline silica dusts, radon, after gases from explosives, exhaust emissions from underground transport and machinery, carbon monoxide (CO), oxides of nitrogen (NO_x)	Noise, ionising radiation, heat, lack of light
Refining of the mineral	Crushed ores, metal fumes, sulphur dioxide (SO_2), arsine	Noise, heat, ? electromagnetic fields (EMFs)
Extracting fossil fuels	Coal dust, radon, drilling muds, petrochemicals, CO	Noise, heat, lack of light, high barometric pressure
Refining fossil fuels	Dust, SO_2, other gases dependent upon process, solvents, metallic catalysts, petrochemical vapours	Noise, heat, ionising radiation
Manufacturing		
Metal smelting	Metal fumes, CO, dust	Noise, heat, EMFs
Founding/forging	Silica dust, metal dusts, metal fumes, CO, phenols, ammonia	Noise, heat, ? EMFs
Plastics	Vinyl chloride, solvent vapours	Noise, heat
Fabrication	Welding fumes including hexavalent chromium (Cr^{VI}), resin vapours, isocyanates, grinding dusts	Noise
Finishing	Solvent vapours, isocyanates, chromic acid mist, acid mists, metal grinding dusts, chlorinated hydrocarbons	Noise
Woodworking	Wood dust, fungicides, phenol–formaldehyde resin	Noise

Continued on p. 10

Table 1.1 *Continued*

Industry	Substance	Main agents
Wood finishing	Solvent vapours, wood dust, biocides, fungicides	Noise
General assembly	Soldering, brazing and welding fumes, adhesive solvent vapours, cutting oils, acids, alkalis	Noise, heat, ? EMFs
Pottery and ceramics	Silica dust, dyes, glazes	Heat
Printing	Solvent vapours, photographic chemicals, acrylates	Noise
Textiles and clothing	Fibres, dyes, mordants, adhesive and stain solvents	Noise
Transfer of materials and process heating	Dusts, vapours, intermediate products, fugitive emissions, sometimes unknown substances	
Transport manufacture (road, rail, sea, air)	Soldering, brazing and welding fumes, adhesive solvent vapours, cutting oils, lead, acids, alkalis	Noise, heat, non-ionising radiation
Health care		
Drug manufacture	Active drug dusts and liquids, aerosol propellants, micro-organisms, food dusts	Extreme cold, noise, ionising and non-ionising radiation
Hospitals	Micro-organisms, sterilisers and preservatives, solvents, pesticides, vaccines, anaesthetic gases, chlorinated hydrocarbons, methyl methacrylate	Noise, ultrasound, ionising and non-ionising radiation
Community	Micro-organisms, pesticides, fungicides	
Research and quality control		
Laboratory work	Solvents, contact with chemicals, mircro-organisms, animal dusts, metals, rock dusts	Ionising radiation

Process	Agents	Physical factors
Food manufacture, preparation and sales		
Milling	Flour and grain dusts	Noise
Baking	Flour, cocoa and spice dusts	Heat
Milk products and fermentation	Protein dust, yeast spores, carbon dioxide (CO_2)	Heat and cold
Food preparation, storage, distribution and sales	Food dusts, vehicle exhaust gases	Heat, cold and extreme cold
Maintenance and repair		
Machinery and transport	Exhaust gases, solvents, welding, brazing and soldering fumes, grinding dusts, fuels, acids, alkalis	Noise, heat, cold, ionising radiation
Construction		
Building and surface works	Cement dust, rock dusts, resin vapours, welding fumes, fibres, paint and adhesive solvent vapours	Noise, cold or heat (geography-dependent)
Tunnelling	Rock dusts, resin vapours, explosive fumes, diesel fumes	Noise, heat, cold, high barometric pressure
Demolition	Welding fumes, surface coating vapours, asbestos and other fibres	Noise, cold
Heat and power generation		
Burning of fuel	Coal, silica and ash dust, CO, SO_2, vanadium, fumes of combustion, tar vapours	Noise, heat
Nuclear generation	Alpha (α) and beta (β) particles	Ionising radiation, heat, noise,
Agriculture		
Arable farming	Pesticides, herbicides, grain dust	Noise, heat, cold
Animal farming and veterinary work	Animal micro-organisms, vaccines, pesticides, animal dusts	Noise, heat, cold
Horticulture	Fungicides, pesticides, herbicides, hormones, vehicle exhaust gases	Heat, noise

....

- management intervention;
- control procedures;
- review and audit effectiveness.

1.6) Summary

The health of the employee at a place of work is the concern of many professional groups. There is a need to identify hazards be they physical, chemical, biological or psychosocial. Once identified, the risks to the workforce must be assessed and measures to control these risks must be instituted. Measuring the effectiveness of this process involves the monitoring of the workplace environment and the health status of the employees. Auditing the effectiveness of these measures and improving the control are never-ending processes.

The bottom line remains the health of the worker. This is what both the workers and employers desire — a healthy workforce at work. It follows that the culture of good health and safety policy and practice must pass from the professionals — and the management — to the workforce. When everyone at the workplace believes that such policies and practice are part of their responsibility, occupational health can be considered to have achieved its main goal.

1.7) The future

Such an ideal of the total 'ownership' of health and safety by all, managers and managed alike, may be some time distant — if it is achieved at all. Nevertheless, the occupational health professional needs to be looking for the newer emphases that will emerge in the next decade, as these will influence the content and style of their work. Apart from the shifts in workforce size, skills and structure mentioned in Section 1.3, there are several other influences that are now beginning to emerge, which could necessitate yet more shifts in the job content of the occupational health practitioner. These are some to start thinking about:

- public safety/consumer protection;
- public risk perceptions (and effective public risk communication);
- environmental impact of workplace process;
- leisure industry risks.

Finally, that which is probably destined to dominate our professional lives into the twenty-first century:

- PSYCHOSOCIAL HEALTH.

2 Occupational Health Services — an International Perspective

2.1 Delivery of occupational health services

Different models exist for the provision of occupational health in various countries, with the differences lying in the mix of occupational health professionals that make up the occupational health team, the range of services that they provide, the legislative requirements and framework and the perceived needs by workers and their employers. Some of the legislative and preventive activities are performed by government departments, whereas the provision of occupational health services for groups of workers is often organised by employers. The training of occupational health professionals is usually offered by academic centres or training institutes.

2.2 Developing countries

In many developing countries, such as in parts of Africa, South America and Asia, occupational health is provided as part of the general medical care for the workforce. In-house medical services are usually only available for larger companies, especially those belonging to multinational organisations. Larger companies employ more workers, have the resources to provide medical facilities for their workforce and often have occupational health policies and standards which apply to all their member companies world-wide. For developing countries, this model often places emphasis on the treatment of illnesses, whether occupational or non-occupational in origin, with fewer resources for occupational health prevention. Some companies even have their own private clinics and hospitals to care for local workers and their families. These clinical facilities also cater for the medical needs of the overseas expatriate staff and their families. One reason why companies often concentrate on treatment services is the limited availability and access to medical facilities in these countries.

Preventive occupational health functions are often organised as a separate safety (or health and safety) department, which increasingly includes environmental aspects in its remit. The model which relies on the availability of doctors, dentists, nurses, care assistants and other clinical staff has been described as providing 'family medicine in industry', rather than providing occupational health cover. Treatment-orientated medical services are the rule in countries such as Chile, where occupational physicians focus on the recognition and treatment of occupational disease, with less emphasis on workplace visits and assessments to identify potential hazards and to recommend corrective action.

2.3) Rapidly industrialising countries, e.g. Malaysia

In countries such as South Korea, Taiwan, Thailand and Malaysia (part of the group of countries often referred to as the 'tiger economies'), there has been rapid economic and industrial development. In these countries, increasing attention is being paid to occupational and environmental health issues. In recent years, especially during 1996 and 1997, many parts of South-East Asia (particularly Malaysia, Singapore and Indonesia) were affected by episodes of environmental haze which enveloped the major cities. This haze was accompanied by an increase in respiratory, eye and other health effects. The source of this haze was thought to be primarily the burning of vegetation and trees during the clearing of tropical forest areas for shifting agriculture, forestry or land development. Other possible contributors include traffic exhaust fumes, industrial activity and the El Niño weather phenomenon. Occupational health professionals in these countries are increasingly involved in advising on such matters of environmental and health concern. Governmental and quasi-governmental organisations have been formed to coordinate activity on occupational and environmental health.

The developments in occupational health in Malaysia can be used as an example of how occupational health services may be provided in an industrialising country. In Malaysia, the Workers and Environmental Health Unit of the Ministry of Health is a central government source for obtaining advice and information, with satellite government occupational health clinics being planned for different parts of the country. The Department of Occupational Safety and Health of the Ministry of Human Resources enforces occupational health and safety legislation. Much of this legislation has been derived from similar UK laws. A National Institute of Occupational Safety and Health has been established to provide training. General practitioners with an interest in occupational health have been appointed by the Social Security Organisation (SOCSO) to evaluate and forward claims for compensating occupational diseases. There are several avenues for training physicians in occupational medicine. These include local academic institutions and training establishments in other countries, such as Australia and Ireland. However, occupational health nursing and occupational hygiene training lag behind. In the private sector, some general practitioners provide clinical cover for factory workers through contracts with employers. The emphasis is on treatment, pre-employment assessments, sickness absence issues and return to work, with fewer opportunities for occupational hygiene assessments or preventive activities at the workplace. With the development of notification schemes for occupational diseases, and the agreement of uniform criteria for diagnosing such diseases, the preventive aspects of occupational health services will have greater emphasis in the future.

2.4 Developed countries

Many Western countries have a legal requirement for the provision of occupational health. The situation in Europe varies from country to country, although there have been attempts by the administration of the European Union (EU) to harmonise occupational exposure standards and requirements for occupational health provisions. Its approach has been to specify minimum standards for compliance by EU member states, but to allow higher standards to be promulgated by individual states if they wish. The EU has also established a European Agency for Health and Safety in Bilbao, Spain. There is also a European Foundation for the Improvement of Living and Working Conditions based in Dublin, Ireland.

In Austria, there is a legal requirement to employ company physicians for companies with 100 or more workers. In The Netherlands, an official occupational health service is mandatory for companies employing more than 500 workers, or those in specifically defined hazardous industries, e.g. the assembly of lead batteries or the manufacture of lead pigments. The occupational health services are mainly preventive in function. The activities are aimed at the early detection of occupational ill health, prevention of occupational disease, rehabilitation, reduction of sickness absence and health surveillance. The multidisciplinary staff employed include occupational physicians, nurses, occupational hygienists and physicians' assistants.

In Portugal, there is a legal requirement (since 1991) to provide occupational safety, hygiene and health services for private and public workplaces employing more than 250 workers. The services include safety officers, nurses, occupational physicians and worker representatives. Occupational hygienists are in short supply, and are rare as team members of these services in Portugal.

Greece has legislative provisions for occupational health services based on occupational health physicians and health visitors. The role and responsibilities of the health visitors are defined under statute. The focus of activity involves the health screening of workers. This includes pre-employment assessments and follow-up, as well as the investigation of workplace conditions.

In Italy, occupational health nursing is not as well developed a field as occupational medicine or occupational safety. The role of nurses in occupational health care is therefore limited. In occupational health services in Australia, physiotherapists are often part of the occupational health team.

In the UK, occupational health nurses and safety practitioners form one of the biggest professional groups in the provision of occupational health. The enforcement of health and safety legislation is the responsibility of a government agency — the Health and Safety Executive (HSE) — which is part of the Department of Environment, Transport and the Regions. It has hygienists, engineers, nurses and physicians amongst its ranks of inspectors. There is no legal requirement for occupational health services, although first aid provisions are mandatory. Recent regulations have required employers to appoint 'competent persons' to assist them in their health and safety duties. Doctors have to be appointed by the HSE for companies with workers exposed to workplace hazards such as lead, asbestos, ionising radiation, compressed air and certain chemicals listed in the Control of Substances Hazardous to Health Regulations 1994. The availability of occupational health services for workers is patchy, and often limited to those employed by larger organisations. More than 90% of workplaces, especially those with small numbers of employees, do not have occupational health cover. Where provided, occupational health services may be an in-house facility, or employers may rely on external contracted providers of occupational health care. Independent group occupational health services are organised on a regional or national level. An area of recent expansion in occupational health services is the National Health Service (NHS). Almost all hospitals in the NHS have some form of occupational health cover, which may be separate from, or may encompass, safety and environmental functions. There has been a gradual expansion of specialist occupational physician-led services for the health-care industry. The activities have still tended to be clinical, with considerable focus on biological hazards. Hygienists and ergonomists, employed as part of the occupational health team for health-care workers, are rare.

In France and Germany, the model used places emphasis on the requirement for the workforce to have periodic access to an occupational health service. The rationale is to allow a review of the health status of the workers, with the aim of detecting ill health early. If there is any indication that illness may be related to workplace factors, investigations and preventive action can follow. German law provides for preventive medical examinations for exposure to a variety of workplace hazards, including noise, ionising radiation and a list of chemical agents. Several million medical examinations are performed annually under these regulations.

The Scandinavian countries, e.g. Finland and Sweden, have systems for occupational health cover that are much admired. Finland has a National Institute for Occupational Health based in Helsinki, with satellite departments in other cities. The activities include research, training, clinical and investigative services. There are also active efforts by this institute to help in occupational health initiatives in developing countries in Africa and Asia. Finland has had an Occupational Health Care Act since 1979. This requires all employers to provide occupational health services for their employees.

In the USA, there is a variation between states in the provision of occupational health. In New York State, private occupational and environmental medicine services predominate, including mobile clinics, multispeciality clinics and other services invariably paid for by employers. New York State's occupational medicine clinics are developed as centres for the diagnosis of occupational disease, some with industrial hygienists attached. The hygienists are in a position to investigate the workplace with the cooperation of the employer and the unions. The diagnosis of a case of occupational disease is treated as a sentinel health event, which indicates a need to assess other coworkers exposed to similar workplace factors. The main government agency for enforcing occupational health and safety legislation in the USA is the Occupational Health and Safety Administration (OSHA) — part of the Department of Labor. Responsibility for research and health hazard evaluations lies with the National Institute for Occupational Safety and Health (NIOSH). This is one of the centres within the Centers for Disease Control and Prevention (CDC) — a public health agency belonging to the Department of Health and Human Services. Occupational exposure standards are produced by several organisations, including NIOSH and OSHA. However, the best-known standards are the threshold limit values and biological exposure indices produced by the American Conference of Governmental Industrial Hygienists (ACGIH) — a non-governmental independent professional organisation (despite its name). The standards are reviewed annually and revised as necessary. They are adopted by many countries outside the USA.

2.5 From clinical care to health promotion

Successful measures have been introduced to reduce workplace exposures and prevent occupational disease in some industries. These have mainly occurred in developed countries, and have resulted in occupational health attention being directed at more difficult targets for prevention, e.g. the reduction of stress, health promotion and activities aimed at strengthening the health status of workers. Occupational health departments in these countries may also place emphasis on general health promotion measures in addition to workplace assessment and health surveillance. Health promotion activities include the provision of facilities for regular exercise at the workplace, campaigns to reduce cigarette smoking, advice on the consumption of alcohol in moderation, safe driving and healthy diet. The rationale proposed for this approach is that, once traditional occupational diseases are prevented, the focus should shift to the improvement of the general health status of the workforce. Unfortunately, in some workplaces health promotion activities have been emphasised at the expense of efforts towards reduction and control of workplace hazards.

Thus, there are different systems available for the provision of occupational health care. Each system has its limitations and advantages, and what works in one industry or country may not be the best model for a different industry or country. The chosen model should be acceptable to both employees and employers, and should take into account the availability of trained occupational health professionals from different disciplines.

2.6 Occupational health services

The range of functions provided by occupational health services is given below.

2.6.1 Clinical occupational health activities

Pre-employment assessments
These vary from the use of a self-completed questionnaire to a full 'hands-on' clinical examination by a physician. The argument against the use of a questionnaire is that job applicants wanting to be employed may be somewhat economical with the truth when answering questions on the state of their health. This is especially the case when the denial of ever experiencing specific health problems is difficult to check and confirm. Full clinical examinations, however, are time consuming and have a low detection rate for relevant abnormalities. A compromise approach is to use an initial screening questionnaire, with a staged evaluation, first by an occupational health nurse, and then by an

occupational physician where indicated (further details of health assessments are discussed in Chapter 7). With legislation against disability discrimination in several countries, the whole issue of pre-employment assessment and its use is being reviewed.

Periodic medical examinations (including health surveillance)

These may be performed because of statutory requirements, or where clinically indicated for groups of workers exposed to specific hazards. In many countries, examples of statutory medical examinations include clinical examination of professional drivers, and examination and blood lead determination for workers exposed to lead compounds. Periodic examinations have also been advocated in health surveillance schemes for workers exposed to respiratory sensitisers, such as isocyanates. The health surveillance of specific groups, e.g. executives, is often in demand from employers and the executives themselves. This is based on the following assumptions: executive staff are expensive to employ, make critical decisions that can affect the success of the company, are time consuming to train and difficult to replace, and therefore should be placed in a system where there is periodic confirmation that they are in good health. Despite this, executive medical examinations are of questionable value. They are costly to perform, with a low detection rate of significant clinical abnormalities. It has also been argued that, if there is clinical value in such periodic assessments, they should be made available to other categories of staff.

Post sickness absence review

The rationale behind reviewing individuals with long-term sickness absence is to ensure that the cause of the illness has not affected their capacity to continue in their present job. It also allows any necessary adjustments to the workplace to be made to accommodate the individual on his/her return to work. For food industries, occupational health services often have the responsibility to ensure that workers are not still infectious before returning to handling food products, especially after a spell of diarrhoea and vomiting.

Immunisation

This is provided by occupational health departments for health-care workers and laboratory and research staff, or where the workforce includes many employees travelling abroad as part of their job duties. Travel to exotic locations requires that the necessary immunisations against communicable diseases are provided. Where this is performed by occupational health departments, it also involves general health advice for other infectious diseases, e.g. sexually transmitted diseases, and food-borne infections.

Health education and counselling

The encouragement of workers to look after their health in terms of healthy lifestyles, proper diets, avoidance of smoking, consumption of alcohol in moderation, adequate exercise and reduction of cardiovascular risk factors has been incorporated into the activities of many occupational health services. These efforts are aimed at using access to the workforce to reduce risk factors for diseases in general, together with steps to prevent occupational disorders.

Treatment

Part of the function of occupational health services may include first aid and minor treatment to the provision of full curative medicine facilities. The extent of clinical services within departments of occupational health varies from non-existent to the availability of dentists, chiropodists and opticians.

Rehabilitation

Occupational health staff can liaise with clinicians and worksite managers for the facilitation of rehabilitation and return to work. Familiarity with the workplace and job alternatives and an understanding of the illness or disability stand the occupational health staff in good stead for this activity.

2.6.2 Workplace assessments

It follows that, without exposure, there is no effect. Therefore, the evaluation of the workplace to eliminate or reduce exposure is critical in achieving the aims of the occupational health department. These tasks are usually carried out by occupational hygienists, who structure their work in terms of recognition, evaluation and control as follows.

Recognition

This is not really a function, but includes the understanding of the toxicology of contaminants or disease aetiology, the industrial process itself (and all of its hazards) and the law.

Evaluation

This often starts at the point of a walk-through survey, where a knowledge of the process/contaminant means that decisions can be made without recourse to measurements, and extends to situations in which sophisticated measurements and/or analytical techniques are necessary to quantify the contaminant with the required accuracy/precision.

Control

The most important attribute of any occupational health professional, but specifically an occupational hygienist, is to be able to improve the work environment. Occupational hygienists use their knowledge of disciplines, such as industrial chemistry, chemical engineering, ventilation design, etc., to try to ensure that the putative agent is either eliminated or controlled.

2.6.3 General advice and support

Advice on compensation

Where an occupational disease has been diagnosed, occupational health services are able to advise the patients on obtaining benefits through workers' compensation schemes.

Disaster planning and advice on dealing with chemical incidents

Planning committees for the development of procedures to deal with chemical spills, road and rail accidents with the discharge of chemicals into the environment and emissions from industrial sites often include staff from occupational health services. Occupational health professionals can facilitate communications with managers of industrial sites, and advise on the nature and extent of exposure, possible health effects and appropriate personal protective equipment for rescue and emergency crew.

Food hygiene

The provision of advice to food handlers and on precautions for the safe handling of food is an important role for occupational health services in the food industry. In addition to the need to ensure the health of the workforce, there is the additional requirement to ensure the safety of the food product.

Advice on environmental issues

Occupational health services are increasingly covering safety and environmental issues, such that some departments are now organised as safety, health and environment (SHE) services.

2.6.4 Other activities

Audit, quality assurance and evaluation
Part of the work of occupational health services involves compliance with internal and external quality standards. An audit or systematic, critical review of the structure, process and outcome can lead to steps to improve the quality of the service (see Chapter 10).

Worker protection and business protection
The challenge for occupational health services is to provide a balance of functions: detect and control workplace hazards early; recognise occupational disease without missing non-occupational illness; provide effective health surveillance; facilitate treatment, rehabilitation and return to work; and ensure that the business of the employer can be conducted safely without detriment to the health of the workforce.

3 Occupational Diseases

3.1

Historical perspective

People were subject to hazards in their daily life long before the Industrial Revolution and the advent of industrial workplaces. The vagaries of climate and food supply, not to mention the menace of the sabre-toothed tiger, provided prehistoric man with quite enough risks to health. True occupational hazards must have arrived, however, by the time of the Stone Age, as the knapping of flints produces small clouds of silica dust. Although our ancestors are unlikely to have lived long enough to die of silicosis, the fashioning of iron tools and the development of mining and smelting certainly increased the dangers for those so engaged.

Indeed, mining was recognised in ancient Egyptian times as being so hazardous that the job was reserved for slaves and criminals. It was not until Agricola (1494–1555) and Paracelsus (1493–1541) formally recorded these risks to employed mediaeval artisans that any real attention was paid to their plight. By the sixteenth century, mining had become a skilled occupation, and Agricola not only described the hazards, but prescribed some remedies, such as improvements to ventilation and mine shaft design, which were necessary to diminish the staggering death rate in the mines of Joachimstal and Schneeberg. The same Carpathian mountains are still mined today, but, instead of silver (used to make the Joachimstaler = taler = dollar), the ore extracted is uranium. This might explain the rampant 'consumption' noted by Agricola, as it was probably lung cancer caused by radioactive gases and dusts.

Nevertheless, the first general and authoritative treatise on diseases related to occupations was written by the physician to the D'Este family in Modena, Bernardino Ramazzini (1633–1714). His book, *De Morbis Artificium*, is still unparalleled as a source of classic descriptions of many occupational diseases, ranging from those of cesspit workers to those of the mirror silverers of Murano. His work was largely unread until the Industrial Revolution in Britain brought occupational diseases to the attention of large numbers of people. Child labour and the atrocious working conditions in the cotton mills of Lancashire shocked many late Georgians and early Victorians, and the first factory legislation was pushed through by philanthropic factory owners, such as Robert Owen, Michael Sadler, Anthony Astley Cooper (Earl of Shaftesbury) and Robert Peel, despite some stiff opposition.

In Britain, the first Act of 1802 was greatly weakened by amendments in Parliament, but it started the process of legislation to protect workers, which culminated in the Health and Safety at Work, etc. Act of 1974. In between these dates, successive Acts reduced the hours of work, particularly of women and young children, and the Act of 1833 established the factory inspectorate. Four inspectors were appointed to cover the whole country. Eleven years later, the inspectors were given the additional power to appoint certifying surgeons in each district to decide on the age of children. The advent of birth certification in 1836 eventually made that role redundant, but an embryonic industrial medical service had been born. Later Acts gave these surgeons other duties, including the investigation of industrial accidents and the certification of fitness for work.

In the USA, the first Child Labour Law was passed in the State of Massachusetts in 1835. Similar legislation followed in most European countries as the Industrial Revolution proceeded apace. By the turn of the twentieth century, the toxic effect of certain materials in widespread use in industry was sufficiently well recognised in Europe and North America to warrant their notification. This provided the power to investigate incidents of disease, with a view to prevention.

In Britain, the first agents so notified in 1895 were lead, phosphorus, arsenic and anthrax. The list later extended to some 16 diseases notifiable by law. The flood of notifications that emanated from the print factories, match works, smelters and slaughterhouses, in the nineteenth century, necessitated the appointment in 1898 of the first medical inspector of factories, Sir Thomas Legge (1863–1932). Legge is famous for many things, not least the furore over his resignation in 1919 due to the government's refusal to ratify an international convention prohibiting the use of white lead for the inside painting of buildings. His aphorisms, although sounding a little paternalistic to late twentieth century ears, are still worth citing.

1 Unless and until the employer has done everything (and everything is a lot), the workman can do little to protect himself.

2 If you bring an influence to bear external to the workman (i.e. one over which he can exercise no control), you will be successful and if you do not, or cannot, you will not be successful.

3 Practically all lead poisoning is due to inhalation.

4 All workers should be told something of the hazards of the materials they work with — if they find out for themselves it may cost them their lives.

5 Influences, useful up to a point but not completely effective when not external but dependent on the will or whim of workers, include respirators, goggles, gloves, etc.

Today, the task of providing occupational health services for all workers is still an unattained ideal, even in developed countries. Furthermore, although many of the older occupational diseases are controlled, new ones continue to surface. The need for continued control is essential, but the registration of occupational diseases and injuries is an imprecise tool, even in the most developed of countries.

3.2 The toll of occupational injuries and disease

3.2.1 Occupational injuries

Accidental injuries at work are common, but the precise numbers are unclear. The incidence of severe permanent injury is of the order of 20–100 per 100 000 employees per year. For high-risk occupations, such as the construction industry, perhaps one-quarter of the workforce has an accident each year. The consequent economic losses in production and work time amount to 3–5% of gross national product. For the 22 European members of the International Labour Organization (ILO), there were a reported 6 000 000 occupational accidents per year between 1987 and 1991, with 25 000 fatalities per year. These numbers are certainly underestimates of the true total, which is probably nearer 10 000 000 than 6 000 000. Clearly, there is much to do to diminish this appalling loss of productivity and quality of life.

3.2.2 Occupational diseases

Even for a seemingly well-developed region of the world, such as Europe, there are great variations in the quality and style of the reporting of occupational diseases, with reported incidences varying by one or even two orders of magnitude. Some of this reflects true differences, but it is believed that most of the variance is due to shortcomings in the reporting procedures. Countries with good registration systems report average rates of occupational disease at a level of 4–12 cases per 1000 employed, but there is great disparity between the lists of registrable occupational diseases between countries. The European Union (EU) is attempting to correct this, and has recently issued, in Recommendation 90/326/EEC, the suggestion that 30 diseases should form the core of reporting procedures (Table 3.1).

The list of 'prescribed' occupational diseases for the UK — which includes the 'Euro 30' — by and large is given in Section 3.5. For most countries with broadly comparable registration procedures, the commonest diseases are:

- musculoskeletal disorders;

Table 3.1 European Union core list of occupational diseases (Euro 30).

Chemical		Biological	Physical	
Inorganic	Organic		Dusts	Others
Cadmium	CS$_2$	Zoonoses	Asbestos†	Ionising
Chromium	Benzene	Viral hepatitis	Silica/silicate (plus	radiation
Mercury	Chlorine	Tuberculosis	lung effects of	Noise-induced
Manganese	Aromatics		sintered metal	hearing loss (NIHL)
Nickel	Polynuclear		Co, Sn, Va, C)	Heat cataract
Lead	aromatics*			Nerve pressure
	Isocyanates			Vibration‡ (plus
				dermatitis and
				asthma)

*Coal distillation. †Fibrogenic/carcinogenic. ‡Osteoarticular and hand–arm vibration syndrome (HAVS).

- noise-induced hearing loss;
- dermatitis;
- asthma;
- pneumoconiosis.

Intoxication or poisoning by metals or solvents is declining, whereas the rates for musculoskeletal disorders are rising. The numbers of new cases of the top 10 compensatable occupational diseases for the UK are listed in Table 3.2.

These numbers are known to be a gross underestimate of the true toll of occupational ill health. For example, for occupational dermatitis, there are about 400 cases reported for Industrial Disablement Benefit each year (Table 3.2), but a national voluntary reporting system for dermatologists and occupational physicians (EPIDERM) reports 10 times this number. A national survey of self-reported ill health for 1990, published 2 years ago (the Labour Force Survey), suggests that the number of dermatitis cases is 54 000 per year in England and Wales alone!

Indeed, the Labour Force Survey, although it might overestimate the real numbers for work-related or work-caused illness, gives a picture of the leading causes of concern in those questioned, and probably gives a reasonably accurate picture of the relative importance of different illnesses (Fig. 3.1). The 1995 survey has just been published (1998) and suggests similar results for the expanded study now including the whole of Great Britain. Moreover, the self-report data has been corroborated to some extent by general practitioner data.

3.2.3 Occupational mortality

In 1995, the latest Decennial Supplement on Occupational Mortality (and

Table 3.2 Top 10 prescribed diseases (new cases 1986–1995). (Source, Health and Safety Commission (HSC), 1996.)

Disease	1986	1987	1988	1989	1990	1991	1992	1993	1994	1995
Vibration white finger	641	1336	1673	1056	2601	5403	2369	1147	1425	1747
Pneumoconiosis	747	652	562	661	709	751	765	853	1006	860
Deafness	1179	1381	1261	1176	1128	1041	972	902	882	763
Tenosynovitis	619	376	322	294	423	556	649	911	800	787
Mesothelioma	305	399	479	441	462	519	551	608	583	685
Asthma	166	220	222	220	216	293	553	510	506	514
Dermatitis	785	464	386	285	301	434	411	419	392	368
Beat conditions	220	57	171	112	95	187	317	256	257	194
Bilateral pleural thickening	111	115	114	125	146	149	160	172	196	188
Cramp hand/forearm	—	—	11	14	18	44	52	116	135	116

Carpal tunnel syndrome, 277 (second year), 2584 (first year). Chronic bronchitis and emphysema, 5087 cases between August 13, 1993 and December 31, 1995.

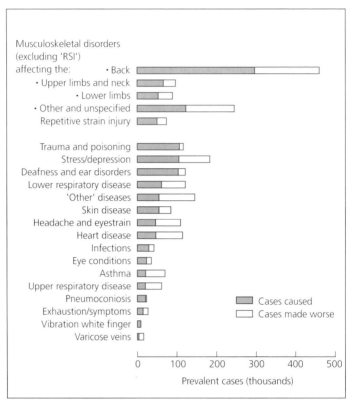

Fig. 3.1 Estimated 12-month prevalence of self-reported work-related illness, by disease category, in England and Wales, Spring 1990. Diseases are ordered by number of cases 'caused'; musculoskeletal conditions are treated as a group.

now cancer registrations) was published in the UK. This series has been produced for over 150 years, and is based on the population at census years, the last one being 1991. The two most important occupational causes of mortality in men were accidental injury and asbestos. Coal mine dust also figured prominently.

For women, the data are less reliable as many women do not have an occupation listed on the death certificate. For teachers, which account for 5% of all women where an occupation is reported, there are excess proportional mortality ratios (PMRs) for certain reproductive cancers, which are probably related to low rates of childbearing. For the health-related professions (10% of occupations reported), suicide rates are high — a comparable finding to men.

For cancer registrations (only 36% had a valid occupational code), some sites show certain occupations in excess as might be expected (e.g. woodworkers and nasal cancer, rubber workers and bladder cancer).

Such tabulations of large volumes of data come into their own as hypothesis generation exercises. For example, for lung cancer — the commonest form of cancer — and excluding PMRs below 125 which might arguably exclude the effect of smoking alone — significant excess PMRs were found for:

Job group	PMR	95% CI
Men		
Shunters and pointsmen	141	109–181
Undertakers	136	101–180
Metal drawers	130	100–166
Women		
Construction workers	269	154–437
Sales representatives	165	124–216
Publicans and bar staff	138	124–156
Plastics workers	306	123–631
Metal polishers	191	109–310
Carpenters	171	105–266
Vocational trainers, social scientists, etc.	180	101–297

CI, confidence interval.

Teachers in higher education (!) had no significantly elevated cancer risks based on registration, but had excess death rates for prostate cancer, brain cancer, lymphoma and certain leukaemias, Parkinson's disease and motor neurone disease. Physicians had excess death rates for viral hepatitis, cirrhosis (men only) and suicide.

3.3 General principles of toxicology

Toxicology is the study of substances that can have adverse health effects in relatively small doses. All substances are capable of causing harm, depending on many factors, including the dose, the route of administration and the susceptibility of the individual. The subject area is of relevance to occupational health professionals as they have a major interest in controlling exposure and preventing ill health from exposure to toxic substances encountered in work situations. Some areas of specialisation in toxicology include forensic toxicology, clinical toxicology, regulatory toxicology, behavioural toxicology and occupational and environmental toxicology.

3.3.1 Hazard and risk

The terms 'hazard' and 'risk' are often confused, or used interchangeably. A clear distinction should be made between the two. 'Hazard' refers to the potential to cause harm. 'Risk' refers to the likelihood of harm occurring, and also takes into account the severity of the effect. Hence, asbestos is a recognised hazard, causing ill effects on the respiratory system. However, the risk of these effects occurring depends on the nature and extent of exposure. If asbestos is present in intact form sealed within roofing material, the risk to health of those who work in the building is very small. On the other hand, attempting to demolish the roof by cutting the roofing material can liberate substantial quantities of asbestos fibres, which can be inhaled or irritate the skin and pose an appreciable risk. The hazard in these two situations is the same, but the risk is different.

3.3.2 Differences in toxicity due to different forms of chemicals

Physical form

Lead ingots do not pose a risk from skin absorption or inhalation (although they could cause injury if dropped from a height). However, if the ingots are heated above the melting point of lead (above 330°C), lead oxide fumes can be produced, and this form of lead, when inhaled and absorbed, causes systemic toxicity.

Spillages of salts of mercury in powder form underneath floorboards may not pose as much of a risk to health as spillages of mercury metal. The metal is liquid and volatile. It vaporises easily at room temperature to produce mercury in a form which can be inhaled to cause mercury poisoning.

The solubility of chemicals in water can determine their bioavailability and rate of clearance. Compounds that are poorly soluble can persist at the site of entry into the body, and may exert long-term pathological effects. This may be the reason why less soluble forms of nickel salts, such as sulphides and oxides of nickel, are respiratory carcinogens, with less evidence for a similar effect from soluble forms.

Chemical form

The cyanide radical (CN^-) is highly toxic to biological enzyme systems, yet hydrocyanic acid (HCN) and sodium cyanide (NaCN) have differing degrees of lethality. HCN is a gas and NaCN is a white crystalline powder, which, although capable of dissolution in water, does not release HCN until it reacts with acid, e.g. gastric hydrochloric acid. Thiocyanate (SCN⁻) contains sulphur linked to the cyanide radical, yet it is relatively non-toxic compared with hydrogen cyanide. Indeed, the rationale behind the administration of sodium thiosulphate in cases of cyanide poisoning is to convert the cyanide to thiocyanate, so that the latter can be safely excreted via the urine.

Organic and inorganic forms

Organic and inorganic compounds of the same metal may have different toxic properties. Inorganic lead poisoning causes colic, constipation, malaise, anaemia and encephalopathy. Poisoning by organic lead compounds, such as tetraethyl lead (TEL), does not produce similar symptoms. The predominant clinical features are those of a toxic organic psychosis — mainly psychiatric symptoms.

Inhalation of inorganic tin, such as tin oxide, leads to a characteristic chest X-ray picture with no functional changes. The effect, referred to as stannosis, is relatively benign, despite the gross radiological picture. Similar effects are seen with the inhalation of barium sulphate dust — causing baritosis — and iron oxide particles — causing siderosis. However, the inhalation of fumes of organic tin compounds, such as tributyl tin, causes irritant effects to the respiratory tract. Other organic tin compounds, such as triethyl tin, have been described as causing cerebral oedema, and triphenyl tin acetate causes hepatic damage.

Valency states

Compounds of metals with different valency states may differ in their toxic and biological properties. For example, chromium compounds may have a valency from 0 to 6. Chromium metal (valency 0) is relatively inert. Trivalent chromium compounds are an essential dietary requirement, Cr(III) having a role in glucose metabolism. Some hexavalent compounds, e.g. calcium chromate, are considered to be pulmonary carcinogens, whereas trivalent compounds are not.

Extent of chlorination

Polychlorinated biphenyls (PCBs) can exist as many different isomers. The extent of chlorination of the biphenyl component affects the properties of the PCB, such as the electrical and thermal resistance. The site and extent of chlorination also affect the toxicity.

The substitution of all four hydrogen atoms on the methane molecule produces carbon tetrachloride, with well recognised hepatotoxic properties. If only three hydrogen atoms on methane are replaced by chlorine, chloroform gas is formed. This has anaesthetic properties and is also hepatotoxic. With only two hydrogen atoms replaced by chlorine, methylene chloride is produced. This agent is used as a paint stripper, and causes an increase in carboxyhaemoglobin when absorbed. Neither carbon tetrachloride nor chloroform has this property.

Similarly, by substituting all four hydrogen atoms on ethylene, tetrachloroethylene (perchloroethylene) is produced, which is used extensively in dry-cleaning. Substituting three hydrogen atoms results in trichloroethylene, used widely as a degreasing agent. When only one hydrogen atom is replaced by chlorine, monochloroethylene (vinyl chloride) is produced. Trichloroethylene and perchloroethylene are hepatotoxic liquids. Vinyl chloride is gaseous, has anaesthetic properties and is the only chlorinated ethylene compound known to cause angiosarcoma of the liver.

3.3.3 Exposure, absorption and metabolism

The main routes of entry for toxic substances into the body are:

- inhalation — for gases, vapours, dusts, fumes and aerosols;
- skin absorption — especially for fat-soluble substances; an 'Sk' notation in the Health and Safety Executive's document, Environmental Hygiene 40 (EH40), indicates those chemicals that can be absorbed through the skin;
- ingestion — rarer for occupational agents, but can result from the consumption of food and drink at process areas in workplaces; inhaled particles trapped on the mucociliary escalator may also be coughed up and then ingested before being cleared via the gastrointestinal tract;
- inoculation — this is important as a means of occupational transmission of blood-borne infections, e.g. hepatitis B.

Toxic agents may have a local effect at the site of entry, or may be distributed via the blood to have effects on other target organs, e.g. liver, lungs, central and peripheral nervous system, bone marrow and kidneys.

- Local effects — include skin and mucous membrane irritation, e.g. to the eyes, nose, throat and lower respiratory tract. The potential for skin contact with chemicals used in the workplace is considerable, and hence contact dermatitis is the commonest occupational disorder. The respiratory tract is the obvious site for effects from inhaled toxic substances. Whether the upper or lower respiratory tract or other target organs are affected by inhaled toxins depends on the speed and efficiency of pulmonary clearance.
- Systemic effects — can be caused by the chemical itself, or by metabolites usually produced on passage through the liver. Metabolites

excreted via the urine can affect the bladder, and those excreted through the bile can affect the lower gastrointestinal tract. Fat-soluble toxic agents are distributed to organs with a high lipid content, e.g. beneath the skin, around the liver and kidneys, to the bone marrow and to the brain and spinal cord. Adipose tissue may act as a depot for the temporary storage and slow release of these fat-soluble agents. Some of these agents, e.g. organic solvents, therefore have a prolonged effect and an extended half-life.

Detoxification

Several enzymatic reactions are responsible for the detoxification of absorbed chemicals. These include enzymes that are part of the cytochrome P450 mixed function oxidase system in the liver microsomes. Other enzymes are dehydrogenases and reductases. The metabolic processes involve phase I reactions, such as oxidation, reduction and hydrolysis, and phase II reactions, such as conjugation with glucuronic acid. The conversion of bilirubin into bilirubin glucuronide is an example of a phase II reaction. This is part of the normal body mechanism for dealing with bilirubin produced by the breakdown of haemoglobin at the end of the 120-day lifespan of red blood cells. Bilirubin is fat soluble, but, on glucuronidation, is converted to a water-soluble form, which is then easily excreted via the bile.

The purpose of detoxification is to produce a less toxic metabolite which can then be excreted. However, the process is imperfect, and at times a more toxic compound or one with carcinogenic or mutagenic properties is produced. Procarcinogens, e.g. polycyclic aromatic hydrocarbons (PAHs), are chemicals that do not directly exert a carcinogenic effect, but, on metabolism, the ultimate or proximate carcinogen is produced. This is believed to be the mechanism by which the urinary bladder becomes the site for malignant change from exposure to PAHs and to β-naphthylamine. PAHs are absorbed via the lungs, where they are transported to the liver. The metabolites produced are excreted via the kidneys and, for the period of contact with the bladder before the urine is voided, there may be a carcinogenic effect from the metabolites on the bladder epithelium.

Excretion

Occupational agents that are systemically absorbed are excreted as the parent chemical compounds or after conversion to other metabolites. The main routes of excretion are:

- via the urine, e.g. aluminium and cobalt;

- through the bile, e.g. silver and copper;
- in the breath, e.g. organic solvents, such as ethanol, toluene and trichloroethylene.

Ingested compounds that are poorly absorbed via the gastrointestinal tract are excreted in the faeces.

Small amounts of absorbed compounds may also be excreted in sweat, milk, tears and saliva. There is a time delay between the systemic absorption of a chemical and its excretion. The clearance of perchloroethylene, for example, occurs in several phases: a rapid phase within hours, and a slow phase over several days or weeks. This information is important for biological monitoring and the interpretation of the results.

Variability of response to toxic agents

Not everyone reacts equally to a given dose of a toxic material. The factors that contribute to individual variability include:

- age;
- sex;
- ethnic group;
- genetic makeup — including inherited differences in speed of metabolism of absorbed chemicals, e.g. slow and fast acetylators of certain drugs;
- immune status;
- atopy — defined as 'an individual or family history of asthma, eczema or hay fever, with increased immunoglobulins and/or positive skin prick tests to recognised allergens';
- nutritional state;
- coexisting disease (and its treatment);
- concomitant exposure to other synergistic or antagonistic chemicals (including prescribed medications, e.g. barbiturates, steroids and alcohol);
- previous exposure to the toxic agent; the administration of halothane has caused toxic hepatitis in some individuals who have had previous exposure to this anaesthetic agent; in addition, previous exposure to allergens may cause sensitisation, so that subsequent exposure to smaller doses can result in severe effects.

3.3.4 Classification of toxic substances

There is no single suitable classification of toxic substances. Various authorities use systems based on physical, chemical, physiological or biological properties or some combination of these.

LD_{50}

One index of acute toxicity in animal studies is the LD_{50}. This is the dose of a test chemical that causes death in 50% of exposed laboratory animals. There is a variation in LD_{50} results depending on the test animal species used, and also on the route of exposure. Hence, LD_{50} data should specify these parameters, e.g. $LD_{50.oral,rat}$ (25 mg kg^{-1} body weight) means 'very toxic if swallowed', and $LD_{50.dermal,rabbit}$ (50 mg kg^{-1} body weight) means 'very toxic following skin contact'.

The following table provides examples of the relative toxicity ratings based on LD_{50} determinations in rats.

Toxicity description	LD_{50} (weight per kilogram single oral dose in rats)
Very toxic	25 mg or less
Toxic	>25–200 mg
Harmful	>200–2000 mg

A variant of the above is the LC_{50}. This refers to the lethal concentration of an aerosol, gas, vapour or particulates which, when administered to a group of test animals by inhalation, causes death in 50% of those animals. Examples of how LC_{50} data are expressed include:

1 $LC_{50.inhalation,rat}$ (0.25 mg l^{-1} per 4 h); this is deemed very toxic by inhalation for aerosols and particulates, under the UK Chemicals (Hazard Information and Packaging for Supply) (CHIP) Regulations 1994;

2 $LC_{50.inhalation,rat}$ (0.5–2 mg l^{-1} per 4 h); this is deemed toxic by inhalation for gases and vapours, under CHIP.

NOAEL (no observable adverse effect level)

A different approach to using animal data for the toxicity rating of chemicals is the determination of the NOAEL. This is the maximum dose that produces no observable adverse effects in a group of test animals. What is sometimes carried out in the setting of occupational exposure standards is to use the NOAEL, adding an appropriate safety factor to produce a standard that protects the majority of exposed workers. The safety factor used seems arbitrary, and may differ depending on the anticipated adverse effects from excessive exposure, or even from one expert committee to another.

Problems with LD_{50} and NOAEL

The above grading systems do not take into account slow or delayed death. The extrapolation of such ranges of toxicity from different animal species to humans must also be exercised with caution, especially when varying results are obtained between different species of test animal. It is important to be aware of the limitations of LD_{50} values. Unfortunately, health and safety standards are sometimes based on such values, and the justification for their use in workplace control criteria is weak. There continues to be an urgent need for the development of methods other than animal testing to determine the toxicity of chemicals to humans.

Risk phrases

For the purpose of classifying and labelling chemicals for supply, safety phrases have been proposed for use in Europe. These phrases are in addition to hazard symbols on packages and transport vehicles. The phrases include those dealing with the properties of chemicals, such as flammability, health effects or environmental effects. Examples include:

- R12 — extremely flammable;
- R45 — may cause cancer;
- R46 — may cause heritable genetic damage;
- R50 — very toxic to aquatic organisms.

Threshold for toxic effect

For toxic chemicals, there is a threshold dose below which there is no observed effect (the NOAEL). Above this threshold, the higher the dose the greater the effect, and/or the greater the number of individuals affected. However, this threshold varies between species, and also within the same species depending on factors such as age, state of health and diet. For some carcinogenic compounds, there may be no threshold. Each exposure, regardless of magnitude, adds to the risk of an effect. Hence, there is a need to control exposures to as low as feasible for carcinogens. For allergens, the threshold for sensitisation may be relatively high, but, once sensitised, the individual can react to minute amounts of the causative agent.

3.3.5 Short-term tests for carcinogenicity

The basis of some short-term tests for carcinogenicity lies in the demonstration that chemical agents have mutagenic properties. The possibility of carcinogenesis is inferred from showing mutagenesis. The development of short-term tests arose because of several factors. These included the costs of performing animal tests, and the time period required before results were obtained. Short-term tests can produce results within several days, whereas animal tests may take several months or years to complete. With the numbers of new chemicals being introduced, there were also insufficient facilities for carrying out animal tests on all new chemicals. Another factor was the interest in developing alternative test systems which do not require animal experiments. Toxicologists explored the development of short-term screening tests, using mainly bacterial systems or cell lines. Many such tests have been produced with varying degrees of success and predictive value. The variety of tests include the Ames test, sister chromatid exchange, the dominant lethal test, the micronucleus test and the Styles cell transformation test. Details of two of these tests are described below.

The Ames test

One variant of this test relies on the use of histidine-dependent *Salmonella typhimurium* on culture plates. The test material is added, and the number of colonies of the bacteria that can grow in the absence of histidine indicates the extent of reverse mutation of the bacteria. A proportion of the bacteria undergoes reverse mutation, so that the bacteria can survive in the absence of the amino acid histidine. The extent of reverse mutation is compared between plates with the test material and control plates without. A significant difference in the number of colonies in test vs. control plates indicates mutagenicity, and therefore inferred carcinogenicity of the test material.

As described, the test is quite good at detecting direct carcinogens, such as alkylating agents. However, for indirect carcinogens, such as aromatic amines and PAHs, an additional step is required to convert the indirect carcinogen to the ultimate carcinogen, before it can cause any mutagenic effect. This step is the addition of liver homogenate from rats or mice, termed the S9 mix, to the test system. The S9 mix refers to the centrifugation of minced liver at 9000 rev min^{-1}. The rationale behind the use of liver homogenate is to supply sufficient enzymes to effect the transformation of procarcinogen to ultimate carcinogen. An additional procedure that can be included is the parenteral administration of phenobarbitone or Aroclor 1254 to the rodents before harvesting the liver for the preparation of the S9 mix. Phenobarbitone or Aroclor enhances the production of liver enzymes, and can increase the enzyme content in the S9 mix. Other variants of the Ames test use strains of *Escherichia coli* instead of *S. typhimurium*.

Sister chromatid exchange (SCE)

The basis of this test is to detect genetic damage by chemicals. The reasoning behind this approach is that chemicals that can cause deoxyribonucleic acid (DNA) damage are likely to possess carcinogenic activity. Cellular genetic material is examined during mitosis after the addition of the test chemical. DNA damage results in the exchange of material between pairs of chromatids at this stage of cell division. The difference in the extent of DNA exchange between cells exposed to the test chemical and those exposed to a control compound indicates whether the test material is carcinogenic.

Detection of adducts

Carcinogens can react with sites on the purine or pyrimidine bases of cellular DNA to produce adducts. These adducts can be detected in urine samples or in haemoglobin or white blood cells. The basis for detecting the presence of such adducts is that they indicate an effect from exposure to a carcinogen and, in theory, this might be of use in a screening programme. However, there are many unanswered questions, such as the specificity and sensitivity of these adducts as an indicator of carcinogen exposure, their persistence, their variability in biological samples, dietary and non-occupational factors that may contribute to adduct formation and the within and between laboratory variability in the detection of adducts. Hence, DNA adducts are interesting research tools, but they currently have little applied value in occupational health practice.

3.4 Target organs

3.4.1 Introduction

In this section, consideration is given to the organs of the body and the way they respond to insult and assault from occupationally related agents. Detailed toxicological and pathological information on each agent cited is given in Chapter 4. However, it is the organ's response to injury that will usually herald the onset of ill health. This is what brings the worker to the attention of physicians. Chronic plumbism, for example, may present itself in a variety of system dysfunctions, and the physician will have to unravel the differential diagnosis: it is a rare event indeed for a patient to complain of overexposure to inorganic lead!

The target organ systems included in this section are:

- respiratory system;
- central and peripheral nervous system;
- genitourinary system;
- cardiovascular system;
- skin;
- liver;

- reproductive system (and endocrine system);
- bone marrow.

3.4.2 Respiratory system

Structure

The upper and lower respiratory tracts are particularly vulnerable to occupationally related noxious agents. Over 80% of these agents gain access to the body through the respiratory system. The effects of such exposure may also be felt in other organ systems, but the brunt of the damage frequently falls on the air passages and lungs.

The system is composed of several anatomically discrete sections:
- the mouth, nasal sinuses, pharynx and larynx;
- the trachea, main and segmental bronchi;
- the bronchioli;
- the alveoli;
- the alveolar–capillary barrier.

The repeated branching of the airways from tracheal bifurcation to alveoli has the effect of greatly increasing the surface area of the respiratory mucosae, whilst reducing the rate of air flow. Thus, the 300 million alveoli offer a surface area of some 70 m^2 for gas exchange, but no alveolus exceeds 0.1 mm in diameter. The thickness of the alveolar epithelial wall, together with the endothelial cell layer of the pulmonary capillaries, is, in health, rarely greater than 0.001 mm and constitutes the blood–gas barrier.

Function

The main function of the lungs is to supply oxygen for uptake by the pulmonary capillaries and to provide the means for removing carbon dioxide diffusing in the opposite direction. The successful achievement of this gas exchange requires three main system functions:
- ventilation;
- gas transfer;
- blood gas transport.

Lung function tests can be similarly grouped.

Ventilatory function is commonly measured by a variety of portable instruments, the most common of which are the peak flow meter and the spirometer. Recent developments in microcomputer analysis have been of great benefit in providing rapid digital and graphical readouts of ventilatory function. Computerised data can also be stored and

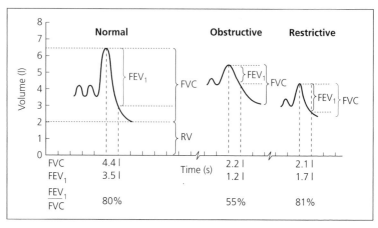

Fig. 3.2 Spirograms to illustrate the difference in forced expiratory volume in 1 s (FEV$_1$) and forced vital capacity (FVC) in health, airways obstruction and restrictive defects (such as diffuse lung fibrosis or severe spinal deformity). Inspiration is upwards and expiration downwards. Although the vital capacity is reduced in both obstructive and restrictive lung disease, the proportion expired in 1 s shows considerable differences. RV, residual volume.

compared with pre-programmed normal values. The main indices determined are:
- forced expiratory volume in 1 s (FEV$_1$);
- forced mid-expiratory flow rate (FMF);
- forced vital capacity (FVC);
- FEV$_1$/FVC ratio;
- flow/volume patterns.

Figure 3.2 illustrates these indices.

Gas transfer and transport measurements require less portable apparatus and are a means of assessing:
- ventilation/perfusion ratios — mainly involving the use of radioactive gases;
- gas diffusion — usually transfer of carbon monoxide T_{LCO};
- red cell gas uptake and transport — usually blood gas levels and pH.

Lung function is altered by a number of non-occupational factors, and tables of 'normal' values take some of these variables into account. They include:
- age;
- sex;
- ethnic group;
- height.

A factor of 0.85 is used to adjust predicted normal values for Caucasians to obtain predicted values for non-Caucasians. Attempts have also been made to derive 'normal' values for specific ethnic groups.

Other factors that affect the results of lung function tests include:

• smoking habits or use of bronchodilator especially within an hour of testing;
• a heavy meal or a chest infection;
• exercise tolerance;
• observer error;
• instrument error;
• diurnal variation;
• ambient temperature.

The chest X-ray

The chest radiograph is a valuable tool for assessing lung effects from exposure to occupationally related dusts. It gives an indication of structural damage. Chest X-rays can be used on the following basis:

1 clinical — to establish the diagnosis and prognosis and as a guide to treatment;

2 epidemiological — to assess the prevalence and progression of disease both in populations and individual members of populations.

To this end, a standard classification of radiographs has been internationally agreed for use in assessing pneumoconiosis. This ILO U/C classification, as it is called, requires a chest radiograph to be taken in a standard fashion, read and classified to a standard format. The main features of this format are listed in Table 3.3.

Profusion relates to the area of spread across the lung fields. Type relates to the size of the opacities. Extent relates to the zones affected. The 1, 2 and 3 profusion groups can be extended to a 12-point system: 0/-, 0/0, 0/1, 1/0, 1/1, 1/2, 2/1, 2/2, 2/3, 3/2, 3/3, 3/4.

Pathology

Occupational lung disorders

Harmful effects to the lung produced by noxious agents can be grouped into the following categories:

• acute inflammation;
• respiratory sensitisation (asthma, ? byssinosis);
• pneumoconiosis;
• extrinsic allergic alveolitis;

Table 3.3 ILO U/C classification of pneumoconiosis.

Feature	Classification
No pneumoconiosis	0
Pneumoconiosis	
Rounded small opacities	
Profusion	1, 2, 3
Type	p, q(m), r(n)
Extent	Zones
Irregular small opacities	
Profusion	1, 2, 3
Type	s, t, u
Extent	Zones
Large opacities	
Size	A, B, C
Type	Well defined/ill defined
Pleural thickening	By site
Diaphragmatic outline	Ill defined: right, left
Cardiac outline	Ill defined: 1, 2, 3
Pleural calcifications	By site and extent

- malignancy (see Chapter 10);
- infections (see Chapter 6).

Acute inflammation. This is primarily caused by the irritant gases and fumes. Their solubility determines whether their effects are most noticeable on the upper or lower respiratory tracts.

Soluble gases that irritate the upper respiratory tract will cause affected individuals to move away from the source of the gas (a protective mechanism). Examples of such gases are:

- ammonia;
- chlorine;
- sulphur dioxide.

Some irritant gases can also cause a delayed pulmonary oedema, with respiratory distress occurring 48–72 h after exposure:

- nitric oxide;
- phosgene;
- fluorine;
- ozone.

Respiratory sensitisation. Occupationally related asthma may be caused by a variety of dusts, either producing an immediate reaction or a late (non-immediate) type. The former may develop within minutes of exposure; the latter may take 4–2 h to develop (usually 4–8 h). It is in this latter group that the suspicion of a work-related cause may be missed, as the effect of the allergenic dust or fume may not be noticed until the evening of the day of exposure. Some people experience a combination of immediate and late effects. A suggested classification for two types of occupational asthma due to agents of different molecular weight is given in Table 3.4.

Occupational asthma has been variously estimated as causing 2–15% of all asthmas, but it is important to realise that atopy is not a predisposing state for more than a few of the known allergenic dusts. Although a good occupational and medical history may settle the diagnosis, some cases are exceedingly difficult to unravel. In these cases, it may be necessary to resort to bronchial challenge testing, which, in competent hands, is a relatively safe procedure. Skin prick testing and serology for immunoglobulin E (IgE) levels may also be of value.

Treatment involves the removal of the sensitised subject from exposure (in some cases, this may necessitate a change in job, or a move to a job with considerably less exposure) and non-specific treatment for the asthmatic symptoms.

Prevention involves several factors:

• efficient and rigorous hygiene control in the workplace;

• substitution with less allergenic materials;

• personal respiratory protection for the worker for specific unavoidable tasks where exposure is anticipated;

• identification of workers at risk — not an easy task; determining atopic individuals is of limited use, as up to 30% of the population have atopic characteristics, and atopy is not necessarily a prognostic feature of occupational asthma;

• periodic medical examinations with pre- and post-shift ventilatory capacity measurements.

Table 3.4 Occupational asthma — possibly two distinct types.

Agent	Examples	Atopy	Exacerbating factors
Large molecular weight protein antigen	Rodent urine Shellfish protein Flour/grain Mite faeces	Yes	Cigarette smoke +
Low molecular weight chemicals	TDI Acid anhydrides Platinum salts Plicatic acid (woods) Abietic acid (colophony)	No	Cigarette smoke ++

TDI, toluene di-isocyanate; +, some; ++, a lot.

The list of potential occupational lung allergens is now extremely long. A few of the more important ones are:

- amoebae ('humidifier fever');
- avian feathers;
- beetles, locusts, cockroaches, grain mites;
- certain reactive dyes;
- colophony — soldering flux;
- drugs, including penicillin, tetracycline and methyldopa;
- enzymes, including *Bacillus subtilis* and pancreatic extracts;
- ethylenediamine;
- formaldehyde and glutaraldehyde;
- fungi;
- grain, flour, hops, tobacco dust;
- isocyanates;
- laboratory animals, e.g. rats and mice, cause 'laboratory animal dander allergy' mainly from proteins in the urine of rodent, cat and dog danders;
- phthalic anhydride (epoxy resin hardener);
- various metal salts, including some platinum, chromium, nickel and vanadium compounds;
- various woods, including cedars, boxwood.

Byssinosis. There is some debate over whether byssinosis should be classified as a type of occupational asthma. The condition is, however, broader and more complex than other forms of asthma. In susceptible individuals, exposure to the dusts of cotton, sisal, hemp or flax can produce acute dyspnoea, with cough and reversible obstruction of the airways. It is first noticed on the first day of the working week, and then subsides on subsequent days. Later, with continued exposure, symptoms recur on subsequent days of the week, until even weekends and holidays are not free of symptoms.

The effects are greatest where the dust concentrations are highest, and are more noticeable with coarser cotton. This has led to the suggestion that the condition is (in part) due to organic contaminants of the cotton boll, such as bracts, and even microbiological agents, such as *E. coli*. Smoking exacerbates the condition and, although irreversible obstruction of the airways may eventually supervene, with possible resulting fatality, no specific pathological features have been identified in the lungs at post-mortem. Chest radiography is unhelpful and treatment is symptomatic.

Studies of Ulster flax workers and Lancashire cotton workers have cast doubt on the ability of this condition to influence mortality rates. Byssinosis, as described today, is probably a mixture of conditions ranging from true asthma to exacerbated chronic bronchitis.

Pneumoconioses. The term 'pneumoconiosis' literally means 'dusty lungs'. For practical purposes, pneumoconiosis is usually restricted to those conditions which cause a permanent alteration in lung architecture following the inhalation of mineral dusts. These dusts include:

- silica (or quartz);
- coal;
- asbestos.

The clinical and radiographic features of silicosis, coal workers' pneumoconiosis and asbestosis are summarised in Fig. 3.3.

Silicosis occurs following the inhalation of 'free' silica, and is most common amongst workers involved in quarrying, mining and tunnelling through quartz-bearing rock, e.g. during gold mining. It is also a recognised hazard of the following processes:

- use of abrasives;
- sand blasting;
- glass manufacture;
- stone cutting and dressing;
- foundry work;
- ceramic manufacture.

Silicosis may present as one of four main clinical types:

- nodular, with hyaline and collagenous lesions in the lungs;
- mixed dust fibrosis, with irregular, stellate, fibrotic lung lesions;
- diatomite — a picture similar to fibrosing alveolitis and usually attributed to diatomaceous earth;
- 'acute' — a rapidly developing alveolar lipoproteinosis with fibrosing alveolitis.

The fibrotic lung lesions frequently calcify to produce a characteristic 'egg-shell' calcification on chest X-rays. There is a progressive restrictive lung disease leading to cor pulmonale. Pulmonary tuberculosis used to be a common complication.

Recent epidemiological studies have suggested that silica may be a lung carcinogen. There seems to be an increased risk of lung cancer in silicotics, and some authorities suggest an additive risk of silica dust exposure and cigarette smoking.

Coal dust produces a somewhat different picture, and frequently has less severe sequelae and is less aggressively fibrotic. Indeed, the distinction between 'simple' and 'complicated' coal pneumoconiosis is often marked, with only a minority of the former progressing to the latter. What factors predispose to this serious turn of events are unknown. At one time, it was thought that workers with rheumatoid

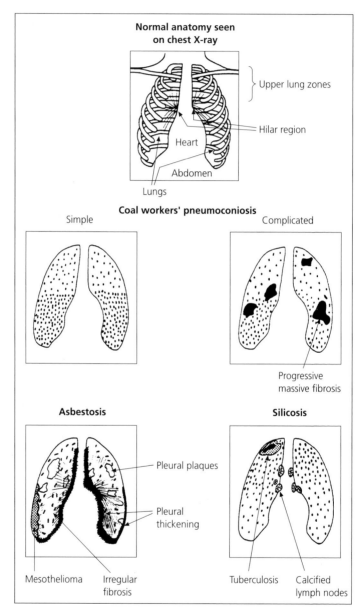

Fig. 3.3 Schematic representation of the chest X-ray appearances of certain dust diseases.

arthritis exposed to coal dust could develop nodules in the lung (Caplan's syndrome), which then progressed to progressive massive fibrosis. The pathogenesis may be immunological. However, Caplan's syndrome is now a rare condition, and the link to massive fibrosis is still uncertain.

In the UK, the prevalence of all categories of coal pneumoconiosis has fallen to less than 5%, with a prevalence of the complicated form (progressive massive fibrosis) of 0.4%. The probability of developing ILO category 2 or 3 simple pneumoconiosis, over a working lifetime in British mines, now stands at between 2 and 12%, if dust levels are maintained at concentrations below the current occupational exposure limits (3 mg m^{-3} for operations where the average quartz level exceeds 0.45 mg m^{-3} to 7 mg m^{-3} for long wall, coal face operations). Indeed, most miners nowadays have little to show radiographically for their work, and, as long as the lung mottling seen remains simple, the worker is usually symptomless. Problems (and symptoms) start if and when the discrete, rounded opacities seen on chest X-rays coalesce, break down or become more fibrotic. Serious pulmonary dysfunction then supervenes, and death is commonly due to cor pulmonale.

Asbestos fibres produce more irregular and more florid fibrotic changes in the lung. The disease is thought to be progressive, and death from restrictive lung disease is common. Clinically, the disease may first be manifested as dyspnoea, non-productive cough, finger clubbing or weight loss. The presence of persistent chest pain frequently heralds a recognised complication of asbestos exposure, namely malignant disease — usually a bronchogenic carcinoma, occasionally a pleural mesothelioma. There is a synergistic effect between asbestos compounds and cigarette smoking in terms of the risk of developing lung cancer.

For completeness, it is worth noting that some dusts seem to produce disturbingly florid lung mottling on chest radiographs, but with little or no evidence of clinical effect or progression. These so-called benign pneumoconioses are associated with the dusts of:
- barium sulphate — baritosis;
- tin — stannosis;
- antimony, zirconium and the rare earths;
- iron — siderosis (although haematite mining is associated with lung cancer, thought to be due to radon gas in the mines).

Extrinsic allergic alveolitis. As noted above, the inhalation of organic materials can give rise to asthma. However, other organic dusts produce alveolitis, with the resultant lowering of gas transfer across the blood–gas barrier. Most of the agents capable of producing this effect are fungal spores, and the most common clinical condition in Britain is farmer's lung. These diseases frequently have acute, influenza-like episodes, which, if exposure is continued, lead to subacute and chronic pulmonary fibrotic disease. The various types of extrinsic allergic alveolitis are summarised in Table 3.5.

Table 3.5 Types of extrinsic allergic alveolitis.

Type	Exposure to	Allergen
Farmer's lung	Mouldy hay	*Micropolyspora faeni, Thermoactinomyces vulgaris*
Bagassosis	Mouldy sugar cane	*T. sacchari*
Suberosis	Mouldy cork	*Penicillium* frequentans
Bird fancier's lung	Droppings and feathers	Avian protein
Malt worker's lung	Mouldy barley	*Aspergillus clavatus*
Humidifier fever	Dust or mist	*T. vulgaris, T. thapophilus* and amoebae (various)
Cheese worker's lung	Mould dust	*P. casei*
Wheat weevil lung	Mouldy grain or flour	*Sitophilus granarius*
Animal handler's lung	Dander, dried rodent urine	Serum and urine proteins
Pituitary snuff taker's lung	Therapeutic snuff	Pig or ox protein

3.4.3 Nervous system

The basic unit of the nervous system is the neuron, which has four components as follows, with the nerve impulse passing from the first to the last:

- the dendrites;
- the cell body itself;
- the axon;
- the synaptic terminal.

The axon is one long nerve fibre with or without myelin sheathing, which speeds nerve conduction. In the normal resting state, the axonal membrane has a resting potential of about −85 mV; this *outside* positive charge is maintained by an active sodium pump mechanism. A nerve impulse is a wave of depolarisation and repolarisation, which runs along the nerve fibre as the membrane permeability to sodium increases, allowing a rapid reversal of polarity, followed by a recovery period as 'normal' permeability is restored. Conduction along the axon is all or nothing, but along the dendrites it is incremental. At the synapse, the electrical energy is transformed into chemical energy by the release of a neurotransmitter, such as acetylcholine. These neurotransmitters may be excitatory or inhibitory.

Occupationally related disorders of peripheral nerves

These may be motor or sensory nerve effects, commonly both. Sensory disturbances are usually distal; motor dysfunction may be proximal or distal. Most toxic substances cause axonal degeneration, usually by a mechanism which is largely unknown. The damage may be limited and reversible, or severe and permanent, depending on the agent, the dose and the duration of exposure. In the case of *n*-hexane and methyl-*n*-butylketone, the effect seems to be due to a common metabolite, 2,5-hexanedione, and leads to giant axonal swelling in the proximal parts of the axon, with peripheral 'dying back'. Apart from the clinical features of peripheral neuropathy, subclinical effects may be detected by nerve conduction studies, which can be useful in the detection of early effects in workers exposed to known neurotoxins.

The most common peripheral neurotoxins are:

- acrylamide and/or dimethylaminoproprionitrile (DMAPN);
- antimony;
- arsenic;
- carbamate pesticides;
- carbon disulphide;
- lead and its compounds (inorganic);
- mercury compounds (inorganic and organic);
- methyl(*o*-methyl)-*n*-butylketone;
- *n*-hexane;
- organophosphate pesticides;
- thallium;
- triorthocresylphosphate.

Occupationally related disorders of the central nervous system (CNS)

Disordered brain function produces a consistent clinical picture, despite the complexity of the organ affected. The primary change is one of disordered consciousness, varying from mild disorientation through to profound coma. Organic psychoses are frequently worst at night, and when the patient is fatigued. These effects may be interspersed with periods of normal mentation. In addition, visual hallucinations may occur, with or without memory disturbance, ideas of reference, paranoia, anxiety and, later, apathy.

Occupational toxins affecting the CNS include organic solvents, heavy metals and CNS depressants, such as anaesthetic gases. Examples include:

- arsenic;

- benzene;
- carbon disulphide (features similar to Parkinsonism);
- carbon monoxide;
- chlorinated hydrocarbons, pesticides such as dieldrin (may manifest as fits);
- compressed air (possibly);
- halothane;
- lead (may manifest as fits);
- manganese (can present as marked psychosis);
- mercury;
- methyl chloroform;
- methylene chloride;
- organic lead compounds;
- perchloroethylene;
- styrene;
- toluene;
- trichloroethylene;
- white spirit.

Screening for CNS effects is not easy and involves a battery of behavioural tests, including cognitive and perceptual psychomotor assessments. Recent international meetings have shown that an agreed battery of psychological tests can be formulated. Examples of such test procedures are available in the larger texts given in 'Further reading' (see Section 13.5).

What remains to be resolved is whether chronic low-dose exposure to various organic solvents can cause organic psychosis. The Danish painters' syndrome — much vaunted in the early 1980s — has not been closely corroborated in American or British studies. The best of these recent studies are, however, not without a measurable effect. It appears that some tests of higher cerebral function show a decremental change following long occupational exposure. The clinical and epidemiological significance of such results remains to be evaluated.

Alcohol abuse may exacerbate the effects of the occupational neurotoxin, but these effects are, nevertheless, relatively rare. In normal clinical practice, diabetes is a more probable diagnosis for the patient with a neuropathy.

3.4.4 Genitourinary system

The kidney plays a crucial role in the excretory and detoxification mechanisms of the body. When a toxic substance is absorbed, the liver will frequently alter its chemical structure. Although it is naive to imagine that the liver 'knows' how to detoxify such foreign material, it is nevertheless a fact that the liver frequently succeeds in increasing the toxin's polarity and/or acidity. Both of these changes will render the material more water soluble, and hence more readily excretable through the kidney. Some toxic substances reach the kidney unchanged; others reach the kidney in the form of a more toxic metabolite; yet others are able to cause damage by either being sequestered in the renal cortex (e.g. cadmium), or by being present in the bladder long enough to cause malignant change (e.g. some of the arylamines, such as 2-naphthylamine and its metabolites).

Common forms of disordered function resulting from occupationally related substances include tubular dysfunction leading to amino aciduria, proteinuria and glycosuria (e.g. mercury) or acute renal failure due to tubular necrosis (e.g. thallium), hypovolaemic shock (arsenic) or tubular blockage by crystalluria (oxalic acid). Cortical necrosis, whilst a rare cause of acute renal failure, occurs more commonly with the toxic nephropathies than with other causes of kidney damage. Furthermore, severe liver damage, due to, for example, organic solvents, may induce a complication of renal failure; it is worth remembering that renal damage caused by drug-induced hypersensitivity can occur not only in those taking the drug therapeutically but also in those making the drug occupationally. The nephrotic syndrome can be occupationally induced if the proteinuria is of sufficient severity. This can occur following exposure to mercury, gold and bismuth.

Renal tract malignancy of occupational origin is an important condition, primarily affecting that part of the genitourinary system in contact with the agent for longest and at the highest concentration, namely the bladder.

Although the prostate possesses the curious ability to concentrate (and excrete) heavy metals, little incontrovertible evidence exists of occupationally induced prostatic disease in workers exposed to heavy metals. The putative link between cadmium exposure and prostatic cancer has not been corroborated by more recent, careful studies.

A short list of the more important occupational factors in nephrotoxicity is given in Table 3.6.

3.4.5 Cardiovascular system

The cardiovascular system is not in the 'front line' when it comes to the onslaught from noxious materials encountered in the workplace. Nevertheless, work may be a risk factor in the pathogenesis of cardiovascular disease, if only as a factor in stress-related illness. The

Table 3.6 Occupational and non-occupational exposures with nephrotoxic effects.

Inorganic	Organic	Miscellaneous
Arsenic	Aniline	Antimicrobials
Bismuth	Carbon tetrachloride	Cantharides
Boron	Chloroform	Chlorinated hydrocarbon
Cadmium	Dimethyl sulphate	insecticides
Gold	Dioxan	Electric shock
Iron salts (in overdose)	Ethylene glycol	Fungi
Lead	EDTA	Horse serum
Mercury	Methoxyfluorane	Trauma
Phosphorus	Methyl alcohol	X-ray contrast media
Potassium chlorate	Methyl chloride	
Thallium	Paraquat	
Uranium	Pentachlorophenol	
	Phenol	
	Turpentine	
	Toluene	

EDTA, ethylenediaminetetra acetic acid.

classical risk factors for cardiovascular disease include:

- age;
- sex;
- weight;
- race;
- smoking;
- blood pressure;
- serum cholesterol concentrations and diet;
- exercise levels;
- personality;
- stress;
- oral contraceptive use;
- family history;
- medical history (e.g. diabetes).

Hazards directly emanating from the workplace tend to have a secondary effect on the cardiovascular system. For example, lead can cause nephropathy, which, in turn, can cause hypertension. Cadmium causes emphysema, which can lead to cor pulmonale; cobalt can cause cardiomyopathy and arsenic is thought to be a factor in peripheral vascular disease.

Certain organic solvents are thought to be capable of inducing cardiac arrhythmias, and vinyl chloride has been linked with Raynaud's phenomenon. Methylene chloride produces carbon monoxide as a metabolite, whilst carbon disulphide seems to possess a direct atherogenic potential. Finally, certain gases can cause hypoxia, directly or at a cellular level, and physical factors, such as vibration, can induce vasospastic disease in the small arteries of the hand.

Thus, the list of occupationally related factors which can cause, induce or exacerbate cardiovascular disease is not inconsiderable and includes:

- antimony;
- arsenic;
- cadmium;
- carbon disulphide;
- carbon monoxide;
- carbon tetrachloride;
- chloroform;
- cobalt;
- electric shock;
- fluorocarbons;
- glyceryl trinitrate and trinitrotoluene;
- halothane;
- lead;
- low atmospheric pressures;
- manganese;
- mercury;
- methylene chloride;
- noise;
- ? shift work;
- temperature;
- trichloroethylene;
- 1,1,1-trichloroethane;
- vibration;
- vinyl chloride.

3.4.6 Skin

The skin consists of two basic elements: an outer epidermis, which acts as a protective armour and is non-wettable, and a dermis, which provides the inherent strength of the skin, largely through its collagen content. The waterproofing capability of the epidermis is, in occupational health terms, a potential problem, as its greasy surface aids the absorption of fat-soluble materials, and is thus a ready route of entry for many organic chemicals.

Skin disease may be characterised by rashes which bear a limited geographical resemblance to the area of external assault. Scratching a rash because of an itch can lead to the extension of the area affected. The use of a variety of ointments in combination may worsen rather than alleviate the symptoms. The use of gloves may protect against further contact with the causative chemicals, but the inappropriate use of gloves may cause chemicals to be trapped between the gloves and the skin of the hands. This can worsen contact dermatitis. Some individuals are also allergic to the ingredients in gloves.

Occupational dermatoses may be broadly divided into two groups:

1 primary irritant contact dermatitis;
2 allergic contact dermatitis.

Primary irritant contact dermatitis

Nearly three-quarters of all occupational dermatoses are of this type. The irritants produce a direct effect on the skin with which they come into contact, and the effect will be more dependent on the dose and duration of exposure than on any inherent response emanating from the individual. For example, concentrated sulphuric acid splashed onto the face of anybody will produce a skin reaction. Soap and water are more variable, but these seemingly harmless materials can cause irritation in non-allergic subjects who carry out frequent hand washing. The degree of effect depends on factors such as:

- skin dryness;
- sweating;
- pigmentation;
- integrity of the epidermis (i.e. whether damaged by trauma);
- presence of hair;
- presence of dirt;
- concurrent or pre-existent skin disease;
- environmental factors, such as temperature, humidity, friction.

Furthermore, some chemicals, such as arsenicals and mercurials, can combine with skin protein and cause skin damage. Hydrofluoric acid and hexavalent chromium compounds can cause deep skin ulcers. Cutting oils and chlorinated naphthalenes can block sebaceous ducts and cause acne — the term 'chloroacne' being used for acne due to chlorinated compounds.

Allergic contact dermatitis

This accounts for 15–20% of all occupational dermatoses. The response is usually specific to one agent, and the skin reaction after contact may be delayed for a week or more. The initial sensitising episode may require substantial concentrations and/or prolonged contact; subsequent reactions can be provoked by shorter/smaller exposures.

The mechanism of the response is a delayed hypersensitivity reaction. The allergen acts as a hapten to combine with protein in the epidermis to provoke a cell-mediated type IV immune exposure. The acute effect is erythema, eruption, vesiculation, oozing and desquamation. In a chronic form, this leads to thickened, fissured skin.

The main occupational contact allergens include:

- dichromates;
- epoxy resins;
- rubber accelerators and antioxidants;
- germicidal agents, such as hexachlorophene;
- dyes, such as paraphenylenediamine;
- topical anaesthetics, such as procaine;
- formaldehyde;
- nickel and its salts;
- mercury and its salts;
- cobalt and its salts.

Diagnosis by patch tests

Patch testing is used to confirm a diagnosis of allergic contact dermatitis. This requires the application of a series of compounds to the skin of the back, followed by assessment of the skin reaction 48–72 h after removal of the test patches. False positives, false negatives and cross-reactions can cause problems in interpretation. Hence, the need for dermatological expertise. The standard series of the test materials may need to be supplemented by additional test substances for specific occupational exposures. In the case of occupational allergic contact dermatitis, familiarity with the work processes and chemicals used is an essential adjunct to patch testing.

Photodermatitis

Exposure to certain agents through skin contact or following ingestion can result in a rash after exposure to ultraviolet light. This includes occupational exposure to tar, pitch and acrylates, e.g. those acrylates used in ultraviolet cured inks, augmented by subsequent exposure to sunlight. Pharmaceutical agents known to cause photodermatitis include griseofulvin and thiazides after ingestion. The non-occupational use of some perfumes and suncreams may lead to photodermatitis.

Occupational vitiligo (leucoderma)

Contact with chemicals can lead to depigmentation of the skin. Examples include hydroquinone and certain substituted phenols and catechols. Hydroquinone is used in photographic film development; p-tert-butylphenol is present in glues, resins, plasticisers and inks. The reversibility of the effect depends on the extent of damage to the melanocytes.

Contact allergens encountered in non-occupational settings include:

- antibiotics;
- colophony;
- vinyl and acrylic resins;
- plants: primula, daffodil, chrysanthemum;
- West African hardwoods;
- pharmaceuticals, such as chlorothiazide, phenothiazines and tolbutamide.

The industries with a recognised risk of occupationally related skin disease are those involved in:

- making leather goods;
- food processing and packing;
- use of adhesive and sealant;
- boat building and repair;
- use of abrasive products;
- agriculture and horticulture.

3.4.7 Liver

The liver is the largest visceral organ. Its mass of parenchymal cells, portal tracts and abundant blood supply is witness to its crucial role as the body's main metabolic factory. The functional unit resides in the lobule and consists of a group of sinusoids running between a terminal portal tract and a few terminal hepatic venules. The liver cells nearest the hepatic venules differ from those near the portal tracts, in that the former receive blood lower in oxygen content. These centrilobular hepatocytes are therefore more vulnerable to toxic (and anoxic) conditions than the periportal cells.

Disordered hepatic function has two main aspects. Firstly, the hepatocytes may be damaged and, secondly, the transport mechanism to, through or from the hepatocytes may be blocked. Both dysfunctions, will, sooner or later, lead to jaundice. The liver's remarkable capacity for hepatocyte regeneration following assault is not matched by its ability to reproduce, faithfully, the basic liver architecture. Thus, major hepatic damage can lead to florid cellular regeneration in a disrupted lobular pattern.

The effects of liver injury are shown in Fig. 3.4.

Pre-existent liver disease may enhance the effects of a new toxic onslaught, and the liver is thus particularly vulnerable to the effects of organic solvents if already reeling under the effects of regular and excessive dosing with ethyl alcohol. Furthermore, it is worth noting that hepatic enzyme induction may alter the liver's ability to handle certain toxins, and the organ itself is occasionally subject to hypersensitivity reaction. The effects of hepatotoxins of occupational origin may be subclassified as shown in Table 3.7.

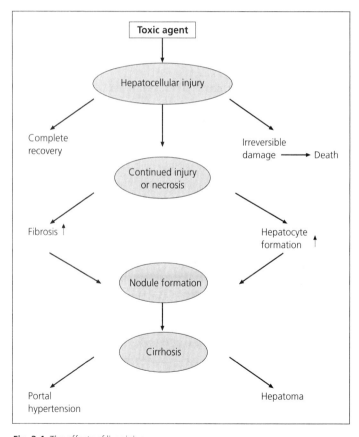

Fig. 3.4 The effects of liver injury.

Table 3.7 Effects of occupationally related hepatotoxins.

Effect	Substance	
	Organic	Inorganic
Centrilobular necrosis	Acrylonitrile	Antimony
	Carbon tetrachloride	Arsenic
	Chlorinated hydrocarbon	Boranes
	insecticides	Phosphorus (yellow)
	Chlorinated naphthylenes	Selenium
	Dimethyl hydrazine	Thallium
	Dimethyl nitrosamine	
	Dinitrophenol	
	Ethyl alcohol	
	Halothane	
	Methyl chloride	
	Nitrobenzene	
	Phenol	
	Polychlorinated biphenyls	
	Tetrachloroethylene	
	1,1,1-Trichloroethane	
	Trichloroethylene	
	Trinitrotoluene	
	Toluene	
	Vinyl chloride	
Hepatic infections	Viral hepatitis (A, B, C)	
	Leptospirosis	
	Q fever	
	Schistosomiasis	
	Amoebiasis	
Cholestatic, cholangiolitic	Methylene dianiline	
	Organic arsenicals	
	Toluene diamine	
	4,4-Diaminodiphenylmethane	

3.4.8 Reproductive system

It was not until the last two decades that serious attention was paid to the possibility that occupational factors could disrupt the normal functioning of the reproductive system (Table 3.8). Anecdotal evidence suggests that women working with lead in the early years of this century became sterile. While the concerns over visual display units and pregnancy outcome have heightened the awareness that reproduction could be disrupted by work exposure, this specific link has been largely discounted.

Now, considerable attention is being paid to the possibility that the health of offspring may be affected by parental exposure. Effects have

Table 3.8 Suspected reproductive effects of occupational exposures.

Agent	Fertility	Spontaneous abortion	Prematurity	Birth defects
Anaesthetic gases	−	?	−	−
Cadmium	+	−	−	−
Carbon disulphide	+	?	−	?
Chlordecone	+	−	−	−
Cytotoxic drugs	+	+	−	−
Dibromochloropropane	+	−	−	−
Ethylene oxide	−	?	−	−
Ethylene glycol ethers	−	?	−	−
Heat	+	−	−	−
Heavy work	−	+	?	−
Infectious agents, e.g. rubella, cytomegalovirus	?	+	+	+
Laboratory work	−	?	−	?
Lead	+	?	−	?
Ionising radiation	+	−	+	+
Mercury	?	?	−	+ (methyl)
Non-ionising radiation	−	?	−	?
Oral contraceptives	+	−	−	−
Organic solvents	−	−	−	?
PCBs	?	−	−	+
Shift work	−	?	?	−
Vinyl chloride	−	?	−	?

+, evidence; −, no evidence.

been reported in children of male parents who smoke, and parental exposure to ionising radiation has been suggested as a cause of childhood malignancy, although the evidence is conflicting. Animal studies have indicated a wide range of chemicals that can disrupt reproductive capacity. For the male, these include steroidal hormones, alkylating agents, antimetabolites, diuretics, psychopharmacological agents, anaesthetics, oral hypoglycaemics, ethyl alcohol, heavy metals, insecticides, herbicides, fungicides, cyclamates, solvents, radiation and heat. For female animals, the list is shorter, but contains many of the same chemicals.

The list for humans is shorter still and more tentative. Nevertheless, the stimulus to look further has come largely from two epidemiological studies of factory populations in the USA, which produced strong evidence that the nematocide, dibromochloropropane, and the chlorinated hydrocarbon insecticide, chlordecone (kepone), could cause human sterility.

It is important to remember that an abnormal pregnancy outcome

spans a wide range of events in the timetable from ovum/sperm to live birth. These include:
- normal gonadal function;
- union of ovum and sperm;
- placental implantation;
- embryonic organogenesis (1–3 months *in utero*);
- fetal development (3–9 months *in utero*);
- normal birth;
- healthy childhood (no cancers).

Furthermore, at least 15–20% of normal conceptions fail to reach full growth and normal delivery. These could be termed 'normal' spontaneous abortions, although most that have been analysed show gross genetic abnormalities. Congenital malformations have been reported in about 3% of all newborn children, with a further 3% reported during postnatal or later development. Some childhood cancers are traceable to maternal exposure during pregnancy, e.g. vaginal carcinoma resulting from mothers treated during pregnancy with diethylstilboestrol. Most abnormal pregnancy outcomes, however, have no known cause.

3.4.9 Endocrine system

The evidence for suggesting that occupational exposure can disrupt other endocrine functions is largely lacking, except for one area: the theoretical possibility that any endocrinologically active pharmaceutical preparation, such as betamethasone, thyroxine and the anticancer drugs, could affect the workers who formulate or synthesise it. There is anecdotal evidence from the industry that such effects can occur, but good epidemiological studies are in short supply.

3.4.10 Bone marrow

The bone marrow contains several important constituents. For the purpose of a review of target organs, two components are of particular note:
- haemopoietic stem cells;
- bone marrow fat.

The stem cell is a remarkable structure, capable of differentiating into most of the major cellular components of the blood. The marrow fat deposits are toxicologically important, because of their inherent ability to absorb fat-soluble compounds, and thereby store these potentially toxic compounds in close proximity to the stem cells.

Whilst some agents are capable of damaging mature red cells (arsenic) or can alter haem synthesis (lead), the most serious effect on the bone marrow is stem cell death (aplastic anaemia) or abnormal division (leukaemia). The two occupational exposures most likely to achieve these disastrous outcomes are:

- benzene;
- ionising radiation.

Benzene exposure has been associated with aplastic anaemia and acute myelogenous leukaemia. There is little doubt that high doses of benzene can cause these effects. What is in dispute is where to place the lower limit of exposure for (relatively) safe working conditions. Ionising radiation can cause many leukaemia cell types, but notably the myeloid series. Chronic lymphatic leukaemia seems not to be radiation induced. Multiple myeloma and other lymphomas have, however, been implicated.

Finally, cytotoxic therapeutic agents, by their very nature, destroy or damage bone marrow cells. These agents are a theoretical risk in pharmaceutical manufacture and a measurable risk in those patients who receive these drugs. Evidence of such effects from other agents, such as ethylene glycol ethers, trinitrotoluene and arsenic, is tenuous and disputed.

3.5) Prescribed diseases in the UK

UK list of prescribed diseases and the occupations for which they are prescribed (April 1997).

A Conditions due to physical agents

Prescribed disease or injury	Any occupation involving:
A1 Inflammation, ulceration or malignant disease of the skin or subcutaneous tissues or of the bones, or blood dyscrasia, or cataract due to electromagnetic radiations (other than radiant heat), or to ionising particles	Exposure to electromagnetic radiations (other than radiant heat) or ionising particles
A2 Heat cataract	Frequent or prolonged exposure to rays from molten or red-hot material
A3 Dysbarism, including decompression sickness, barotrauma and osteonecrosis	Subjection to compressed or rarefied air or other respirable gases or gaseous mixtures

Continued on p. 66

Conditions due to physical agents *Continued*

Prescribed disease or injury	Any occupation involving:
A4 Cramp of the hand or forearm due to repetitive movements	Prolonged periods of handwriting, typing or other repetitive movements of the fingers, hand or arm
A5 Subcutaneous cellulitis of the hand	Manual labour causing severe or prolonged friction or pressure on the hand
A6 Bursitis or subcutaneous cellulitis arising at or about the knee due to severe or prolonged external friction or pressure at or about the knee	Manual labour causing severe or prolonged external friction or pressure at or about the knee
A7 Bursitis or subcutaneous cellulitis arising at or about the elbow due to severe or prolonged external friction or pressure at or about the elbow	Manual labour causing severe or prolonged external friction or pressure at or about the elbow
A8 Traumatic inflammation of the tendons of the hand or forearm, or of the associated tendon sheaths (tenosynovitis)	Manual labour, or frequent or repeated movements of the hand or wrist
A9 Miner's nystagmus	Work in or about a mine
A10 Sensorineural hearing loss amounting to at least 50 dB in each ear, being the average of hearing losses at 1, 2 and 3 kHz frequencies, and being due in the case of at least one ear to occupational noise ('occupational deafness')	**a** The use of powered (but not hand-powered) grinding tools on cast metal (other than weld metal) or on billets or blooms, or work wholly or mainly in the immediate vicinity of those tools whilst they are being so used; or **b** the use of pneumatic percussive tools on metal, or work wholly or mainly in the immediate vicinity of those tools whilst they are being so used; or **c** the use of pneumatic percussive tools for drilling rock in quarries or underground or in mining coal or in sinking shafts or for tunnelling in civil engineering works, or work wholly or mainly in the immediate vicinity of those tools whilst they are being so used; or **c(a)** the use of pneumatic percussive tools on stone in quarry works, or work wholly or mainly in

Continued

Conditions due to physical agents *Continued*

Prescribed disease or injury	Any occupation involving:
	the immediate vicinity of those tools whilst they are being so used; or
	d work wholly or mainly in the immediate vicinity of plant (excluding power press plant) engaged in the forging (including drop stamping) of metal by means of closed or open dies or drop hammers; or
	e work in textile manufacturing where the work is undertaken wholly or mainly in rooms or sheds in which there are machines engaged in weaving man-made or natural (including mineral) fibres or in the high-speed false twisting of fibres; or
	f the use of, or work wholly or mainly in the immediate vicinity of, machines engaged in cutting, shaping or cleaning metal nails; or
	g the use of, or work wholly or mainly in the immediate vicinity of, plasma spray guns engaged in the deposition of metal; or
	h the use of, or work wholly or mainly in the immediate vicinity of, any of the following machines engaged in the working of wood, that is to say: multicutter moulding machines, planing machines, automatic or semi-automatic lathes, multiple cross-cut machines, automatic shaping machines, double-end tenoning machines, vertical spindle moulding machines (including high-speed routing machines), edge banding machines, band sawing machines with a blade width of not less than 75 mm and circular sawing machines in the operation of which the blade is moved towards the material being cut; or

Continued on p. 68

....

Conditions due to physical agents *Continued*

Prescribed disease or injury	Any occupation involving:
	i the use of chain saws in forestry; or
	j air arc gouging or work wholly or mainly in the immediate vicinity of air arc gouging; or
	k the use of band saws, circular saws or cutting discs for cutting metal in the metal founding or forging industries, or work wholly or mainly in the immediate vicinity of those tools whilst they are being so used; or
	l the use of circular saws for cutting products in the manufacture of steel, or work wholly or mainly in the immediate vicinity of those tools whilst they are being so used; or
	m the use of burners or torches for cutting or dressing steel-based products, or work wholly or mainly in the immediate vicinity of those tools whilst they are being so used; or
	n work wholly or mainly in the immediate vicinity of skid transfer banks; or
	o work wholly or mainly in the immediate vicinity of knock out and shake out grids in foundries; or
	p mechanical bobbin cleaning or work wholly or mainly in the immediate vicinity of mechanical bobbin cleaning; or
	q the use of, or work wholly or mainly in the immediate vicinity of, vibrating metal moulding boxes in the concrete products industry; or
	r the use of, or work wholly or mainly in the immediate vicinity of, high-pressure jets of water or a mixture of water and abrasive material in the water jetting industry (including work under water); or
	s work in ships' engine rooms; or

Continued

Conditions due to physical agents *Continued*

Prescribed disease or injury	Any occupation involving:
	t the use of circular saws for cutting concrete masonry blocks during manufacture, or work wholly or mainly in the immediate vicinity of those tools whilst they are being so used; or **u** burning stone in quarries by jet channelling processes, or work wholly or mainly in the immediate vicinity of such processes; or **v** work on gas turbines in connection with: (i) performance testing on test bed; (ii) installation testing of replacement engines in aircraft; (iii) acceptance testing of Armed Service fixed-wing combat planes; or **w** the use of, or work wholly or mainly in the immediate vicinity of: (i) machines for automatic moulding, automatic blow moulding or automatic glass pressing and forming machines used in the manufacture of glass containers or hollow ware; (ii) spinning machines using compressed air to produce glass wool or mineral wool; (iii) continuous glass toughening furnaces
A11 Episodic blanching, occurring throughout the year, affecting the middle or proximal phalanges or, in the case of a thumb, the proximal phalanx, of: **a** in the case of a person with 5 fingers (including thumbs) on one hand, any 3 of those fingers, or **b** in the case of a person with only 4 such fingers, any 2 of those fingers, or **c** in the case of a person with less than 4 such fingers, any one of those fingers or, as the case may be the one remaining finger (vibration white finger)	**a** The use of hand-held chain saws in forestry; or **b** the use of hand-held rotary tools in grinding or in the sanding or polishing of metal, or the holding of material being ground, or metal being sanded or polished, by rotary tools; or **c** the use of hand-held percussive metal-working tools, or the holding of metal being worked upon by percussive tools, in riveting, caulking, chipping, hammering, fettling or swaging; or

Continued on p. 70

Conditions due to physical agents *Continued*

Prescribed disease or injury	Any ocupation involving:
	d the use of hand-held powered percussive drills or hand-held powered percussive hammers in mining, quarrying, demolition or on roads or footpaths, including road construction; or **e** the holding of material being worked upon by pounding machines in shoe manufacture
A12 Carpal tunnel syndrome	The use of hand-held vibrating tools whose internal parts vibrate so as to transmit that vibration to the hand, but excluding those which are solely powered by hand

B Conditions due to biological agents

Prescribed disease or injury	Any occupation involving:
B1 Anthrax	Contact with animals infected with anthrax or the handling (including the loading or unloading or transport) of animal products or residues
B2 Glanders	Contact with equine animals or their carcasses
B3 Infection by *Leptospira*	**a** Work in places which are, or are liable to be, infested by rats, field mice or voles, or other small mammals; or **b** work at dog kennels or the care or handling of dogs; or **c** contact with bovine animals or their meat products or pigs or their meat products
B4 Ankylostomiasis	Work in or about a mine
B5 Tuberculosis	Contact with a source of tuberculous infection
B6 Extrinsic allergic alveolitis (including farmer's lung)	Exposure to moulds or fungal or heterologous proteins by reason of employment in:

Continued

Conditions due to biological agents *Continued*

Prescribed disease or injury	Any occupation involving:
	a agriculture, horticulture, forestry, cultivation of edible fungi or malt-working; or **b** loading or unloading or handling in storage mouldy vegetable matter or edible fungi; or **c** caring for or handling birds; or **d** handling bagasse
B7 Infection by organisms of the genus *Brucella* (brucellosis)	Contact with; **a** animals infected by *Brucella*, or their carcasses or parts thereof, or their untreated products; or **b** laboratory specimens of vaccines of, or containing, *Brucella*
B8 Viral hepatitis	Contact with: **a** human blood or human blood products; or **b** a source of viral hepatitis
B9 Infection by *Streptococcus suis* (rare form of meningitis from pigs)	Contact with pigs infected by *Streptococcus suis*, or with the carcasses, products or residues or pigs so infected
B10 **a** Avian chlamydiosis	Contact with birds infected with *Chlamydia psittaci*, or with the remains or untreated products of such birds
b Ovine chlamydiosis	Contact with sheep infected with *Chlamydia psittaci*, or with the remains or untreated products of such sheep
B11 Q fever	Contact with animals, their remains or their untreated products
B12 Orf	Contact with sheep, goats or with the carcasses of sheep or goats
B13 Hydatidosis	Contact with dogs

C Conditions due to chemical agents

Prescribed disease or injury	Any occupation involving:
C1 Poisoning by lead or a compound of lead	The use or handling of, and exposure to the fumes, dust or vapour of, lead or a compound of lead, or a substance containing lead
C2 Poisoning by manganese or a compound of manganese	The use or handling of, or exposure to the fumes, dust or vapour of, manganese or a compound of manganese, or a substance containing manganese
C3 Poisoning by phosphorus or an inorganic compound of phosphorus or poisoning due to the anti-cholinesterase or pseudo-anti-cholinesterase action of organic phosphorus compounds	The use or handling of, or exposure to the fumes, dust or vapour of, phosphorus or a compound of phosphorus, or a substance containing phosphorus
C4 Poisoning by arsenic or a compound of arsenic	The use or handling of, or exposure to the fumes, dust or vapour of, arsenic or a compound of arsenic, or a substance containing arsenic
C5 Poisoning by mercury or a compound of mercury	The use or handling of, or exposure to the fumes, dust or vapour of, mercury or a compound of mercury, or a substance containing mercury
C6 Poisoning by carbon disulphide	The use or handling of, or exposure to the fumes or vapour of, carbon disulphide or a compound of carbon disulphide, or a substance containing carbon disulphide
C7 Poisoning by benzene or a homologue of benzene	The use or handling of, or exposure to the fumes of, or vapour containing benzene or any of its homologues
C8 Poisoning by a nitro or amino or chloro derivative of benzene or of a homologue of benzene, or poisoning by nitrochlorobenzene	The use or handling of, or exposure to the fumes of, or vapour containing a nitro or amino or chloro derivative of benzene, or of a homologue of benzene, or nitrochlorobenzene
C9 Poisoning by dinitrophenol or a homologue of dinitrophenol or by substituted	The use or handling of, or exposure to the fumes of, or vapour

Continued

Conditions due to chemical agents *Continued*

Prescribed disease or injury	Any occupation involving:
dinitrophenols or by the salts of such substances	containing dinitrophenol or a homologue or substituted dinitrophenols or the salts of such substances
C10 Poisoning by tetrachloroethane	The use or handling of, or exposure to the fumes of, or vapour containing tetrachloroethane
C11 Poisoning by diethylene dioxide (dioxan)	The use or handling of, or exposure to the fumes of, or vapour containing diethylene dioxide (dioxan)
C12 Poisoning by methyl bromide	The use or handling of, or exposure to the fumes of or vapour containing methyl bromide
C13 Poisoning by chlorinated naphthalene	The use or handling of, or exposure to the fumes of or dust or vapour containing chlorinated naphthalene
C14 Poisoning by nickel carbonyl	Exposure to nickel carbonyl gas
C15 Poisoning by oxides of nitrogen	Exposure to oxides of nitrogen
C16 Poisoning by *Gonioma kamassi* (African boxwood)	The manipulation of *Gonioma kamassi* or any process in or incidental to the manufacture of articles therefrom
C17 Poisoning by beryllium or a compound of beryllium	The use or handling of, or exposure to the fumes, dust or vapour of, beryllium or a compound of beryllium, or a substance containing beryllium
C18 Poisoning by cadmium	Exposure to cadmium dust or fumes
C19 Poisoning by acrylamide monomer	The use or handling of, or exposure to, acrylamide monomer
C20 Dystrophy of the cornea (including ulceration of the corneal surface) of the eye	**a** The use or handling of, or exposure to, arsenic, tar, pitch, bitumen, mineral oil (including paraffin), soot or any compound, product or residue of any of these substances, except quinone or hydroquinone; or

Continued on p. 74

Conditions due to chemical agents *Continued*

Prescribed disease or injury	Any occupation involving:
	b exposure to quinone or hydroquinone during their manufacture
C21 **a** Localised new growth of the skin, papillomatous or keratotic (warts and scaliness) **b** Squamous cell carcinoma of the skin (form of skin cancer — chimney sweep's cancer)	The use or handling of, or exposure to, arsenic, tar, pitch, bitumen, mineral oil (including paraffin), soot or any compound, product or residue of any of these substances, except quinone or hydroquinone
C22 **a** Carcinoma of the mucous membrane of the nose or associated air sinuses **b** Primary carcinoma of a bronchus or of a lung	Work in a factory where nickel is produced by decomposition of a gaseous nickel compound which necessitates working in or about a building or buildings where that process or any other industrial process ancillary or incidental thereto is carried on
C23 Primary neoplasm (including papilloma, carcinoma-in-situ and invasive carcinoma) of the epithelial lining of the urinary tract (renal pelvis, ureter, bladder and urethra) (cancer of the lining of the bladder)	**a** Work in a building in which any of the following substances is produced for commercial purposes: (i) α-naphthylamine, β-naphthylamine or methylene-bis-orthochloroaniline; (ii) biphenyl substituted by at least one nitro or primary amino group or by at least one nitro and primary amino group (including benzidine); (iii) any of the substances mentioned in subparagraph (ii) above if further ring substituted by halogeno, methyl or methoxy groups, but not by other groups; (iv) the salts of any of the substances mentioned in subparagraphs (i) to (iii) above; (v) auramine or magenta; or **b** the use or handling of any of the substances mentioned in subparagraph **a** (i) to (iv), or work in a process in which any such substance is used, handled or liberated; or

Continued

Conditions due to chemical agents *Continued*

Prescribed disease or injury	Any occupation involving:
	c the maintenance or cleaning of any plant or machinery used in any such process as is mentioned in subparagraph **b**, or the cleaning of any plant or machinery used in any such process as is mentioned in subparagraph **b**, or the cleaning of clothing used in any such building as is mentioned in subparagraph **a** if such clothing is cleaned within the works of which the building forms a part in a laundry maintained and used solely in connection with such works; or **d** exposure to coal tar pitch volatiles produced in aluminium smelting involving the Soderberg process (the method of producing aluminium by electrolysis in which the anode consists of petroleum coke and mineral oil which is baked *in situ*)
C24 **a** Angiosarcoma of the liver **b** Osteolysis of the terminal phalanges of the fingers **c** Non-cirrhotic portal fibrosis	**a** Work in or about machinery or apparatus used for the polymerisation of vinyl chloride monomer, a process which, for the purposes of this provision, comprises all operations up to and including the drying of the slurry produced by the polymerisation and the packaging of the dried product; or **b** work in a building or structure in which any part of that process takes place
C25 Occupational vitiligo	The use or handling of, or exposure to, *p*-tert-butylphenol, *p*-tert-butylcatechol, paramyl-phenol, hydroquinone or the monobenzyl or monobutylether of hydroquinone
C26 Damage to the liver or kidneys due to exposure to carbon tetrachloride	The use of or handling of, or exposure to the fumes of, or

Continued on p. 76

....

Conditions due to chemical agents   *Continued*

Prescribed disease or injury	Any occupation involving:
	vapour containing carbon tetrachloride
C27 Damage to the liver or kidneys due to exposure to trichloromethane (chloroform)	The use of or handling of, or exposure to the fumes of, or vapour containing trichloromethane (chloroform)
C28 Central nervous system dysfunction and associated gastrointestinal disorders due to exposure to chloromethane (methyl chloride)	The use of or handling of, or exposure to the fumes of, or vapour containing chloromethane (methyl chloride)
C29 Peripheral neuropathy due to exposure to *n*-hexane or methyl-*n*-butylketone	The use of or handling of, or exposure to the fumes of, or vapour containing *n*-hexane or methyl-*n*-butylketone
C30 Chrome dermatitis, or ulceration of the mucous membranes or the epidermis, resulting from exposure to chromic acid, chromates or dichromates	The use or handling of, or exposure to, chromic acid, chromates or dichromates

D Miscellaneous conditions

Prescribed disease or injury	Any occupation involving:
D1 Pneumoconiosis (includes silicosis and asbestosis)	**a** Set out in Part II of Schedule 1 of the Social Security (Industrial Injuries) (Prescribed Diseases) Regulations 1985 **b** Specified in Regulation 2(b)(ii) of the Social Security (Industrial Injuries) (Prescribed Diseases) Regulations 1985
D2 Byssinosis	Work in any room where any process up to and including the weaving process is performed in a factory in which the spinning or manipulation of raw or waste cotton or of flax, or the weaving of cotton or flax, is carried on
D3 Diffuse mesothelioma (primary neoplasm of the mesothelium of the pleura or of the pericardium or of the peritoneum) (cancer of the lining of the lung)	Exposure to asbestos, asbestos dust or any admixture of asbestos at a level above that commonly found in the environment at large

Continued

Miscellaneous conditions *Continued*

Prescribed disease or injury	Any occupation involving:
D4 Allergic rhinitis which is due to exposure to any of the following agents: **a** isocyanates; **b** platinum salts; **c** fumes or dusts arising from the manufacture, transport or use of hardening agents (including epoxy resin curing agents) based on phthalic anhydride, tetrachlorophthalic anhydride, trimellitic anhydride or triethylene-tetramine; **d** fumes arising from the use of rosin as a soldering flux; **e** proteolytic enzymes; **f** animals including insects and other arthropods used for the purpose of research or education or in laboratories; **g** dusts arising from the sowing, cultivation, harvesting, drying, handling, milling, transport or storage of barley, oats, rye, wheat or maize, or the handling, milling, transport or storage of meal or flour made therefrom; **h** antibiotics; **i** cimetidine; **j** wood dust; **k** ispaghula; **l** castor bean dust; **m** ipecacuanha; **n** azodicarbonamide (occupational asthma) **o** animals including insects and other arthropods, or their larval forms, used for the purposes of pest control or fruit cultivation or the larval forms of animals used for the purposes of research, education or in laboratories; **p** glutaraldehyde; **q** persulphate salts or henna; **r** crustaceans or fish or products arising from these in the food processing industry; **s** reactive dyes; **t** soya bean; **u** tea dust; **v** green coffee bean dust; **w** fumes from stainless steel	Exposure to any of the agents set out in column 1 of this paragraph

Continued on p. 78

Miscellaneous conditions   *Continued*

Prescribed disease or injury	Any occupation involving:
D5 Non-infective dermatitis of external orgin (excluding dermatitis due to ionising particles or electromagnetic radiations other than radiant heat)	Exposure to dust, liquid or vapour or any other external agent except chromic acid, chromates or dichromates capable of irritating the skin (including friction or heat, but excluding ionising particles or electromagnetic radiations other than radiant heat)
D6 Carcinoma of the nasal cavity or associated air sinuses (nasal carcinoma)	**a** Attendance for work in or about a building where wooden goods are manufactured or repaired; or **b** attendance for work in a building used for the manufacture of footwear or components of footwear made wholly or partly of leather or fibre board; or **c** attendance for work at a place used wholly or mainly for the repair of footwear made wholly or partly of leather or fibre board
D7 Asthma which is due to exposure to:	**a** isocyanates; **b** platinum salts; **c** fumes or dusts arising from the manufacture, transport or use of hardening agents (including epoxy resin curing agents) based on phthalic anhydride, tetrachlorophthalic anhydride, trimellitic anhydride or triethylene-tetramine; **d** fumes arising from the use of rosin as a soldering flux; **e** proteolytic enzymes; **f** animals including insects and other arthropods used for the purpose of research or education or in laboratories; **g** dusts arising from the sowing, cultivation, harvesting, drying, handling, milling, transport or storage of barley, oats, rye, wheat or maize, or the handling, milling, transport or storage of meal or flour made therefrom;

Continued

Miscellaneous conditions   *Continued*

Prescribed disease or injury	Any occupation involving:
	h antibiotics; **i** cimetidine; **j** wood dust; **k** ispaghula; **l** castor bean dust; **m** ipecacuanha; **n** azodicarbonamide (occupational asthma); **o** animals including insects and other arthropods, or their larval forms, used for the purposes of pest control or fruit cultivation or the larval forms of animals used for the purposes of research, education or in laboratories; **p** glutaraldehyde; **q** persulphate salts or henna; **r** crustaceans or fish or products arising from these in the food processing industry; **s** reactive dyes; **t** soya bean; **u** tea dust; **v** green coffee bean dust; **w** fumes from stainless steel welding; **x** any other sensitising agent
D8 Primary carcinoma of the lung where there is accompanying evidence of one or both of the following: **a** asbestosis; **b** unilateral or bilateral diffuse pleural thickening extending to a thickness of 5 mm or more at any point within the area affected as measured by a plain chest radiograph (not being a computerised tomography scan or other form of imaging) which: (i) in the case of unilateral diffuse pleural thickening, covers 50% or more of the area of the chest wall of the lung affected; or (ii) in the case of bilateral diffuse pleural thickening, covers 25% or more of the combined area of the chest wall of both lungs	**a** The working or handling of asbestos or any admixture of asbestos; or **b** the manufacture or repair of asbestos textiles or other articles containing or composed of asbestos; or **c** the cleaning of any machinery or plant used in any of the foregoing operations and of any chambers, fixtures and appliances for the collection of asbestos dust; or **d** substantial exposure to the dust arising from any of the foregoing operations

Continued on p. 80

Miscellaneous conditions *Continued*

Prescribed disease or injury	Any occupation involving:
D9 *Unilateral or bilateral diffuse pleural thickening* extending to a thickness of 5 mm or more at any point within the area affected as measured by a plain chest radiograph (not being a computerised tomography scan or other form of imaging) which: (i) in the case of unilateral diffuse pleural thickening, covers 50% or more of the area of the chest wall of the lung affected; or (ii) in the case of bilateral diffuse pleural thickening, covers 25% or more of the combined area of the chest wall of both lungs	**a** The working or handling of asbestos or any admixture of asbestos; or **b** the manufacture or repair of asbestos textiles or other articles containing or composed of asbestos; or **c** the cleaning of any machinery or plant used in any of the foregoing operations and of any chambers, fixtures and appliances for the collection of asbestos dust; or **d** substantial exposure to the dust arising from any of the foregoing operations
D10 Primary carcinoma of the lung	**a** Work underground in a tin mine; or **b** exposure to bis(chloromethyl)ether produced during the manufacture of chloromethyl methyl ether; or **c**. exposure to zinc chromate, calcium chromate or strontium chromate in their pure forms
D11 Primary carcinoma of the lung where there is accompanying silicosis	Exposure to silica dust in: **a** glass or pottery manufacture; **b** tunnelling in, quarrying sandstone or granite; **c** metal ore mining; **d** slate quarrying or the manufacture of artefacts from slate; **e** clay mining; **f** using siliceous materials as abrasives; **g** stone cutting; **h** stone masonry; **i** foundry work

Continued

Miscellaneous conditions *Continued*

Prescribed disease or injury	Any occupation involving:
D12 Chronic bronchitis or emphysema Except in the circumstances specified in Regulation 2(d): **a** chronic bronchitis; or **b** emphysema; or **c** both where there is accompanying evidence of a forced expiratory volume in 1 s (measured from the position of maximum inspiration with the claimant making maximum effort) which is: (i) at least 1 l below the mean value predicted in accordance with JE Cotes, *Lung Function: Assessment and Application in Medicine*, 5th edn. Oxford: Blackwell Scientific Publications, 1994, for a person of the claimant's age, height and sex; or (ii) less than 1 l	Exposure to coal dust by reason of working underground in a coal mine for a period or periods amounting in aggregate to at least 20 years (whether before or after July 5, 1948) and any such period or periods shall include a period or periods of incapacity while engaged in such an occupation

4 Chemicals, Gases, Dusts and Particles

Introduction

This chapter aims to provide an abridged account of the sources/uses, health effects and measurement requirements for a number of substances.

In terms of the types of activity that generate the majority of exposures in the working environment (gases/vapours and dusts/fibres), the following is an abridged list of periodic and/or continuous processes.

1 Material handling which gives rise to dust, gases or vapours:
- debagging;
- pouring of liquids;
- transfer from one container to another;
- transfer from one mode of transport to another;
- blending;
- stirring or agitating;
- screening or sieving;
- crushing or grinding;
- emptying;
- recharging;
- sampling.

2 Processes causing emission of (mainly) vapours, but also particles:
- stirring and agitating;
- surface coating;
- drying;
- spraying;
- dipping;
- curing;
- baking;
- welding;
- sampling.

3 Processes producing mainly dust, but also some fume or gas:
- machining;
- drilling;
- planing;
- sanding;
- milling;
- cutting;
- sawing;
- dismantling;
- demolition.

Fugitive emissions produce gases, liquids and vapours, and occur as a result of leaks from:
- fractured or corroded pipes, vessels and containers;
- poorly made joints or the breakdown of seals on joints;
- along the shafts of valves;
- along the shafts of pumps;
- spills and collisions.

Each year, the Health and Safety Executive (HSE) in the UK publishes a document, Environmental Hygiene 40 (EH40), which contains occupational exposure limits (OELs) for use with the Control of Substances Hazardous to Health (COSHH) Regulations 1994. Under COSHH, there are two types of OEL for hazardous substances: occupational exposure standards (OESs) and maximum exposure limits (MELs). Both types of limit are concentrations of hazardous substances in the air, averaged over a specified period of time, referred to as a time-weighted average (TWA). Two time periods are used: long-term (8-h) and short-term (15-min) periods.

These UK exposure figures (OESs and MELs) are set on the recommendations of the Health and Safety Commission's (HSC) Advisory Committee of Toxic Substances (ACTS) and its Working Group on the Assessment of Toxic Chemicals (WATCH). Following a detailed review and consideration of all the relevant information, these committees consider, first, what type of limit should be set following specific rules and, second, the level at which the limit should be set.

An OES is set at a level that (based on current scientific knowledge) will not damage the health of workers exposed to it by inhalation day after day. MELs are set for substances which may cause serious health effects, such as cancer and occupational asthma, and for which 'safe' levels of exposure cannot be determined, or for substances for which safe levels may exist, but control to these levels is not reasonably practicable.

The indicative criteria for occupational exposure limits

For a substance to be assigned an OES, it must meet all of the following three criteria.

Criterion 1. The available scientific evidence allows for the identification, with reasonable certainty, of a concentration, averaged over a reference period, at which there is no indication that the substance is likely to be injurious to employees if they are exposed by inhalation day after day to that concentration.

Criterion 2. Exposures to concentrations higher than that derived under criterion 1, and which could reasonably occur in practice, are unlikely to produce serious short- or long-term effects on health over the period of time it might reasonably be expected to take to identify and remedy the cause of excessive exposure.

Criterion 3. The available evidence indicates that compliance with the OES, as derived under criterion 1, is reasonably practicable.

For a substance to be assigned an MEL, it must meet either of the following criteria.

Criterion 4. The available evidence on the substance does not satisfy criterion 1 and/or 2 for an OES, and exposure to the substance has, or is liable to have, serious health implications for workers.

Criterion 5. Socioeconomic factors indicate that, although the substance meets criteria 1 and 2 for an OES, a numerically higher value is necessary if the controls associated with certain uses are to be regarded as reasonably practicable.

The HSE's list of OELs quotes airborne concentrations either volumetrically as parts per million (ppm) or gravimetrically as milligrams of the substance per cubic metre of air (mg m^{-3}). For many gases and vapours, both units are used, with the relationship between them being defined by the equation:

$$\text{OEL in mg m}^{-3} = \frac{\text{OEL in ppm} \times \text{MW}}{24.05526}$$

where MW is the molecular weight (molar gas in g mol^{-1}) of the substance. (Note that 24.05526 l mol^{-1} is the molar volume of an ideal gas at 20°C and 1 atm pressure (760 mmHg, 101 325 Pa, 1.01325 bar).)

For substances assigned both an 8-h TWA and a short-term reference period, the total duration of peak exposures above the 8-h TWA values should be limited to 1 h in a 24-h period, but without prejudice to the generality of the 8-h TWA. For those substances for which no short-term limit is specified, it is recommended that a figure of three times the long-term limit should be used as a guideline for controlling short-term excursions in exposure.

Unfortunately, it is rare for an individual to be exposed to only a single substance. Mixed exposures are much more common. The ways in which the constituent substances of a mixed exposure interact vary considerably. Some mixed exposures involve substances that act on different body tissues or organs, by different toxic mechanisms or by causing various effects which are independent of each other. Other mixtures will include substances that act on the same organs, or by similar mechanisms, so that the effects reinforce each other, and the substances are additive in their effect. In some cases, the overall effect is considerably greater than the sum of the individual effects, and the system is synergistic. This may arise from the mutual enhancement of the effects of the constituents because one substance potentiates another.

The main types of interaction are given below.

1 *Synergistic substances*. Cases of synergism (asbestos and smoking) and potentiation (methylethylketone (MEK) and *n*-hexane) are rare, but serious. Seek specialist advice.

2 *Additive substances*. Where there is reason to believe that the effects of the constituents are additive, and where the exposure limits are based on the same health effects, the mixed exposure should be assessed by means of the formula:

$$C_1/L_1 + C_2/L_2 + C_3/L_3 \ldots < 1$$

where C_1, C_2, etc., are the TWA concentrations of the constituents in air and L_1, L_2, etc., are the corresponding exposure limits. The use of this formula is only applicable where the additive substances have been assigned OESs and L_1, L_2, etc., relate to the same reference period in the list of approved OESs. Where the sum of the *C/L* fractions does not exceed unity, the exposure is considered not to exceed the notional exposure limits. If one of the constituents has been assigned an MEL, the additive effect should be taken into account in deciding the extent to which it is reasonably practicable to reduce exposure further.

3 *Independent substances*. Where no synergistic or additive effects are known or considered to be likely, the constituents can be regarded as acting independently. It is then sufficient to ensure compliance with each of the exposure limits individually.

Complicating factors

Several factors that complicate the assessment and control of exposure to individual substances will also affect cases of mixed exposures and will require similar special consideration. These factors include:

1 exposure to a substance for which there is no established limit (see Guidance on Regulation 7 of COSHH in the General COSHH Approved Code of Practice) or for which an MEL has been set;

2 the relevance of factors such as alcohol, medication or smoking;

3 absorption via the skin or by ingestion, as well as by inhalation;

4 substances in mixtures may mutually affect the extent of their absorption, as well as their health effects, at a given level of exposure.

To appreciate how much or how little information has been used in deciding upon a particular value, EH64: Summary Criteria for Occupational Exposure Limits (updated annually — including summaries for all MELs and around 100 substances with OESs) and Documentation of the Recommended TLVs, published by the American Conference of Governmental Industrial Hygienists (ACGIH), should be consulted.

4.2 Monitoring of the workplace environment

Basic techniques for measuring the airborne concentration of a specific chemical or particle are therefore only briefly mentioned in this chapter, under the particular substance. It must be pointed out that these are not necessarily the definitive techniques, as often more than one is available, and new methods are continually being developed. Many analytical chemists also have their own preferences, and they should always be consulted before embarking upon a particular method of sampling. The HSE publishes guidance for the analysis of certain substances in the series Methods for the Determination of Hazardous Substances (MDHS). Where appropriate, the MDHS numbers are quoted.

4.3 Inorganic chemicals

4.3.1 Aluminium (Al)

Occurrence. Metalliferous ores, mainly as alumina, bauxite (Al_2O_3).
Properties. Light, white metal.
Uses. Alloys, engine and aircraft components, window frames and food containers. Oxides used as abrasives. Insoluble salts, such as hydroxide, used in antacid preparations.
Metabolism. Ingested aluminium salts are poorly absorbed from the gastrointestinal tract. Can interfere with phosphate absorption. Excreted in the faeces. Lung retention is also possible.
Health effects. Acute: massive oral doses cause gastrointestinal irritation, but whether long-term sequelae, such as encephalopathy, can occur is disputed (some of those affected by the Camelford water supply incident in the UK continue to complain of a range of symptoms a decade after the event). Chronic: Shaver's disease (a form of pulmonary fibrosis) was described in 1947 in workers who inhaled aluminium, but this effect has not been described in subsequent studies. Workers in the aluminium smelting and refining industries can develop 'pot room asthma' and have an increased risk of bladder cancer. However, none of these effects is considered to be due to aluminium or aluminium salts. Fluorosis used to occur in such workers and those in neighbouring areas from fluoride ore smelting. The putative association between aluminium absorption and Alzheimer's disease is unresolved.

Biological monitoring. Body burden of aluminium appears to be little affected by non-dietary intake.

Treatment. Non-specific and usually not relevant.

Measurement. Sampled onto cellulose ester membrane filters using SIMPEDS/Higgins and Dewell cyclones at 2.2 l min^{-1} for respirable dust, and the Institute of Occupational Medicine (IOM)/7-hole United Kingdom Atomic Energy Authority (UKAEA) head for total inhalable dust. If necessary, acid (HNO$_3$) digestion and atomic absorption spectrophotometry (National Institute for Occupational Safety and Health (NIOSH) 7013).

Occupational exposure limits. HSE OES: 8-h TWA: total inhalable, 10 mg m^{-3}; respirable dust, 4 mg m^{-3}.

4.3.2 Antimony (Sb)

Occurrence. Metalliferous ores, usually as sulphide (Sb$_2$S$_3$).

Properties. Silvery-white, soft metal with properties very similar to arsenic. Stibine (SbH$_3$) is a gas (p. 133) formed from antimony on reaction with nascent hydrogen (haemolytic agent).

Uses. Alloys, paint pigment, rubber compounding.

Metabolism. Few severe poisonings — probably similar to arsenic.

Health effects. Similar to arsenic, although vomiting and eye and mucous membrane irritation may be more severe. Cardiac arrhythmias and mild jaundice have been reported.

Health surveillance. Periodic review of cardiac symptoms.

Treatment. British anti-lewisite (BAL, dimercaprol), intramuscularly (i.m.).

Measurement. Antimony and compounds (particulate): sampled onto cellulose acetate filter (pore size, 0.8 µm) at an air flow rate of around 2 l min^{-1} for subsequent analysis for Sb using atomic absorption spectrophotometry.

Occupational exposure limits. Antimony and compounds as Sb, HSE MEL: 8-h TWA, 0.5 mg m^{-3}.

HSE guidance. EH19 — Antimony: Health and Safety Precautions.

4.3.3 Arsenic (As)

Occurrence. Widely dispersed in nature, usually in association with metalliferous ore, e.g. FeAsS. It is therefore a by-product of both ferrous and non-ferrous smelting, mainly as the trioxide As$_2$O$_3$.

Properties. Arsenic is a steel-grey brittle metal. Compounds of arsenic include As$_2$O$_3$, a crystalline solid, trivalent and pentavalent forms and arsine (AsH$_3$) gas (p. 133).

Uses. Alloys, insecticides, fungicides, rodenticides, pigments, decoloriser in glass and paper making.

Metabolism. Normal body constituent due to wide dispersion in nature. Stored in keratin. Excretion slow in the urine.

Health effects. Acute: severe respiratory irritation, headache, abdominal pain, diarrhoea and vomiting — shock. Skin irritation and allergy are possible. See also arsine (p. 133). Chronic: gastrointestinal symptoms occasionally; peripheral neuropathy — mainly sensory; dermatitis, with or without areas of depigmentation. Equivocal evidence of liver damage — vascular or parenchymal in type. Carcinogenic changes in skin and lungs.

Health surveillance and biological monitoring. Periodic review of skin, respiratory and other symptoms. Arsenic levels in urine, hair and nails less reliable. 'Normal' levels: urine, 70 nmol mmol^{-1} creatinine; hair, 5 ppm.

Treatment. Non-specific for skin and respiratory disturbances. BAL, i.m.

Measurement. Arsenic and compounds (particulate): sampled onto a treated cellulose ester filter (pore size, 0.8 µm) at an air flow rate of around 2 l min^{-1} for subsequent analysis for As using atomic absorption spectrophotometry.

Occupational exposure limits. Arsenic and compounds (except arsine and lead arsenate) as As, HSE MEL: 8-h TWA, 0.1 mg m^{-3}. Lead arsenate as Pb, HSE: 0.15 mg m^{-3}.

HSE guidance. Arsenic and compounds: EH8 — Arsenic: Health and Safety Precautions. MDHS 41.

4.3.4 Beryllium (Be)

Occurrence. Mainly as beryllium aluminium silicate, $3BeO.Al_2O_3.6SiO_2$. Emerald (with chromium oxide), aquamarine and chrysoberyl are three varieties.

Properties. A very light, hard, non-corrosive, grey metal.

Uses. Alloys, nuclear reactors (fission moderator, neutron source, with uranium), aerospace, ceramics, formerly used in fluorescent light tubes.

Metabolism. Absorption is poor from the gut, but good from the lungs. Protein bound with liver, spleen and skeleton deposition. Urinary excretion variable.

Health effects. Acute: chemical pneumonitis, cough, chest pain, dyspnoea, pneumonia. Conjunctivitis, rhinitis, pharyngitis. Skin irritant. Chronic: sarcoid-like granulomata — mainly in the lungs, but occasionally subcutaneous. The lung lesions can lead to progressive interstitial fibrosis with hilar lymphadenopathy resulting in cor pulmonale. Beryllium is probably a lung carcinogen. Chest radiography in severe cases shows widespread nodules, 1–5 µm in size, which may coalesce. Kveim test will distinguish berylliosis from sarcoidosis.

Health surveillance. Chest radiography. Pulmonary function tests.
Treatment. Non-specific management of pulmonary fibrosis. Chelation therapy with ethylenediaminetetra acetic acid (EDTA) has been used with some success in acute poisoning, and corticosteroids may be helpful in chronic fibrotic lung disease.
Measurement. Sampled onto cellulose acetate filter (pore size, 0.8 µm) at an air flow rate of around 1 l min^{-1} for subsequent analysis after treatment for Be using atomic absorption spectrophotometry (30 min at 0.025 mg m^{-3}). MDHS 29/2.
Occupational exposure limits. HSE MEL: 8-h TWA, 0.002 mg m^{-3}.
HSE guidance. EH13 — Beryllium: Health and Safety Precautions. MDHS 29/2.

4.3.5 Cadmium (Cd)

Occurrence. Cadmium sulphide (CdS), usually in association with zinc ore.
Properties. Soft, ductile, silvery-white metal, which is corrosion resistant and electropositive.
Uses. Alloys, electroplating, alkaline storage batteries, pigments, nuclear reactors (neutron absorber).
Metabolism. Mainly absorbed through inhalation. Bound to plasma globulin, with accumulation in the kidney and lesser amounts in the liver. Urinary excretion poor in the absence of renal damage.
Health effects. Acute: increased salivation, nausea, vomiting → shock (ingestion). Cadmium fumes can cause a severe chemical pneumonitis which can lead to pulmonary oedema and death. Mucous membrane irritation may also occur. Chronic: non-specific features include gastrointestinal disturbance, yellow rings on the teeth and anosmia. The main target organs are, however, the lungs and kidneys. Emphysema can be severe and is usually focal (? due to reduced α-antitrypsin). Nephrotoxicity is usually manifested as tubular damage with proteinuria (especially β_2-microglobulins), glycosuria and amino aciduria. Hypertension has been implicated as a sequela of chronic cadmium exposure. Lung carcinoma is thought by many to follow chronic exposure, but the case for prostate cancer is weak.
Health surveillance and biological monitoring. Lung function tests, urinalysis for β_2-microglobulins and cadmium. Cadmium in urine is indicative of exposure, but is a poor estimate of effect. Renal cortical cadmium levels are more reliable, but difficult to measure (neutron activation analysis).

Treatment. Calcium EDTA is useful in acute poisoning. Chronic renal and pulmonary effects are often discovered at a late and irreversible stage.
Measurement. Sampled onto cellulose acetate filter (pore size, 0.8 μm) at an air flow rate of 2 l min^{-1} for subsequent analysis after treatment for Cd using atomic absorption spectrophotometry (MDHS 10/2 and 11).
Occupational exposure limits. Cadmium dust and salts, cadmium oxide fume as Cd, HSE MEL: 8-h TWA, 0.025 mg m^{-3}.
HSE guidance. MDHS 10/2 and 11.

4.3.6 Chromium (Cr)

Occurrence. Chromite ore (FeO.Cr$_2$O$_3$).
Properties. Hard, corrosion-resistant, grey metal. Several valency states including divalent, trivalent and hexavalent.
Uses. Stainless steel and other alloys, electroplating, pigments, leather tanning.
Metabolism. Essential trace element. Better absorption for hexavalent than trivalent forms. Hexavalent forms enter cells and are reduced intracellularly to trivalent chromium. Excretion mainly in the urine in trivalent form.
Health effects. Hexavalent salts are irritant and corrosive, causing chronic skin and nasal (chrome ulcers) and respiratory tract irritation. Chromate ore workers have an increased incidence of lung carcinoma, thought to be due to the slightly soluble hexavalent chromium compounds of strontium, calcium and zinc. Chromium platers, exposed to chromic acid mist, have also been reported to have an excess of lung cancer.
Biological monitoring. None of value, although attempts have been made to use blood and urinary chromium.
Treatment. Remove chromium salts from skin. EDTA ointment for skin contact. Ascorbic acid may assist conversion of hexavalent to less toxic trivalent form.
Measurement. Chromium, chromates, soluble chromic and chromous salts: sampled onto cellulose acetate filter (pore size, 0.8 μm) at an air flow rate of around 1.5 l min^{-1} for subsequent analysis for Cr using atomic absorption spectrophotometry. Chromic acid and chromates: sampled onto polyvinyl chloride (PVC) filter (pore size, 5 μm) at an air flow rate of around 1 l min^{-1} for subsequent colorimetric analysis.
Occupational exposure limits. Chromium metal, Cr(II) and Cr(III) compounds as Cr, HSE OES: 8-h TWA, 0.5 mg m^{-3}. Chromium(VI) compounds as Cr, HSE MEL: 8-h TWA, 0.05 mg m^{-3}.
HSE guidance. EH2 — Chromium: Health and Safety Precautions.

EH6 — Chromic Acid Concentrations in Air. Chrome Ulceration: Epitheliomatous-Ulceration Order 1919 (S, R and O 1919 No. 1775). MDHS 12/2 and 13.

4.3.7 Lead (Pb)

Occurrence. Mainly as the sulphide (PbS), in association with other metallic sulphates.

Properties. Soft, bluish-grey metal. Heavy, malleable, ductile. Inorganic and organic compounds.

Uses. Pipes, sheet metal, foil, ammunition, pigments, solders, anti-knock additive to petrol (organic compound only).

Metabolism. Poorly absorbed through the gut (10%), but dependent on the calcium and iron content of the diet. Pulmonary absorption more effective. Transported in form bound to red cell membrane and stored mainly in bone. Excretion mainly urinary.

Health effects. Inorganic. Acute: non-specific with lassitude, abdominal cramps and constipation, myalgia and anorexia. Chronic: peripheral motor neuropathy (especially wrist drop, although this is rarely seen nowadays) and anaemia are the main late manifestations. Disturbances of haem synthesis and a slowing of motor nerve conduction times can be detected soon after excessive absorption has commenced. Renal damage and encephalopathy are rare and usually confined to children. Organic. Differs from inorganic in being primarily associated with psychiatric manifestations, such as insomnia, hyperexcitability and even mania.

Biological monitoring. Blood lead UK suspension level: 70 µg per 100 ml. Urinary δ-aminolaevulinic acid and red cell (free erythrocyte) zinc protoporphyrin concentration. (For organic lead absorption, urinary lead estimation is more useful.)

Treatment. If necessary, calcium EDTA or penicillamine can be given. The latter can be given orally and is therefore the treatment of choice. Organic lead poisoning does not respond to such chelation therapy.

Measurement. Inorganic lead: sampled onto cellulose acetate filter (pore size, 0.8 µm) in single-hole holder at an air flow rate of around 1 l min^{-1} for subsequent analysis after treatment for Pb using atomic absorption spectrophotometry. Note that filters should be partially covered, as with UKAEA-type holders. Organic lead: sampled through charcoal tube at an air flow rate of 1000 ml min^{-1} for subsequent analysis of Pb using atomic absorption spectrophotometry.

'Lead in air standard'. Inorganic lead as Pb, 8-h TWA: 0.15 mg m^{-3}. Tetraethyl lead as Pb, 8-h TWA: 0.10 mg m^{-3}.

Legal requirements and HSE guidance. Control of Lead at Work

Regulations 1980 (SI 1980 No. 1248). Control of Lead at Work Code of Practice, revised June 1985. EH28 — Control of Lead: Air Sampling Techniques and Strategies. EH29 — Control of Lead: Outside Workers. MDHS 6/2, 7, 8 and 18.

4.3.8 Manganese (Mn)

Occurrence. Widely occurring as MnO_2, $MnSiO_3$.

Properties. Reddish-grey, hard metal. Decomposes in water.

Uses. Alloys, dry-cell batteries, potassium permanganate, glass and ceramics, matches.

Metabolism. Essential trace element. Poorly absorbed from the gut, somewhat better from the lungs. Accumulates in the kidney, liver and bone. Excretion largely through the gut. Transport in body is intracellular, with surprisingly low cerebral concentrations.

Health effects. Acute: manganese oxide fume is a respiratory and mucous membrane irritant. Chronic: slow onset (1–2 years) with headache, asthenia, poor sleep and disturbed mental state. Neurological signs are primarily of the basal ganglia $\rightarrow$ Parkinsonism.

Health surveillance and biological monitoring. Assessment of central nervous system (CNS) symptoms, especially extrapyramidal system. No special tests.

Treatment. Calcium EDTA before permanent brain damage has occurred. Thereafter, L-dopa has been shown to be useful, at least in the short term.

Measurement. Sampled onto cellulose acetate filter (pore size, 0.8 µm) at an air flow rate of 1.5 l min^{-1} for subsequent analysis for Mn using atomic absorption spectrophotometry (NIOSH 7300).

Occupational exposure limits. Manganese and compounds (except fume, tetraoxide and organic manganese) as Mn, HSE OES: 8-h TWA, 5 mg m^{-3}. Manganese fume as Mn, HSE OES: 8-h TWA, 1 mg m^{-3}; 15-min short-term exposure limit (STEL), 3 m m^{-3}. Trimanganese tetraoxide, HSE OES: 8-h TWA, 1 mg m^{-3}. Tricarbonyl (β-cyclopentadienyl) manganese as Mn, OES: 8-h TWA, 0.1 mg m^{-3}; 15-min STEL, 0.3 mg m^{-3} (Sk). Tricarbonyl (methylcyclopentadienyl) manganese as Mn, OES: 8-h TWA, 0.2 mg m^{-3}; 15-min STEL, 0.6 mg m^{-3} (Sk).

4.3.9 Mercury (Hg)

Occurrence. Mainly as sulphide ore (HgS), rarely as liquid metal.

Properties. Liquid at normal temperature and pressure. Therefore has a measurable vapour pressure. Mixes in unique fashion with other metals (amalgams).

Uses. Scientific instruments, amalgams, 'silvering', solders, pharmaceuticals, paints, seed dressings (organic compounds only), explosives.

Metabolism. Salts rapidly absorbed by all routes (metallic mercury poorly absorbed from the gut). Inorganic salts more readily absorbed through the gut and excreted by kidneys than organic compounds. Organics have predilection for the CNS.

Health effects. Acute: rare in industry. Febrile illness with pneumonitis. If severe, can cause oliguric renal failure. Chronic: slow onset with peculiar neuropsychiatric disorder (erethism) with features of anxiety neurosis, timidity and paranoia. Accompanied by gingivitis, excessive salivation, intention tremor, dermatographia, scanning speech. Upper motor neurone lesions and visual field constriction more commonly associated with organic mercurialism. Anterior capsule of the lens of the eye may be discoloured. Nephrotic syndrome.

Biological monitoring. Mercury in urine (preferably 24-h specimen) for longer term exposure or blood for acute exposure. The biological exposure index is 20 mmol mol^{-1} creatinine for urinary mercury and 75 nmol l^{-1} for blood mercury. Electromyography.

Treatment. BAL, calcium EDTA — both more effective for inorganic mercurialism.

Measurement. Mercury vapour: measured with a direct reading instrument using ultraviolet light (interfered with by the presence of oil mist of vapour). Organic compounds: sampled through adsorbent tube (hopcolite) at an air flow rate of 50 ml min^{-1} for subsequent analysis for Hg using atomic absorption spectrophotometry (MDHS 16). By diffusive sample (see MDHS 58).

Occupational exposure limits. Mercury and compounds (except organic alkyls) as Hg, HSE OES: 8-h TWA, 0.025 mg m^{-3} (biological monitoring guidance value, Bmgv). Mercury alkyls as Hg, HSE OES: 9-h TWA, 0.01 mg m^{-3}; 15-min STEL, 0.03 mg m^{-3} (Sk).

HSE guidance. EH17 — Mercury: Health and Safety Precautions. Medical Series (MS) 12 — Mercury: Medical Surveillance. MDHS 16 and 58.

4.3.10 Nickel (Ni)

Occurrence. Sulphide ore extracted by separation or Mond process (unique reaction of nickel with carbon monoxide to produce nickel carbonyl Ni(CO)$_4$) (see p. 130).

Properties. Hard, ductile, magnetic, silvery-white metal. Low corrosion.

Uses. Alloys (especially with steel), electroplating, oil catalyst, coins, ceramics, batteries.

Metabolism. Poor absorption with wide bodily distribution, especially the brain and lungs. Rapid excretion in the urine and faeces.

Health effects. Acute: allergic contact dermatitis. Fume can cause pneumonitis. Chronic: carcinoma of the nose and nasal sinuses associated with exposure to nickel, although exact aetiological agent is unknown — nickel oxides and sulphides, or even nickel arsenide.

Health surveillance. Review of allergies, previous respiratory problems.

Treatment. Non-specific. Disulphiram has been used for nickel carbonyl poisoning.

Measurement. Sampled onto cellulose acetate filter (pore size, 0.8 μm) at an air flow rate of around 2 l min^{-1} for subsequent analysis for Ni using atomic absorption spectrophotometry (MDHS 42/2).

Occupational exposure limits. Nickel compounds as Ni: soluble compounds, HSE MEL: 8-h TWA, 0.1 mg m^{-3}; insoluble compounds, HSE MEL: 8-h TWA, 0.5 mg m^{-3}. Nickel carbonyl as Ni, HSE OES: 15-min STEL, 0.24 mg m^{-3} (0.1 ppm). Nickel organic compounds as Ni, HSE OES: 8-h TWA, 1 mg m^{-3}; 15-min STEL, 3 mg m^{-3}.

HSE guidance. MDHS 42/2.

4.3.11 Phosphorus (P)

Occurrence. Wide, usually as phosphates of calcium.

Properties. Three allotropic forms — yellow (spontaneously ignites), red and black. Can form a gaseous hydride (PH$_3$) (p. 133), as well as organic compounds (p. 116).

Uses. Agriculture, baking powder, detergents, explosives, paper and printing. Phosphoric acid is an anti-rust agent.

Metabolism. Rapid absorption by ingestion or inhalation.

Health effects. Acute: phosphorus oxides cause severe pneumonitis. Yellow phosphorus can cause severe burns and liver damage. Chronic: 'phossy jaw' — now virtually unknown. A severe, painful necrotic disease of the bone — usually the mandible.

Health surveillance. Dental surveillance, including radiography for early phossy jaw.

Treatment. Wound debridement.

Measurement. Phosphoric acid: sampled onto solid sorbent tube (Tenax) for subsequent analysis using gas chromatography flame ionisation detector (FID) (NIOSH 7905). Phosphoric acid: sampled onto solid orbent tube (washed silica gel) for subsequent analysis using ion chromatography (NIOSH 7903). Phosphorus compounds: bubbled into distilled water for subsequent colorimetric analysis (NIOSH 6402).

Occupational exposure limits. Orthophosphoric acid, HSE OES: 15-min STEL, 2 mg m^{-3}. Phosphorus (yellow), HSE OES: 8-h TWA, 0.1 mg m^{-3}; 15-min STEL, 0.3 mg m^{-3}. Diphosphorus pentachloride, HSE OES: 8-h TWA, 0.89 mg m^{-3} (0.1 ppm). Phosphorus pentasulphide, HSE OES: 8-h TWA, 1 mg m^{-3}; 15-min STEL, 3 mg m^{-3}. Diphosphorus pentoxide: HSE OES: 15-min STEL, 2 mg m^{-3}. Phosphorus trichloride, HSE OES: 8-h TWA, 1.1 mg m^{-3} (0.2 ppm); 15-min STEL, 2.9 mg m^{-3} (0.5 ppm). Phosphoryl trichloride, HSE OES: 8-h TWA, 1.3 mg m^{-3} (0.2 ppm); 15-min STEL, 3.8 mg m^{-3} (0.6 ppm).

4.3.12 Platinum (Pt)

Occurrence. Alluvial deposits.

Properties. Soft, ductile, malleable, non-corrosive, white metal.

Uses. Electrical contacts, catalyst, alloys, jewellery, photography.

Health effects. Acute: nasal irritation. Chronic: platinum asthma (especially after exposure to chloroplatinic acid or one of its salts). Dry, scaly skin irritant or allergic dermatitis.

Health surveillance. Pulmonary function tests. Some advocate pre-employment allergy testing (prick tests).

Treatment. Non-specific.

Measurement. Sampled onto cellulose acetate filter (pore size, 0.8 μm) at an air flow rate of around 2 l min^{-1} for subsequent analysis using atomic absorption spectrophotometry (MDHS 46).

Occupational exposure limits. Platinum metal, HSE OES: 8-h TWA, 5 mg m^{-3}. Platinum salts, soluble as Pt, HSE OES: 8-h TWA, 0.002 mg m^{-3} (except halogeno-platinum compounds in which a platinum atom or ion is directly coordinated to one or more halide ions; these compounds are subject to an MEL). Halogeno-platinum compounds: HSE MEL: 8-h TWA, 0.002 mg m^{-3}.

HSE guidance. MDHS 46.

4.3.13 Thallium (Tl)

Occurrence. As a complex with copper, silver and selenium, $(TlCuAg)_2Se$.

Properties. Soft, malleable, silvery-grey metal. Soluble in acids. Oxidises in air.

Uses. Rodenticide, insecticide, optical equipment, alloys, fireworks, dyes, depilatory agent.

Metabolism. Readily absorbed by all routes. Excretion is slow, poisoning is cumulative.

Health effects. Acute: vomiting, diarrhoea, abdominal pain, anxiety state.

Acute ascending polyneuritis. Chronic: polyneuritis, alopecia, albuminuria, ocular lesions.

Health surveillance. Medical surveillance of peripheral and central nervous system. Hair loss is a significant sign.

Treatment. None.

Measurement. Sampled onto cellulose acetate filter (pore size, 0.8 µm) at an air flow rate of around 2 l min^{-1} for subsequent analysis using atomic absorption spectrophotometry (NIOSH 7300).

Occupational exposure limits. Thallium, soluble compounds as Tl, HSE OES: 8-h TWA, 0.1 mg m^{-3}.

4.3.14 Vanadium (V)

Occurrence. Vanadinite ($9PbO.3V_2O_5PbCl_2$). Also a by-product of oil-burning furnaces, when vanadium pentoxide is deposited in the flues.

Properties. Grey–white lustrous powder.

Uses. Alloys with steel increase the hardness and malleability of products. Catalyst, insecticide, dyes.

Metabolism. Inhalation is main route of entry. Rapid renal excretion.

Health effects. Acute: severe pneumonitis (usually due to exposure to flue dust) with mucous membrane irritation and gastrointestinal disturbances. Chronic: chronic bronchitis; eczematous skin lesions; fine tremor of extremities; greenish discolouration of tongue.

Biological monitoring. Urinary vanadium.

Treatment. Non-specific.

Measurement. Vanadium oxides sampled onto PVC filter in a Higgins and Dewell cyclone for subsequent analysis using X-ray powder diffraction.

Occupational exposure limits. Divanadium pentoxide as V, HSE OES: 8-h TWA: total inhalable dust, 0.5 mg m^{-3}; fume and respirable dust, 0.04 mg m^{-3}.

4.3.15 Welding fume

Welding fume cannot be easily classified as the composition is dependent upon the alloy being welded and the method of welding being used, and is invariably a mixture of substances. There is suggestive evidence of an increased risk of lung cancer in welders. Arc welding fume, in particular, must be analysed for individual constituents, both particulate and gaseous, to determine whether specific recommended limits are exceeded. Under the heading of 'Mixed exposures' in EH40/98, Appendix 4, the HSE refers the reader to Guidance Note EH54: Assessment of Exposure to Fume from Welding and Allied Processes. In the ACGIH limit recommendation book, a useful paragraph on the

complex nature of welding fume is appended.
HSE guidance. MS15 Welding. EH54 and EH55.

4.3.16 Zinc (Zn)

Occurrence. As sulphide or carbonate.
Properties. High corrosion resistance. Poor conductor.
Uses. Galvanising, brass (5–40% Zn), dyes, electroplating.
Metabolism. Essential trace element, e.g. carbonic anhydrase is a zinc-containing enzyme. Also thought to be an important factor in wound healing. Poorly absorbed. Faecal excretion.
Health effects. Acute: metal fume fever. Can occur with fume of other metals, but zinc is the most common. Symptoms resemble influenza and come on within 12 h of exposure. Recovery is rapid with no sequelae. Zinc chloride is a skin and lung corrosive.
Health surveillance. Review of symptoms and pulmonary function tests where indicated.
Treatment. Non-specific management of pulmonary disorders. Acute skin contact with zinc chloride benefits from irrigation with calcium EDTA solution.
Measurement. Zinc fume: sampled onto cellulose acetate filter (pore size, 0.8 µm) at an air flow rate of around 2 l min^{-1} for subsequent analysis using atomic absorption spectrophotometry. Zinc stearate: sampled onto a weighed glass fibre filter for gravimetric analysis. Zinc chloride fume, HSE OES: 8-h TWA, 1 mg m^{-3}. Zinc oxide fume, HSE OES: 8-h TWA, 5 mg m^{-3}; 15-min STEL, 10 mg m^{-3}. Zinc distearate, HSE OES: 8-h TWA, total inhalable dust, 10 mg m^{-3}; 15-min STEL, 20 mg m^{-3}; respirable dust, 4 mg m^{-3}.

4.4 Organic chemicals

In general, organic chemicals are carbon-containing compounds. Carbon has a valency of 4, and a unique ability to form chain or ring structures with itself. Aliphatic compounds are hydrocarbons with a chain structure, e.g. *n*-hexane. Aromatic compounds have ring structures based on benzene.

e.g. *n*-hexane

Aromatic compounds are rings:

e.g. benzene

The two groups have differing properties, depending not only on their configuration, but also on the elements attached to the 'unoccupied' valency arms.

Organic compounds that are important for industrial processes are frequently hydrocarbons (methane and benzene) or hydrocarbons with some hydrogen atoms replaced by halogens, such as chlorine. The chlorinated hydrocarbons are fat soluble and are often non-flammable, non-combustible and non-explosive, but *not* safe.

As a *general* rule, increasing the chlorination of aliphatic hydrocarbons leads to increasing toxicity, whereas the reverse is true of aromatic hydrocarbons. Many chlorinated hydrocarbons are hepatotoxic and, on combustion at high temperatures, release the toxic irritant gas, phosgene $(COCl_2)$.

4.4.1 Acrylamide

Properties. White, crystalline powder. Readily undergoes polymerisation, water soluble. Molecular weight (MW), 71.08.

Uses. Manufacture of flocculators, dyes, leather substitutes, paper, pigments; used in soil stabilisation, mining and removal of industrial wastes.

Metabolism. Absorbed mainly through the skin, but also by inhalation and ingestion. Metabolism largely unknown. Monomer is neurotoxic, polymer is harmless.

Health effects. Acute: eye and mucous membrane irritation. Chronic: peripheral neuropathy and mid-brain lesions. Numbness, paraesthesia and weakness of limbs (legs more than arms). Ataxia, slurred speech, lethargy, increased sweating.

Health surveillance. Electromyography and nerve conduction studies.

Treatment. Wash contaminated skin thoroughly. No specific treatment for neurotoxic effects, but further exposure may produce a more severe reaction dose for dose.

Measurement. Sampled through midget impinger containing distilled water. The aqueous solution is injected directly into a high-pressure liquid chromatograph (HPLC) (MDHS 57).

Occupational exposure limits. HSE MEL: 8-h TWA, 0.3 mg m^{-3} (Sk).

HSE guidance. MDHS 57.

4.4.2 Acrylonitrile

$$H_2C = CH$$
$$|$$
$$C \equiv N$$

Properties. Explosive, flammable liquid. Readily polymerised. MW, 53.06.

Uses. Manufacture of synthetic rubber, acrylic resins and fibres.

Metabolism. Skin and lung absorption. Toxicity due to the release of cyanide radical (CN$^-$). Excreted as thiocyanate in urine.

Health effects. Acute: vapour is severe eye irritant and skin vesicant. Headache, sneezing, weakness, dizziness → asphyxia and death. Chronic: epidemiological studies in humans support animal experiments suggesting that acrylonitrile is carcinogenic (probably lung, colon (?)).

Biological monitoring. Cyanomethaemoglobin levels, blood pH and bicarbonate.

Treatment. Must be rapid as for any cyanide poisoning. Amyl nitrite (inhalation). Dicobalt edetate (intravenously (i.v.)). Hydroxycobalamine (?) (i.v.).

Measurement. Sampled onto a charcoal tube at an air flow rate of 200 ml min^{-1} for subsequent gas chromatographic analysis. Colorimetric detector tubes are also available (MDHS 1).

Occupational exposure limits. HSE MEL: 8-h TWA, 4.4 mg m^{-3} (2 ppm) (Sk).
HSE guidance. EH27 — Acrylonitrile: Personal Protective Equipment. MDHS 1, 2 and 55.

4.4.3 Anaesthetic gases

There are a number of gases in current use (and a number that have been discontinued for a variety of reasons — mainly due to toxicity — such as chloroform and trichloroethylene). The main gases of note for occupational exposure purposes are nitrous oxide, halothane, enflurane and isoflurane.

By definition, anaesthetic gases are toxic agents in that they induce unconsciousness. The fluoride groups, as in methoxyflurane and isoflurane, are metabolised to fluoride compounds, which can be nephrotoxic (to the patient). However, the greatest concern over occupational exposure and health effects has centred on reproductive outcome. An increased rate of spontaneous abortions in female anaesthetists was first reported in 1968, but, many studies later, the matter has not been completely resolved. It appears that birth defect reports were not substantiated by later, more careful, studies, but the link with spontaneous abortion does appear to be quite persuasive — especially in studies where the ambient levels of gases in the operating room were well in excess of current standards. Levels of nitrous oxide above 100 ppm and of halothane above 10 ppm also lead to impaired mood and cognitive function in operating room staff.

Occupational exposure limits. Nitrous oxide: HSE OES: 8-h TWA, 183 mg m^{-3} (100 ppm). Halothane: HSE OES: 8-h TWA, 82 mg m^{-3} (10 ppm). Enflurane and isoflurane: HSE OES: 8-h TWA, 383 mg m^{-3} (50 ppm).

4.4.4 Aniline

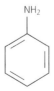

Properties. Colourless, oily liquid with aromatic odour. MW, 93.13.
Uses. Dyes, perfumes, explosives, pharmaceuticals, rubber processing.
Metabolism. Skin and lung absorption. Converts haemoglobin (where

iron is in ferrous state) to methaemoglobin (where iron is in ferric form) with a resulting diminution of the oxygen-carrying capacity of the blood.
Health effects. Acute: mild skin irritant. Moderate exposure may only cause some cyanosis. Severe poisoning results in anoxia and death, which may be delayed for a few hours after exposure.
Biological monitoring. Methaemoglobin levels must be monitored during treatment.
Treatment. Remove all traces of aniline from the skin and all contaminated clothing. Methylene blue (i.v.) is justified for comatose patients with methaemoglobin levels above 60%. Methylene blue reduces methaemoglobin to haemoglobin.
Measurement. Sampled onto a silica gel tube at an air flow rate of 200 ml min^{-1} for subsequent analysis using gas chromatography (NIOSH 2002). Colorimetric detector tubes are also available.
Occupational exposure limits. HSE OES: 10 mg m^{-3} (2 ppm) (Sk) (under review).

4.4.5 Benzene

(C_6H_6)

Occurrence. By-product of petroleum and coke-oven industries.
Properties. Colourless, flammable liquid. The fat solvent *par excellence*. MW, 78.11.
Uses. The initial compound is used in the production of numerous organic aromatics, including styrene, phenol and cyclohexane, as well as many plastics, paints, glues, dyes and pharmaceuticals.
Metabolism. Lung and skin absorption with ready transportation and uptake by fatty tissue. Excretion is slow through the lungs, with a little appearing in the urine as conjugated phenols.
Health effects. Chronic: bone marrow depression with a delayed effect, in some cases, of many years. The early symptoms and signs are vague, but, later, tiredness and spontaneous bleeding may occur as anaemia, pancytopenia and/or thrombocytopenia become more severe. Aplastic anaemia, acute myeloblastic leukaemia and acute erythroleukaemia are the most feared effects of chronic exposure.
Health surveillance. Periodic red and white cell counts of questionable value, but may detect early haemopoietic effects. Urinary phenol has been used for biological monitoring.

Treatment. Acute intoxication will usually respond to removal from exposure and respiratory system support measures. The development of aplastic or leukaemic effects augurs ill. Treatment is as for other causes of these conditions, but the prognosis is poor.

Measurement. Sampled onto a charcoal tube at an air flow rate of 200 ml min^{-1} for subsequent analysis using gas chromatography (MDHS 17). Colorimetric detector tubes are also available.

Occupational exposure limits. HSE MEL: 8-h TWA, 16 mg m^{-3} (5 ppm).

HSE guidance. MDHS 17 and 50.

4.4.6 Carbon disulphide

Properties. Colourless liquid. MW, 76.16.

Uses. Solvent for fats, sulphur, rubber oils. Insecticide. Preparation of viscose rayon.

Metabolism. Absorbed through the lungs and skin. Slow metabolism and excretion with main concentration build-up in the brain.

Health effects. Acute: severe skin and mucous membrane irritant. Dizziness, headaches, psychosis, drowsiness. Chronic: four distinct syndromes: (i) Parkinsonian-like affection due to damage to the corpus striatum and globus pallidus; (ii) peripheral neuropathy affecting motor and sensory nerves as well as ocular nerves; (iii) psychotic conditions (rarely seen nowadays, but lesser neuropsychiatric states are still described); (iv) cardiovascular disease — possibly due to increased blood cholesterol and β-lipoprotein leading to ischaemic heart disease and peripheral vascular damage. However, recent research suggests that part (at least) of this cardiovascular effect may be due to an acute myotoxic effect on cardiac muscle leading to fatal arrhythmias.

Biological monitoring. The iodine–azide reaction with urine will detect organic sulphate metabolites of carbon disulphide, but the reaction is not specific for CS_2.

Treatment. Symptomatic treatment only.

Measurement. Sampled onto a charcoal tube at an air flow rate of 200 ml min^{-1} for subsequent analysis using gas chromatography (MDHS 15). Colorimetric detection tubes are also available.

Occupational exposure limits. HSE MEL: 8-h TWA, 32 mg m^{-3} (10 ppm) (Sk).

HSE guidance. MDHS 15, EH 45.

4.4.7 Carbon tetrachloride

$$
\begin{array}{c}
Cl \\
| \\
Cl - C - Cl \\
| \\
Cl
\end{array}
$$

Properties. Colourless, non-flammable liquid with characteristic smell. Burning yields phosgene and hydrogen chloride gas. MW, 153.82.

Uses. Solvent, degreaser, manufacture of refrigerants, such as Freon, in fire extinguishers and as grain fumigant.

Metabolism. Absorbed through the lungs, skin and gut and stored in fatty tissues. Excreted unchanged through the lungs, although some is metabolised and excreted in the urine.

Health effects. Acute: nausea, vomiting, drowsiness, dizziness. Chronic: dry, scaly dermatitis. Centrilobular necrosis with or without fatty degeneration of the liver. Acute oliguric renal failure. There is a synergistic effect if there is concomitant exposure to alcohol.

Biological monitoring. Blood concentration is of limited value.

Treatment. Non-specific. Most cases recover, but renal and hepatic damage may be permanent.

Measurement. Sampled onto a charcoal tube at an air flow rate of 1000 ml min^{-1} for subsequent analysis using gas chromatography (MDHS 28). Colorimetric detection tubes are also available.

Occupational exposure limits. HSE OES: 8-h TWA, 13 mg m^{-3} (2 ppm) (Sk).

HSE guidance. MDHS 28.

4.4.8 Chlorinated naphthalenes

$$C_{10}H_{(8-n)}Cl_n$$

Properties. A group of compounds with varying degrees of chlorination. The higher the chlorine content, the higher the melting point.

Uses. Wire insulation and flame resistance in condensers.

Metabolism. Inhalation of fumes and percutaneous absorption of liquids.

Health effects. Acute: little effect. Chronic: two distinct effects: (i) chloroacne from skin contact; (ii) liver damage from inhalation.

Health surveillance. Reporting of skin symptoms by those exposed and skin examination. Liver function tests where liver damage is suspected.

Treatment. Non-specific.

4.4.9 Chloroform

$$Cl - \underset{\underset{Cl}{|}}{\overset{\overset{H}{|}}{C}} - Cl$$

Properties. Clear, colourless, non-flammable liquid with characteristic odour. MW, 119.38.

Uses. Fat solvent, manufacture of fluorocarbons, plastics. Abandoned as an anaesthetic agent due to its hepatotoxicity.

Metabolism. Absorbed through the lungs (and skin). Stored in fatty tissue and slowly excreted through the lungs and, to a lesser extent, the kidneys.

Health effects. Acute: skin irritant. Potent anaesthetic. Chronic: liver enlargement and damage potentiated by alcohol abuse (causes hepatic tumours in rodents). Oliguric renal failure. Chronic dry, scaly dermatitis.

Treatment. Non-specific.

Measurement. Sampled onto a charcoal tube at an air flow rate of 1000 ml min^{-1} for subsequent analysis using gas chromatography (MDHS 28).

Occupational exposure limits. HSE OES: 8-h TWA, 9.9 mg m^{-3} (12 ppm) (Sk).

HSE guidance. MDHS 28.

4.4.10 1,1,1-Trichloro-2,2-bis-(*p*-chlorophenyl)ethane (DDT)

2 isomers

Properties. White, crystalline solid. MW, 354.49.

Uses. Insecticide. Effective in malaria control for destroying mosquito vector, although concern regarding bioaccumulation in the environment.

Metabolism. Absorbed through the gut and intact skin. Metabolised slowly to 1,1'-(2,2-dichloroethenylidene)-bis[4-chlorobenzene] (DDE) and 2,2-bis(4-chlorophenyl) acetic acid (DDA) with storage in fatty tissues and excretion in the urine.

Health effects. In high doses (10 mg kg^{-1} body weight), DDT causes CNS effects, including paraesthesia, tremors and convulsions. Occupational exposure studies have been remarkable for their lack of evidence of long-term CNS or hepatic effects, despite animal evidence of hepatic tumours and the widespread banning of the use of the compound.

Treatment. Clear skin contamination. Diazepam for convulsions. Otherwise, non-specific.

Measurement. Airborne particulate is sampled onto a glass fibre filter at an air flow rate of around $1.5 \, l \, min^{-1}$, is subsequently removed by isooctane and the aliquot is analysed by gas chromatography.

Occupational exposure limits. HSE OES: 8-h TWA, $1 \, mg \, m^{-3}$; 15-min STEL, $3 \, mg \, m^{-3}$.

4.4.11 Dinitrobenzene

3 isomers:

ortho-   meta-   para-

Properties. Solid, colourless, odourless flakes. Three isomeric forms. MW, 168.11.

Uses. Dyes, explosives.

Metabolism. Inhalation and skin absorption cause methaemoglobinaemia.

Health effects. Acute: headache, dizziness, vomiting and weakness. Hypotension, tachycardia, hyperpnoea. Chronic: weakness, fatigue, cyanosis and pallor. Symptoms may be exacerbated by alcohol or sunlight. Liver damage (acute necrosis) is rare.

Health surveillance. Methaemoglobin levels. Occasionally patients exhibit albuminuria or porphyrinuria.

Treatment. Remove all traces of dinitrobenzene from the skin. Methylene blue may be justified in severe methaemoglobinaemia; otherwise, oxygen and other respiratory supportive measures usually suffice.

Measurement. Air is drawn through a cellulose acetate filter in series with a bubbler containing 10 ml of ethylene glycol at a flow rate of $1.5 \, l \, min^{-1.}$ At the end of the sampling period, the filter is added to the bubbler liquid. The resulting sample is analysed by high-pressure liquid chromatography.

Occupational exposure limits. HSE OES: 8-h TWA, 1 mg m^{-3} (0.15 ppm); 15-min STEL, 3.5 mg m^{-3} (0.5 ppm) (Sk).

4.4.12 Dinitrophenol

(2 isomers)

Properties. Explosive, yellow, crystalline solid. MW, 184.11.
Uses. Explosive, dyes, timber preservative.
Metabolism. Absorbed through the gastrointestinal tract, skin and respiratory tract. Effects enhanced by heat and alcohol. Excretion is slow, urine becomes orange and skin is turned yellow. Dinitrophenol and its homologue dinitroorthocresol interfere with temperature regulation by the uncoupling of oxidative phosphorylation. This leads to an increase in metabolic rate.
Health effects. Acute: sudden onset of chest pain and dyspnoea with or without hyperpyrexia, profuse sweating and thirst. Chronic: similar to acute effects with or without liver tenderness and jaundice. Cataract formation. Neutropenia and albuminuria were noted when dinitrophenol was in vogue for weight reduction therapy.
Biological monitoring. Urine analysis for dinitrophenol or its metabolite 2-amino-4-nitrophenol has limited use.
Treatment. Cooling, oxygen, sedation.

4.4.13 Ethylene oxide

Properties. Colourless, flammable gas (odour detection, 500 ppm). Heavier than air.
Uses. Chemical intermediate in the production of ethylene glycol and polyester fibres with dichlorodifluoromethane (to lower the risk of explosion and fire). It is used as a general purpose gaseous sterilising agent, particularly in hospitals.

Metabolism. Soluble in water; it is a highly reactive epoxide and an alkylating agent.

Health effects. Acute: narcotic properties with CNS depression. In high concentrations (several hundred parts per million), it can cause nausea, vomiting, headache, mucous membrane and eye irritation. Chronic: probably capable of causing peripheral neuropathy and encephalopathy. More seriously, the alkylating properties result in good evidence of animal carcinogenicity and reprotoxicity. It is a probable human carcinogen — particularly for the haemopoietic system.

Biological monitoring. None of relevance.

Treatment. Remove from (acute) exposure. Oxygen and respiratory support measures.

Measurement. Sampled onto a charcoal tube with an optimum volume of just less than 5 l (10 ml min^{-1} for 8 h; maximum, 200 ml min^{-1}). Desorbed with CS_2 for subsequent analysis using gas chromatography (MDHS 26).

Occupational exposure limits. HSE MEL: 8-h TWA, 9.2 mg m^{-3} (5 ppm).

4.4.14 Formaldehyde

$$H \underset{}{-} \overset{\overset{\textstyle O}{\|}}{C} \underset{}{-} H$$

Properties. Colourless gas with a pungent odour. Commonly used as an aqueous solution (formalin) of 34–38% formaldehyde. MW, 30.03.

Uses. Plastics and resin manufacture, preservative, intermediate in chemical manufacture. Used also in textile industry as a crease-resistant agent.

Metabolism. Mainly by inhalation. Metabolised in the liver and excreted in the urine and exhaled air. Converted to formate in many tissues, including red blood cells.

Health effects. Acute: severe mucous membrane irritation. Chronic: potent allergen for skin, (?) respiratory tract. Probable animal carcinogen (nasal tumours in rats). Limited evidence to date of human carcinogenic effect, but formaldehyde and hydrochloric acid can produce bis(chloromethyl)ether (BCME), a proven human lung carcinogen.

Biological monitoring. None in common use.

Treatment. Symptomatic for acute overexposure.

Measurement. Air is bubbled through a 0.5% solution of 3-methyl-2-

benzothiazolone hydrazone in a bubbler at a flow rate of 1 l min^{-1}. The resulting solution is analysed by colorimetric means. Colorimetric detector tubes are also available (MDHS 19).

Occupational exposure limits. HSE MEL: 8-h TWA and 15-min STEL, 2.5 mg m^{-3} (2 ppm).

4.4.15 Glutaraldehyde

(OHC–(CH$_2$)$_3$–CHO)

Properties. An oily clear liquid, usually mixed with water at approximately 2%. MW, 100.12.

Uses. Disinfectant. Before use, glutaraldehyde has to be activated by the addition of sodium bicarbonate. Used in hospitals for sterilising endoscopes.

Metabolism. Little is known about the metabolism following systemic absorption in humans.

Health effects. Acute: respiratory irritant. Splashes onto the skin cause irritant dermatitis. Chronic: causes asthma. Skin contact can lead to allergic dermatitis.

Health surveillance. Pre-employment examination to include assessment of specific allergies and baseline lung function tests. Periodic respiratory symptom review, with serial peak flow readings and repeat lung function tests being indicated if respiratory symptoms develop. Further dermatological assessment if rashes develop.

Management and treatment. Removal from further exposure if exposed worker has asthma. Control measures for reduction of exposure essential.

Measurement. Sampled onto solid sorbent tube of silica gel (coated with 2,4-dinitrophenyl HCl, 300 mg/150 mg) at a flow rate of 0.05–0.5 l min^{-1}. Analysed by high-pressure liquid chromatography, ultraviolet detection (NIOSH 2532).

Occupational exposure limits. HSE OES: 15-min STEL, 0.83 mg m^{-3} (0.2 ppm).

4.4.16 Isocyanates

(e.g. toluene diisocyanate (TDI), two isomers)
Properties. Colourless liquid. MW, 174.16.
Uses. Polyurethane production varying from flexible form (TDI) to rigid types (diphenylmethane diisocyanate, MDI).

(Toluene diisocyanate
two isomers)

Metabolism. Poorly understood. Effects proportional to volatility (TDI > MDI).
Health effects. Acute: respiratory irritation in all exposed at high concentrations, and irritation with or without sensitisation on contact, especially in atopics. Chronic: permanent pulmonary disability may cause decrease in forced expiratory volume in 1 s (FEV_1) in absence of symptoms, postulated but disputed.
Health surveillance. Serial peak flow spirometric readings and periodic review of symptoms.
Treatment. Symptomatic. Avoid further exposure in sensitised individuals.
Measurement. Air is drawn through an impregnated tape. The resulting stain is photometrically examined. Proprietary instrument available. A colorimetric detection tube for TDI is available. Alternatively, a measured volume of sample air is drawn through a glass impinger (bubbler) containing 1-(2-methoxyphenyl)-piperazine for subsequent analysis using high-pressure liquid chromatography (MDHS 25). In another method, a measured volume of sample air is drawn through a glass impinger containing dimethylformamide and dilute hydrochloric acid for subsequent colorimetric analysis (MDHS 49).
Occupational exposure limits. HSE MEL for all isocyanates in air (as –NCO): 8-h TWA, 0.02 mg m^{-3}; 15-min STEL, 0.07 mg m^{-3}.
HSE guidance. EH 16 — Isocyanates: Toxic Hazards and Precautions. MS8 — Isocyanates: Medical Surveillance. MDHS 25 and 49.

4.4.17 Ketones and ethers

Ketones and Ethers

Uses. Solvents (especially dimethylketone (acetone), methylethylketone (MEK), methylbutylketone (MBK), diethylether methyl-*n*-butylketone (MnBK) and methylisobutylketone (MIBK)).

Health effects. Acute: upper respiratory tract irritants. Cause dermatitis. Chronic: narcotic. MnBK can cause peripheral neuropathy. Neurotoxic effects potentiated by concomitant exposure to MEK and/or MIBK. Bis(chloromethyl)ether (BCME) is a strong alkylating agent and a potent lung carcinogen.

Biological monitoring. Non-specific. Exceptions: MEK and MIBK in urine.

Treatment for acute overexposure. Non-specific. Symptomatic. Remove to fresh air.

Measurement. Ethers and ketones are sampled by drawing air through a Tenax tube at a flow rate of 200 ml min^{-1} for subsequent analysis using gas chromatography.

Occupational exposure limits.

Allyl glycidylether (AGE), HSE OES: 8-h TWA, 24 mg m^{-3} (5 ppm); 15-min STEL, 47 mg m^{-3} (10 ppm).

n-Butyl glycidylether (BGE), HSE OES: 8-h TWA, 135 mg m^{-3} (25 ppm).

Bis(chloromethyl)ether (BCME), HSE MEL: 8-h TWA, 0.005 mg m^{-3} (0.001 ppm).

Diethylether, HSE OES: 8-h TWA, 1230 mg m^{-3} (400 ppm); 15-min STEL, 1540 mg m^{-3} (500 ppm).

Diglycidylether (DGE), HSE OES: 8-h TWA, 0.54 mg m^{-3} (0.1 ppm).

Diisopropylether, HSE OES: 8-h TWA, 1060 mg m^{-3} (250 ppm); 15-min STEL, 1310 mg m^{-3} (310 ppm).

Ethylene glycol monobutylether (2-butoxyethanol), HSE OES: 8-h TWA, 123 mg m^{-3} (25 ppm) (Sk).

Ethylene glycol monomethylether (2-methoxyethanol), HSE MEL: 8-h TWA, 16 mg m^{-3} (5 ppm) (Sk).

Glycol monoethylether (2-ethoxyethanol), HSE MEL: 8-h TWA, 37 mg m^{-3} (10 ppm) (Sk).

Isopropyl glycidylether (IGE), HSE OES: 8-h TWA, 241 mg m^{-3} (50 ppm); 15-min STEL, 362 mg m^{-3} (75 ppm).

Propylene glycol dinitrate (PGDN), HSE OES: 8-h TWA, 1.4 mg m^{-3} (0.2 ppm); 15-min STEL, 1.4 mg m^{-3} (0.2 ppm) (Sk).
Propylene glycol monomethylether, HSE OES: 8-h TWA, 375 mg m^{-3} (100 ppm); 15-min STEL, 1120 mg m^{-3} (300 ppm).
Diethylketone (pentan-3-one), HSE OES: 8-h TWA, 716 mg m^{-3} (200 ppm); 15-min STEL, 895 mg m^{-3} (250 ppm).
2,6-Dimethylheptan-4-one, HSE OES: 8-h TWA, 148 mg m^{-3} (25 ppm).
Ethylamylketone (5-methylheptan-3-one), HSE OES: 8-h TWA, 133 mg m^{-3} (25 ppm).
Ethylbutylketone (heptan-3-one), HSE OES: 8-h TWA, 237 mg m^{-3} (50 ppm); 15-min STEL, 475 mg m^{-3} (100 ppm) (Sk).
Methyl-*n*-amylketone (heptan-2-one), HSE OES: 8-h TWA, 237 mg m^{-3} (50 ppm); 15-min STEL, 475 mg m^{-3} (100 ppm) (Sk).
Methylbutylketone (hexan-2-one) (MBK), HSE OES: 8-h TWA, 21 mg m^{-3} (5 ppm) (Sk).
Methylethylketone (butan-2-one) (MEK), HSE OES: 8-h TWA, 600 mg m^{-3} (200 ppm); 15-min STEL, 899 mg m^{-3} (300 ppm) (Sk).
2-Methylcyclohexanone, HSE OES: 233 mg m^{-3} (50 ppm); 15-min STEL, 350 mg m^{-3} (75 ppm) (Sk).
Methylisoamylketone (5-methylhexan-2-one), HSE OES: 8-h TWA, 237 mg m^{-3} (50 ppm); 15-min STEL, 475 mg m^{-3} (100 ppm) (Sk).
Methylisobutylketone (methylpentan-2-one) (MIBK), HSE OES: 8-h TWA, 208 mg m^{-3} (50 ppm); 15-min STEL, 416 mg m^{-3} (100 ppm) (Sk).
Methylisopropylketone (MIPK), ACGIH recommended limit: 705 mg m^{-3} (200 ppm).
Methylpropylketone (pentan-2-one), HSE OES: 8-h TWA, 716 mg m^{-3} (200 ppm); 15-min STEL, 895 mg m^{-3} (250 ppm).
HSE guidance: MDHS 23.

4.4.18 Methyl alcohol (methanol)

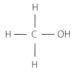

Properties. Colourless liquid which smells like ethanol. MW, 32.04.
Uses. Celluloid manufacture, paint remover, varnishes, antifreeze, cements.
Metabolism. Absorbed by all routes and slowly metabolised to formaldehyde and formic acid.
Health effects. Acute: headache, dizziness, dermatitis, conjunctivitis.

Chronic: optic nerve damage and blindness from ingestion. Cases of eye damage due to consumption of home-made alcoholic beverages inadvertently — or illicitly — containing methanol.

Biological monitoring. Urine methanol levels at end of the shift.

Treatment. Treatment of acidosis. Blindness is irreversible.

Measurement. Sampled onto a silica gel tube at an air flow rate of 50 ml min^{-1} for subsequent analysis using gas chromatography. A general alcohol detector tube is available.

Occupational exposure limits. HSE OES: 8-h TWA, 266 mg m^{-3} (200 ppm); 15-min STEL, 323 mg m^{-3} (250 ppm) (Sk).

4.4.19 Methyl bromide (bromomethane)

Properties. Colourless, odourless gas. MW, 92.95.

Uses. Fire extinguishers, refrigerant, insecticide and fumigant.

Metabolism. Rapidly absorbed by inhalation, and toxic either directly or through metabolites such as bromide.

Health effects. Acute: late onset (several hours' delay) of acute respiratory tract irritation. Nausea, vomiting, headaches and convulsions may also occur. Chronic: recovery from the acute attack is usual, but prolonged exposure or delayed treatment can cause peripheral neuropathy, tremor, renal failure and psychiatric disorders.

Treatment. Non-specific. Treat convulsions with diazepam or phenobarbitone; bromide in blood may be useful for assessing extent of acute exposure.

Measurement. Sampled onto two large charcoal tubes in series at an air flow rate of 1000 ml min^{-1} for subsequent analysis using gas chromatography. Colorimetric detection tubes are also available.

Occupational exposure limits. HSE OES: 8-h TWA, 20 mg m^{-3} (5 ppm); 15-min STEL, 59 mg m^{-3} (15 ppm).

4.4.20 Methylene chloride (dichloromethane)

Properties. Non-flammable, colourless liquid. MW, 84.93.

Uses. Paint and varnish remover, insecticide, fumigant, solvent, fire extinguisher.

Metabolism. Skin and lung absorption. Metabolised with the production of carbon monoxide.

Health effects. Acute: skin and mucous membrane irritant. Acute intoxication with stupor, numbness and tingling of limbs following inhalation. Chronic: dry, scaly dermatitis. Can precipitate cardiac insufficiency due to increase in carboxyhaemoglobin.

Biological monitoring. Carboxyhaemoglobin levels in blood and carbon monoxide in exhaled air. Smoking affects biological monitoring results.

Treatment. Non-specific. Maintain adequate oxygenation.

Measurement. Sampled onto a charcoal tube at an air flow rate of 1000 ml min^{-1} for subsequent analysis using gas chromatography. Colorimetric detection tubes are also available. (NIOSH 1012).

Occupational exposure limits. HSE MEL: 8-h TWA, 350 mg m^{-3} (100 ppm); 15-min STEL, 1060 mg m^{-3} (300 ppm).

4.4.21 Methyl isocyanate

$$CH_3 \text{---} CNO$$

Properties. Was the agent released in the Bhopal incident (1984). Resulted in several thousand deaths and many more suffering ill health in those exposed in the workplace and the surrounding community.

Uses. Polyurethane foams, plastics and pesticide production.

Metabolism. Little is known about the metabolism following systemic absorption in humans.

Health effects. Skin, mucosal and respiratory tract irritant. High exposures lead to pulmonary oedema, pulmonary fibrosis, neurological and behavioural effects and effects on pregnancy outcome. Cataracts and delayed ocular symptoms have also been reported.

Management and treatment. Removal from further exposure. Administer oxygen. Monitor for development of delayed pulmonary oedema.

Measurement. See Section 4.4.16 (p. 112).

HSE guidance. See Section 4.4.16 (p. 112).

Occupational exposure limits. HSE MEL (as –NCO): 8-h TWA, 0.02 mg m^{-3}; 15-min STEL, 0.07 mg m^{-3}.

4.4.22 Organophosphates

Organophosphates (OPs) are a group of carbon-based compounds with phosphorus in the general chemical formula. They are used as pesticides, e.g. in sheep dip to control sheep scab and other parasites. Examples include Malathion, Parathion, Dichlorvos and triorthocresylphosphate (TOCP). Unfortunately, ingestion of OP pesticides is common as a means of suicide in some developing countries, such as Sri Lanka.

$$(C_2H_5O)_2 \longrightarrow P \longrightarrow O \longrightarrow \bigcirc \longrightarrow NO_2$$

Parathion

Metabolism and toxicity. Organophosphates which are absorbed systemically inactivate acetylcholinesterase at synapses in the nervous system by phosphorylation of the enzyme. This inactivation of the cholinesterase allows prolonged action of acetylcholine released at synapses and nerve endings. Effects of OP poisoning are therefore those of excessive cholinergic activity. Organophosphates are metabolised to dialkyl phosphates which are then excreted in the urine.

Health effects. Acute: cholinergic effects, such as chest tightness, wheezing, slurred speech, blurred vision, sweating, salivation, abdominal cramps, diarrhoea and vomiting. Chronic: there is some evidence indicating decrement of neurophysiological function following long-term exposure to OPs used in sheep dip. It has also been suggested that the use of a variety of chemical agents, including OPs, may have contributed to the ill-defined 'Gulf War syndrome'. Some OPs, such as TOCP, can cause a delayed, sometimes irreversible, peripheral neuropathy.

Biological monitoring. Plasma or red cell cholinesterase levels can be determined. Plasma cholinesterase measures pseudo-cholinesterase activity. Red blood cell cholinesterase is preferred for biological monitoring as it determines true acetylcholinesterase levels. Red cell cholinesterase reduced to less than 70% of an individual's baseline level indicates substantial exposure. Biological monitoring programmes for pesticide applicators often include several pre-application determinations and a post-application determination of cholinesterase activity. Field kits are available for such analysis. Blood levels of the pesticides and urinary dialkyl phosphate levels can be used as indicators of the extent of exposure.

Management and treatment. Rapid removal away from further exposure and removal of contaminated clothing are essential. Aldoximes, such as Pralidoxime chloride (2-PAM), are used as antidotes for the treatment of OP poisoning. It appears to be less effective for Malathion than other OPs. Pralidoxime is administered as a single dose by slow intravenous infusion. In addition, atropine is also used to block excessive cholinesterase action (2–4 mg every 5–10 min, until signs of atropinisation appear). Atropine is also used for carbamate (a non-OP cholinesterase inhibitor) poisoning, but aldoximes are contraindicated for this group of pesticides.

Measurement. Sampled onto solid sorbent tube for subsequent analysis using gas chromatography FPD (NIOSH 5600).

Occupational exposure limits. Dichlorvos: HSE OES: 8-h TWA, 0.92 mg m^{-3} (0.1 ppm); 15-min STEL, 2.8 mg m^{-3} (0.3 ppm) (Sk). Malathion: HSE OES: 8-h TWA, 10 mg m^{-3} (Sk). Parathion: HSE OES: 8-h TWA, 0.1 mg m^{-3}; 15-min STEL, 0.3 mg m^{-3} (Sk). TOCP: HSE OES: 8-h TWA, 0.1 mg m^{-3}; 15-min STEL, 0.3 mg m^{-3}.

HSE guidance. MS17.

4.4.23 Phenol

Properties. Colourless crystals. In solution, was used by Lister in his historic carbolic disinfectant sprays. MW, 94.11.

Uses. Insecticides, disinfectants, pharmaceuticals, perfumes, explosives.

Metabolism. Readily absorbed by all routes. Oxidised to quinones and excreted in the urine, which darkens on standing due to homogentisic acid.

Health effects. Acute: powerful skin corrosive. Headache, dizziness, weakness, convulsions. Chronic: chronic dermatitis from low concentrations following repeated skin contact; severe scarring from phenol splashes. Renal failure. Weight loss, gastrointestinal disturbances.

Biological monitoring. Following systemic absorption — total phenol in the urine at the end of the shift.

Treatment. Liberal flushing with water of contaminated skin. Sedatives for convulsions. The use of polyethylene glycol eye irrigation for splashes into the eye has been advocated by some authorities.

Measurement. Air is drawn through a 0.1 N solution of sodium hydroxide in a bubbler at an air flow rate of 1000 ml min^{-1}; the acidified solution is analysed using a gas chromatograph. Colorimetric detection tubes are also available.

....

Occupational exposure limits. HSE OES: 8-h TWA, 20 mg m^{-3} (5 ppm) and 15-min STEL, 39 mg m^{-3} (10 ppm) (Sk).

4.4.24 Styrene

Properties. Colourless liquid. MW, 104.15.

Uses. Solvent for synthetic rubber, chemical intermediate, manufacture of polymerised synthetics and glass-reinforced plastics (in boat building). Also ingredient in acrylonitrile–butadiene–styrene (ABS) copolymer.

Metabolism. Absorbed through the lungs and skin. Rapidly metabolised to mandelic acid and, to a lesser extent, phenylglyoxylic acid and excreted in the urine.

Health effects. Acute: acute mucous membrane irritation. Drowsiness, diminished cognitive and perceptual skills. Chronic: fissured dermatitis and other features of CNS depression.

Biological monitoring. Urinary mandelic acid and phenylglyoxylic acid concentrations. Styrene in blood.

Treatment. Non-specific.

Measurement. Sampled onto a charcoal tube at an air flow rate of 200 ml min^{-1} for subsequent analysis using gas chromatography (MDHS 44).

Occupational exposure limits. HSE MEL: 8-h TWA, 430 mg m^{-3} (100 ppm); 15-min STEL, 1080 mg m^{-3} (250 ppm).

HSE guidance. MDHS 43 and 44.

4.4.25 Tetrachloroethane

Properties. Heavy, non-flammable liquid. The most toxic of the chlorinated hydrocarbons. MW, 167.85.

Uses. Solvent, artificial pearl production, chemical intermediate.

Metabolism. Rapid absorption from the skin and lungs. Slowly metabolised and excreted in the urine. Main metabolite oxalic acid (?).

Health effects. Acute: gastrointestinal and upper respiratory tract irritation. CNS depression. Chronic: hepatic: hepatomegaly and hepatic failure; neurological: polyneuropathy, particularly of the extremities; renal: albuminuria; dermatological: dry, scaly dermatitis.

Health surveillance and biological monitoring. Non-specific. Organ function tests may be valuable.

Treatment. Non-specific. Severe hepatic or neurological damage may be irreversible or even fatal.

Measurement. Sampled onto a charcoal tube at an air flow rate of 200 ml min^{-1} for subsequent analysis using gas chromatography (NIOSH 1019).

Occupational exposure limits. ACGIH threshold limit value (TLV): 8-h TWA, 6.9 mg m^{-3} (1 ppm) (Sk).

4.4.26 Tetrachloroethylene (perchloroethylene)

Properties. Non-flammable liquid with characteristic odour. MW, 165.8.

Uses. Solvent widely used as dry-cleaning agent, fumigant.

Metabolism. Readily absorbed through the lungs and skin. Metabolised to trichloroacetic acid (TCA), and excreted in small amounts in the urine, but mainly excreted unchanged in the breath.

Health effects. Acute: powerful narcotic. Can cause mucous membrane and skin irritation as well as liver damage. Chronic: CNS depression and liver damage. Rodent carcinogen.

Biological monitoring. Urine TCA (end of working week sample) and breath sample analysis for perchloroethylene.

Treatment. Non-specific.

Measurement. Sampled onto a charcoal tube at an air flow rate of 1000 ml min^{-1} for subsequent analysis using gas chromatography.

Occupational exposure limits. HSE OES: 8-h TWA, 345 mg m^{-3} (50 ppm); 15-min STEL, 689 mg m^{-3} (100 ppm).

HSE guidance. MDHS 28.

....

4.4.27 Toluene (methyl benzene)

Properties. Colourless liquid. MW, 92.14.

Uses. Benzene manufacture, paint solvent, component of petrol.

Metabolism. Rapidly absorbed through the lungs and skin, and excreted as hippuric acid in the urine.

Health effects. Acute: narcotic. Conjunctival irritation and ulceration. Cardiac arrhythmias (has caused deaths in 'sniffers'). Chronic: liver (?), kidney and bone marrow (probably due to benzene as a contaminant). Toluene exposure is rarely pure, exposure frequently including benzene with or without xylene.

Biological monitoring. Urinary hippuric acid levels. A biological exposure index of 2.5 g g^{-1} creatinine has been suggested by ACGIH (1997). Note: hippuric acid is not a metabolite specific to toluene. It can be produced from dietary sources, such as food preserved with benzoic acid.

Treatment. Non-specific.

Measurement. Sampled onto a charcoal tube at an air flow rate of 1000 ml min^{-1} for subsequent analysis using gas chromatography. Colorimetric detection tubes are also available.

Occupational exposure limits. HSE OES: 8-h TWA, 191 mg m^{-3} (50 ppm); 15-min STEL, 574 mg m^{-3} (150 ppm) (Sk).

HSE guidance. MDHS 40, 64 and 69.

4.4.28 1,1,1-Trichloroethane

Properties. Non-flammable liquid. MW, 133.4. Trade name: Genklene. Causes damage to the ozone layer.

Uses. Solvent, degreasing agent.

Metabolism. Readily absorbed through the lungs and, to some extent, through the skin. Metabolised to TCA and excreted in the urine.

Health effects. Acute: mucous membrane and skin irritant, narcotic, capable of sensitising the myocardium to adrenaline, thereby causing arrhythmias. Chronic: dry, scaly dermatitis.

Biological monitoring. Urinary TCA estimations.
Treatment. Non-specific.
Measurement. Sampled onto a charcoal tube at an air flow rate of 1000 ml min^{-1} for subsequent analysis using gas chromatography. NIOSH 1003.
Occupational exposure limits. HSE OES: 8-h TWA, 1110 mg m^{-3} (200 ppm); 15-min STEL, 2200 mg m^{-3} (400 ppm).
HSE guidance. MDHS 28.

4.4.29 Trichloroethylene

Properties. Non-flammable liquid. MW, 133.41.
Uses. Degreasing agent, anaesthetic gas.
Metabolism. Readily absorbed through the lungs and, to a lesser extent, the skin. Metabolised to chloral hydrate and then to TCA or its glucuronide, and trichloroethanol excreted in the urine.
Health effects. Acute: powerful narcotic, action exacerbated by ethanol. Consistent exposure to trichloroethylene and alcohol consumption responsible for 'degreasers flush'. Mild respiratory and skin irritant. Chronic: peripheral neuropathy has been reported. Addictive.
Biological monitoring. Urinary TCA estimations.
Treatment. Non-specific.
Measurement. Sampled onto a charcoal tube at an air flow rate of 1000 ml min^{-1} for subsequent analysis using gas chromatography.
Occupational exposure limits. HSE MEL: 8-h TWA, 550 mg m^{-3} (100 ppm); 15-min STEL, 820 mg m^{-3} (150 ppm) (Sk).
HSE guidance. MDHS 28.

4.4.30 Trinitrotoluene (TNT)

Properties. Colourless, explosive crystals. MW, 227.14.
Uses. Explosives.

Metabolism. Absorbed through the skin and enhanced by sweating.
Health effects. Acute: cyanosis, mild anaemia. Irritant dermatitis and
gastritis. Chronic: yellow- or orange-stained skin. Toxic jaundice is rare,
but when it occurs is frequently fatal. Aplastic anaemia.
Biological monitoring. Coproporphyrinuria is proportional to the severity
of poisoning. Red blood cell and platelet count reduced.
Treatment. Thorough flushing of contaminated skin with water. The
addition of potassium sulphate to the water is useful, as contact with TNT
produces a red colour. This can be used as an indicator of the
effectiveness of decontamination. Otherwise, non-specific.
Measurement. Sampled onto a cellulose acetate filter (pore size, 0.8 µm)
at an air flow rate of around 2 l min^{-1} for subsequent colorimetric
analysis.
Occupational exposure limits. HSE OES: 8-h TWA, 0.5 mg m^{-3} (Sk).

4.4.31 Vinyl chloride (monochloroethylene)

Properties. Flammable gas with pleasant odour. MW, 62.5.
Uses. Polymerised to plastics, solvent in rubber manufacture. Previously
used as aerosol propellant, and has anaesthetic properties.
Metabolism. Rapidly absorbed by inhalation and partially excreted by the
same route. Rapid clearance from the blood through poorly understood
metabolic pathways, but it is possible that some of the health effects are
related to the body reaction to vinyl chloride–protein complexes, which
are considered 'foreign'.
Health effects. Acute: narcotic. Chronic: fatigue, lassitude, abdominal
pain. Raynaud's phenomenon, which can be severe. Acro-osteolysis of
fingertips leading to pseudo-clubbing and scleroderma-like changes.
Angiosarcoma of the liver — rare, but invariably fatal. Occurred
following high exposures in workers clearing vinyl chloride monomer
(VCM) polymerisation chambers.
Health surveillance. Radiography of the hands. Liver function monitoring
has been disappointing.
Treatment. Non-specific.
Measurement. Sampled onto two charcoal tubes in series at an air flow
rate of 50 ml min^{-1} for subsequent analysis using gas chromatography
(NIOSH 1007). Colorimetric detector tubes are also available.

Occupational exposure limits. HSE MEL: 3 ppm averaged over 1 year. The annual maximum exposure limit is supplemented by an 8-h TWA MEL of 7 ppm for personal exposure with the proviso that the annual limit is not exceeded.

4.4.32 Xylene

3 isomers:

ortho-   meta-   para-

Properties. Colourless liquid. MW, 106.17. Three isomers.
Uses. Solvent. Chemical intermediate.
Metabolism. Rapidly absorbed from the lungs; metabolised and excreted in the urine as methyl hippuric acid.
Health effects. Acute: mucous membrane irritation. Narcotic. Chronic: aplastic anaemia has been postulated, but may be due to benzene contamination (as with toluene).
Biological monitoring. Urinary methyl hippuric acid.
Treatment. Non-specific.
Measurement. Sampled onto a charcoal tube at an air flow rate of 1 l min^{-1} for subsequent analysis using gas chromatography (NIOSH 1501).
Occupational exposure limits. HSE OES: 8-h TWA, 441 mg m^{-3} (100 ppm); 662 mg m^{-3} (150 ppm) (Sk).

4.5 Toxic gases

Although many organic compounds may be inhaled in vapour or gaseous form, the toxic gases *per se* are usually deemed to include compounds such as methane, sulphur dioxide and hydrocyanic acid.

In general, these gases may be classified as:
• simple asphyxiants, e.g. nitrogen, carbon dioxide and methane;
• chemical asphyxiants, e.g. carbon monoxide, hydrogen sulphide and hydrogen cyanide;
• upper respiratory tract irritants, e.g. ammonia and sulphur dioxide;
• lower respiratory tract irritants, e.g. oxides of nitrogen and phosgene.

4.5.1 Simple asphyxiants

These gases are only likely to be a danger when their concentration in inhaled air is sufficient to cause a diminution in oxygen levels. Levels of oxygen below 14% lead to pulmonary hyperventilation and tissue anoxia.

Nitrogen

Nitrogen is the main constituent of air and is also present in high concentrations in some mines ('chokedamp'). Indeed, the miners' canary and safety lamp were, in the main, introduced to detect such asphyxiating underground environments. In addition, nitrogen has industrial uses in ammonia production, as an inert atmosphere and as a freezing agent (boiling point, −195.8°C). In hyperbaric work, such as diving, nitrogen becomes toxic, causing narcosis. Nitrogen bubbles are thought to be responsible for symptoms of 'bends' in divers. It is normally detected chemically by eliminating other gases: what remains as an inert gas is assumed to be nitrogen.

Methane

Methane is the product of the anaerobic decay of organic matter. Hence, it is found in sewers and wherever biodegradable organic matter is stored or dumped. It is also a natural constituent of fossil fuel reserves, and is frequently found in coal mines and, occasionally, in other mines. Natural gas, used as a fuel in the UK, contains a large percentage of methane. It is explosive and lighter than air, and therefore, in a concentrated form, will rise to make layers in unventilated ceilings and roofs which pose an explosive hazard. Explosive concentrations depend upon the percentage of oxygen present, but, in fresh air, 5.2% is the lower explosive limit and 14% is the upper explosive limit. Methods of detection started with the simple Davy lamp introduced in 1816, which, in modified form, is still used underground in coal mines today. The principle of detection involves a 'halo' of blue above the wick of a lowered flame, the shape of which indicates the concentration of methane. A double wire gauze prevents the heat igniting methane outside the lamp. The latest instruments use solid-state sensors.

Carbon dioxide

Carbon dioxide occurs naturally as a product of combustion and of gradual oxidation, and hence can occur wherever combustible or organic materials are to be found. Industrially, it is found as a by-product of brewing, coke ovens, blast furnaces and silage dumps. It has a wide use as an industrial gas, e.g. in the carbonisation of drinks, brewing and

4 Chemicals, Gases, Dusts and Particles

4.5 Toxic gases

....

refrigeration. It is heavier than air and, in concentrated form, can produce 'pools' of inert atmosphere in low, unventilated places such as sumps and sewers. It occurs in mines in conjunction with nitrogen as a gas known as 'blackdamp', and in the aftermath of explosions as a gas known as 'afterdamp'.

Occupational exposure limits. HSE OES: 8-h TWA, 9150 mg m^{-3} (5000 ppm); 15-min STEL, 27 400 mg m^{-3} (15 000 ppm).

Carbon dioxide, unlike methane and nitrogen, is capable of stimulating the medullary respiratory centre to produce hyperpnoea. This begins to occur at a concentration of 3%, whilst, at 10% or more, loss of consciousness is rapid. It is also important to remember that, although the toxic effects of simple asphyxiants are readily reversed if removal from exposure and oxygenation are rapid, the 'weights' of the gases will determine the least hazardous approach by the rescue team to the stricken patient.

Methane is lighter than air, carbon dioxide is heavier, and nitrogen, comprising 80% of normal air, is approximately the same density as air. This characteristic of nitrogen, plus its inability to stimulate the respiratory centre, makes it a clinically inappropriate replacement for carbon dioxide as an inert gas for the transportation of other products. Nevertheless, this is exactly what is happening in many industries today.

4.5.2 Chemical asphyxiants

Carbon monoxide (CO)

Occurrence. Produced by the incomplete combustion of carbonaceous compounds; also from the metabolism of methylene chloride.

Properties. Colourless, odourless gas; burns with a blue flame. MW, 28.0.

Uses. By-product of mining, smelting, foundry work, petrochemical processes and many processes involving combustion.

Metabolism. High affinity of absorbed gas for haemoglobin, leading to elevated carboxyhaemoglobin levels and diminished oxygen-carrying capacity of blood. Excreted through the lung. Non-cumulative poison.

Health effects. Acute: insidious onset with giddiness, headache, chest tightness, nausea. Unconsciousness rapidly supervenes at concentrations in excess of 3500 ppm. No cyanosis (indeed, the patient (at post-mortem!) frequently has a deceptive healthy pink complexion due to carboxyhaemoglobin). Chronic: headache. Organic brain damage if asphyxiation is prolonged.

Biological monitoring. Carboxyhaemoglobin levels in blood.

Treatment. Remove from exposure and give 95% O_2, 5% CO_2.

Measurement. Normally an immediate indication of concentration is required for safety reasons, and hence it is measured by direct reading instruments, using a variety of principles. It can be sampled over a long period by slowly filling a container for subsequent analysis through a direct reading instrument. Colorimetric detector tubes are also available.

Occupational exposure limits. HSE OES: 8-h TWA, 58 mg m^{-3} (50 ppm); 15-min STEL, 349 mg m^{-3} (300 ppm).

Legal requirements. Coal and Other Mines (Locomotives) Regulation 1956 (SI 1956 No. 1771).

Hydrogen cyanide (HCN)

Occurrence. Gas emanates from contact of cyanide salts with acid.

Properties. Colourless gas with (apparently!) a bitter almond smell.

Uses. Precious metal extraction, particularly the plating industry. Fumigant and steel hardener.

Metabolism. Inhibits the action of cytochrome oxidase, thus disrupting cellular respiration.

Health effects. Acute: rapid onset of headache, hypopnoea, tachycardia, hypotension, convulsions and death. The rapidity of the onset of symptoms necessitates treatment statim. Chronic: none.

Biological monitoring. Blood cyanide concentrations.

Treatment. Remove contaminated clothing and wash skin. Administer amyl nitrite by inhalation and 100% oxygen if the patient is breathing spontaneously. Amyl nitrite induces the formation of methaemoglobin, and this has an affinity for circulating cyanide. It mops up the cyanide before it can reach the cells. The same rationale applies for administering sodium nitrite i.v. as an antidote. The indication of methaemoglobinaemia is a safer alternative to cyanide poisoning. Sodium thiosulphate can also be given i.v. following sodium nitrite. This converts the cyanide to the less toxic sodium thiocyanate, which is cleared via the urine. Dicobalt edetate (Kelocyanor) is a chelating agent, and is advocated for the unconscious patient with a definite history of cyanide exposure. If in doubt, dispatch the patient immediately to hospital. Recent industrial experience suggests that the potentially toxic dicobalt edetate need not be given immediately, even in the unconscious patient, unless vital signs are deteriorating.

Measurement. Sampled through a filter (to remove particulate cyanide interference) into a midget bubbler containing 0.1 mol l^{-1} potassium hydroxide at an air flow rate of 2 l min^{-1}. The solution is analysed using a cyanide ion-selective electrode. Colorimetric detection tubes are also available.

Occupational exposure limits. HSE MEL: 15-min STEL, 11 mg m^{-3} (10 ppm) (Sk).

Hydrogen sulphide (H$_2$S)

Occurrence. Wherever sulphur and its compounds are being used or disposed.

Properties. Colourless gas with the smell of rotten eggs, and a toxicity akin to hydrogen cyanide.

Uses. None of major importance.

Metabolism. Inhibits cytochrome oxidase (cf. HCN) and causes increase in sulphmethaemoglobin.

Health effects. Acute: lacrimation, photophobia and mucous membrane irritation in low concentrations. In high concentrations, paralysis of the respiratory centre can cause sudden unconsciousness. Chronic: keratitis. Skin vesicles. No cumulative effects.

Biological monitoring. None of great relevance.

Treatment. Removal from exposure. Administer oxygen and consider using amyl or sodium nitrite to convert haemoglobin to methaemoglobin, for combination with H$_2$S, thereby lowering the effective H$_2$S concentrations.

Measurement. Sampled onto a molecular sieve tube via a desiccant tube of sodium sulphate at an air flow rate of 150 ml min^{-1} for subsequent analysis using gas chromatography. Colorimetric detection tubes are also available.

Occupational exposure limits. HSE OES: 8-h TWA, 14 mg m^{-3} (10 ppm); 15-min STEL, 21 mg m^{-3} (15 ppm).

4.5.3 Irritants

The irritant gases, as their name implies, are not respirable without embarrassment. The somewhat artificial division into upper and lower respiratory tract irritants is largely on the basis of solubility. Thus, the highly soluble gases, such as ammonia, sulphur dioxide and chlorine, exert their irritant effect on the upper respiratory tract, which, unless the exposure is prolonged and severe, saves the lungs. Conversely, gases of low solubility, such as oxides of nitrogen and phosgene, have little effect on the upper respiratory tract; their effect is delayed and the main brunt of the damage is borne by the lungs.

Ammonia (NH$_3$)

Properties. Colourless gas with pungent odour. Lighter than air.

Uses. Widely used industrial gas. Manufacture of fertilisers, refrigerants and as a catalyst and reagent.

Metabolism. Extremely soluble in water, producing a caustic alkaline solution of ammonium hydroxide. Detectable to most humans at 30–50 ppm.

Health effects. At concentrations above 50 ppm, the gas is an irritant to the eyes, mucous membrane and upper respiratory tract. Exposure is not voluntarily tolerated above 500 ppm. At 5000–10 000 ppm, severe, and often fatal, respiratory tract damage occurs, with denuded bronchial epithelium and pulmonary oedema. There is some evidence of long-term respiratory damage following acute exposure.

Biological monitoring. None of relevance.

Treatment. Remove from exposure. Oxygen and respiratory support measures.

Measurement. Sampled onto silica gel treated with sulphuric acid at a flow rate between 0.1 and 0.2 l min^{-1}. Extracted with deionised water and analysed with visible absorption (NIOSH 6015).

Occupational exposure limits. HSE OES: 8-h TWA, 18 mg m^{-3} (25 ppm); 15-min STEL, 25 mg m^{-3} (35 ppm).

Chlorine (Cl$_2$)

Properties. Greenish-yellow gas of pungent odour, over twice as heavy as air.

Uses. Chemical and pharmaceutical production, water disinfection in swimming pools, plastics manufacture.

Metabolism. Releases nascent oxygen from water and forms hydrochloric acid, which can cause severe protoplasmic damage in high concentrations.

Health effects. Acute: severe upper respiratory tract irritation leading to pulmonary oedema and death in those unable to escape its effects. Recovery from an acute exposure may be prolonged. Chronic: chronic bronchitis.

Biological monitoring. None of relevance.

Treatment. Remove from exposure. Oxygen and respiratory support measures.

Measurement. Sampled by passing air through a fritted bubbler, containing 100 ml of dilute methyl orange, at an air flow rate of around 1.5 l min^{-1} for subsequent colorimetric analysis. Colorimetric detector tubes are also available.

Occupational exposure limits. HSE OES: 8-h TWA, 1.5 mg m^{-3} (0.5 ppm); 15-min STEL, 2.9 mg m^{-3} (1 ppm).

Fluorine (F$_2$)

Properties. A greenish-yellow gas with a pungent odour. One of the most chemically active elements.

Uses. Fluorides are used as metal fluxes; uranium hexafluoride is used to separate isotopes of uranium. Glass etching, pottery, refrigeration (organic fluorides). Fluorides added to drinking water prevent dental caries.

Health effects. Acute: severe, penetrating, painful skin burns. Severe inhalational effects including laryngeal spasm, oedema and haemoptysis. Chronic: skin scarring. Pulmonary fibrosis. Fluorosis of the bones. Systemic effects of hydrofluoric acid exposure are related to the disturbance of calcium and magnesium metabolism. Cardiac arrhythmias may follow lowered levels of these elements in the blood. Serum electrolyte estimation may indicate the need for calcium supplements.

Biological monitoring. Blood fluoride levels.

Treatment. Hydrofluoric acid. Burns must be treated immediately with copious quantities of ice-cold water, followed by benzalkonium chloride (for 2–4 h) and then magnesium oxide/glycerine paste. Massaging calcium gluconate gel into the burn or infiltration of calcium gluconate solution at the site of the injury is considered by some to be the treatment of choice. Large burns require hospitalisation and surgical debridement. Respiratory tract irritation by fluorine gas requires intensive supportive measures.

Occupational exposure limits. HSE OES: 15-min STEL, 1.6 mg m^{-3} (1 ppm).

Nickel carbonyl (Ni(CO)$_4$)

Occurrence. Generated during nickel refining (Mond process).

Properties. Colourless, odourless gas.

Uses. The unique properties of nickel carbonyl enable nickel to be extracted from the ore and subsequently released from the carbonyl gas in nearly 100% pure form.

Metabolism. Similar to carbon monoxide.

Health effects. Acute: headache, nausea, vomiting, unconsciousness. These symptoms may subside and be followed up to 36 h later with pulmonary irritation and oedema. Chronic: cancer of nasal sinuses and lungs (?).

Biological monitoring. Urinary nickel after acute exposure to nickel carbonyl.

Treatment. Remove from exposure. Administer oxygen. Observe for at least 48 h after initial exposure. Sodium diethyl-dithiocarbamate

(Dithiocarb), orally or parenterally, depending on the severity of symptoms.
Measurement. Sampled through an impinger containing a reagent at an air flow rate of 2 l min^{-1} for subsequent analysis using atomic absorption spectrophotometry. Colorimetric detector tubes are also available.
Occupational exposure limits. HSE OES: 15-min STEL, 0.24 mg m^{-3} (0.1 ppm).

Oxides of nitrogen (N_2O, NO, NO_2)

Properties. NO_2 is the gas of greatest occupational health importance here and is reddish-brown with a pungent odour. Nitrous oxide (N_2O) is an anaesthetic gas. Nitric oxide (NO) is a colourless gas, with little known effect in humans.
Uses. NO_2 is used in the manufacture of nitric acid, explosives and jet fuel. It is generated during welding (some types), silo storage, blasting operations and diesel engine operation.
Health effects. NO_2 exposure. Acute: insidious, due to slow progression of pulmonary irritation some 8–24 h after exposure. Severe exposure can result in death from pulmonary oedema within 48 h. NO_2 is the aetiological agent in silo-filler's disease. Chronic: brown discoloration of teeth. Transient patchy lung opacities on chest radiography.
Biological monitoring. None of relevance.
Treatment. Non-specific. Observe all those exposed for at least 48 h and admit to hospital anyone developing signs of respiratory irritation.
Measurement. Sampled onto impregnated molecular sieve tubes in tandem, at an air flow rate of between 25 and 50 ml min^{-1}, for subsequent spectrophotometric analysis. Colorimetric detector tubes are available for nitrogen dioxide and nitrous fumes (NO + NO_2).
Occupational exposure limits. Nitric oxide (NO), HSE OES: 8-h TWA, 31 mg m^{-3} (25 ppm); 15-min STEL, 44 mg m^{-3} (35 ppm). Nitrogen dioxide (NO_2), HSE OES: 8-h TWA, 5.7 mg m^{-3} (3 ppm); 15-min STEL, 9.6 mg m^{-3} (5 ppm).
Legal requirements. The Coal and Other Mines (Locomotives) Regulations 1956 (SI 1956 No. 1771).

Ozone (O_3)

Properties. Gas generated during arc welding (especially when the weld creates very little fume i.e. MIG and aluminium) and from the photochemical oxidation of automobile exhaust gases. Ozone layer in the stratosphere said to protect against global warming.
Uses. Oxidising agent, water fumigant, bleaching agent.

Health effects. Respiratory tract and mucosal irritant. Exposure to high concentrations can lead to pulmonary oedema.

Management and treatment. Removal from further exposure. Administer oxygen. Steroids may be indicated for severe effects on the lungs.

Measurement. Colorimetric detection tubes are available.

HSE guidance. EH38.

Occupational exposure limits. HSE OES: 15-min STEL, 0.4 mg m^{-3} (0.2 ppm).

Phosgene (carbonyl chloride) (COCl$_2$)

Properties. Sweet-smelling, highly toxic gas. MW, 98.93.

Uses. Source of chlorine, war gas. Evolution of phosgene is a hazard of burning chlorinated hydrocarbons, including many plastics.

Health effects. Acute: mild early symptoms followed by insidious onset of severe pulmonary oedema within succeeding 24–48 h. Chronic: no permanent lung damage in survivors.

Treatment. Hospital treatment of respiratory effects is obligatory.

Measurement. Air is drawn into a midget impinger containing nitrobenzylpyridine, at an air flow rate of 1000 ml min^{-1}, for subsequent colorimetric analysis. Colorimetric detector tubes are available.

Occupational exposure limits. HSE OES: 8-h TWA, 0.08 mg m^{-3} (0.02 ppm); 15-min STEL, 0.25 mg m^{-3} (0.06 ppm).

Sulphur dioxide (SO$_2$)

Properties. Colourless gas with pungent odour and a density twice that of air. Constituent of air pollution.

Uses. Chemical and paper industries, bleaching, fumigation, refrigeration, preservative. A common by-product of smelting sulphide ores.

Metabolism. Produces sulphurous acid on solution in water, leading to acidosis. Can be detected at concentrations as low as 3 ppm.

Health effects. Acute: acute mucous membrane irritant. The respiratory tract irritation is so severe that escape from the gas is imperative. Failure to escape leads to severe pulmonary oedema and death. May trigger asthmatic attacks in susceptible individuals. Corneal ulceration and scarring following prolonged eye irritation. Chronic: diminution in olfactory and gustatory senses. Chronic bronchitis.

Biological monitoring. None of relevance.

Treatment. Remove from exposure, oxygen, respiratory support.

Measurement. Sampled onto an impregnated cellulose filter, containing

....

potassium hydroxide, through a cellulose acetate pre-filter to collect particulate sulphates and sulphites, at an air flow rate of 1.5 l min^{-1}. The impregnated filter is extracted with deionised water for subsequent anion exchange chromatography. Direct reading instruments and colorimetric detector tubes are also available, and can also be sampled using a bubbler containing hydrogen peroxide for wet chemical analysis.

Occupational exposure limits. HSE OES: 8-h TWA, 5.3 mg m^{-3} (2 ppm); 15-min STEL, 13 mg m^{-3} (5 ppm).

Arsine (AsH$_3$), phosphine (PH$_3$) and stibine (SbH$_3$)

Arsenic, phosphorus and antimony are unique among the elements in producing hydride gases. Apart from the use of arsine in semiconductor technology, all are of little or no commercial importance, but are evolved when the elements are exposed to nascent hydrogen, as when metal dross is in contact with acidic water.

Arsine and stibine are both powerful haemolytic agents, and can cause massive intravascular haemolysis leading to acute oliguric renal failure. Phosphine produces gastrointestinal and neurological symptoms. Long-term sequelae may be the result of the effects of the hydrides or the release of the elements themselves due to oxidation.

Measurement. Because of the acute nature of the toxic effects, emergency medication is normally required. Arsine is associated with a mild smell of garlic (odour threshold, 0.5 ppm, or 10 times OEL), but stibine and phosphine odours cannot be described. Detection tubes are available for arsine and phosphine. Arsine can be collected on a charcoal tube at an air flow rate of 200 ml min^{-1} for subsequent analysis using atomic absorption spectrophotometry. Phosphine and stibine can be collected on an impregnated silica gel tube at an air flow rate of 200 ml min^{-1} for subsequent colorimetric analysis.

Occupational exposure limits. Arsine: HSE OES: 8-h TWA, 0.16 mg m^{-3} (0.05 ppm). Phosphine: HSE OES: 15-min STEL, 0.42 mg m^{-3} (0.3 ppm). Stibine: HSE OES as Sb: 8-h TWA, 0.52 mg m^{-3} (0.1 ppm); 15-min STEL, 1.6 mg m^{-3} (0.3 ppm).

Legal requirements and HSE guidance. Arsine (as a component of arsenic): The Factories (Notification of Diseases) Regulations 1966 (SI 1966 No. 1400). Arsine and phosphine (as compounds of arsenic and phosphorus): Factories Act 1961, Section 82. EH11 — Arsine: Health and Safety Precautions. EH12 — Stibine: Health and Safety Precautions. EH20 — Phosphine: Health and Safety Precautions.

4.6 Dusts and particles

4.6.1 Introduction

Many occupational hazards occur as airborne particles: dust, fibres, mists, fume, radioactive particles, bacteria and viruses. A dispersed suspension of solid or liquid particles in a gas or mixture of gases (normally air) is known as an *aerosol*. The health risks from inhaling such an aerosol depend upon the nature and size of the particles, their airborne concentration and the part of the respiratory system in which they are deposited. The particle size and the position in the lung are related.

In order to define the size of particles found in the workplace, which are mainly irregular in shape, a convention is adopted that assigns a diameter to a particle based upon its aerodynamic properties, in particular its settling velocity in still air. A particle is assigned an *aerodynamic diameter*, which is defined as the diameter of a unit density sphere, i.e. water, which settles at the same velocity as the particle in question.

This dimension is relevant to the way in which the particle is deposited in the lung, the method of sampling and air cleaning.

Typical airborne particles

- Dusts: 1–75 μm in diameter; sources: from attrition, e.g. cutting, grinding, sanding, finishing, transport, sieving, crushing, screening, blasting, etc.
- Fibres: 1 : 3 aspect ratio; sources: natural mineral (asbestos), natural vegetable (jute, cotton), synthetic mineral (glass fibre, rockwool, ceramic), synthetic organic (nylon, terylene).
- Fume: usually below 1 μm; from the sublimation and oxidation of molten metal, e.g. lead, cadmium, chromium, iron, nickel, etc.
- Mists: atmospheric: above 20 μm; water droplets condensed on a particle nucleus from surfaces of open tanks.
- Smoke: mixture of particles and gases usually below 1 μm; sources: combustion.
- Biological: bacteria, viruses, fungi.
- Radiation: radioactive particles, α and β, from: mining, manufacturing, power generation, research and investigations; also occurs naturally.

Particle size and respiratory penetration

Ill health from the inhalation of aerosols can be divided into three groups, depending upon the region of the respiratory system into which the particles are deposited:

1 extrathoracic (upper respiratory tract);

2 thoracic (bronchi and bronchioles);

3 alveolar (alveoli).

Extrathoracic. Certain bacteria, fungi and allergens may deposit in the upper respiratory tract, which may lead to inflammation of mucous membranes, e.g. rhinitis; particles such as wood dust, nickel and radioactive particles may lead to ulceration and nasal cancer.

Thoracic. Many particles that reach the tracheobronchial region (i.e. bronchi and bronchioles) may lead to bronchoconstriction, bronchitis and bronchial carcinoma.

Alveolar. Certain particles that reach the gas exchange region of the lung (i.e. alveoli) may lead to pneumoconiosis, emphysema, alveolitis and pulmonary carcinoma. Particles reaching this part of the lung are known as *respirable*. Certain fibres may be carried to the pleura to cause mesothelioma.

International collaboration has recently led to agreement on the definitions of health-related aerosol fractions in the workplace, defined as: *inhalable*, *thoracic* and *respirable*. These are published in British Standard BS 6069, EN 481 and are summarised in Fig. 4.1, which relates the aerodynamic diameter of the particle with the percentage of particles penetrating the three regions.

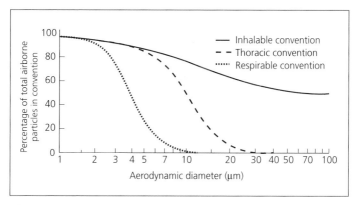

Fig. 4.1 International Standards Organization (ISO)/Comitée Européen de Normalisation (CEN)/American Conference of Governmental Industrial Hygienists (ACGIH) sampling conventions for health-related controls.

The respirable curve has a median aerodynamic diameter of 4.25 µm and the thoracic curve of 11.64 µm. The inhalable curve has an indeterminate endpoint at the larger end and has no median diameter. *Respirable fibres* are defined as having an aspect ratio (length to width) of 3 : 1, a length of more than 5 µm and a diameter of less than 3 µm.

4.6.2 Dusts and particles

Asbestos (see also section on lung diseases, p. 43)
Occurrence. Naturally occurring fibrous silicates — either serpentine (chrysotile) or amphibole (crocidolite, amosite and anthophyllite).
Properties. Highly resistant to temperature, pressure and acids, but these properties vary with the variety of asbestos. Serpentine varieties are also capable of being woven into cloth.
Uses. Many and varied, including asbestos cement, building and insulation materials, brake lining and fire-proofing devices.
Metabolism. Induces severe and possibly irreversible fibrosis in body tissues.
Health effects. Acute: none of note. Chronic: chronic fibrotic lung disease — asbestosis. Pleural plaque formation and calcification. Carcinoma of the lung (synergistic effect with cigarette smoking). Malignant mesothelioma of the pleura and peritoneum. Skin corns. Carcinoma of the larynx (?) and (possibly) ovary and gastrointestinal tract.
Health surveillance. Asbestos bodies in the sputum. Pulmonary function tests including spirometry and gas diffusion. Serial chest radiography.
Treatment. Removal from exposure. Management of chronic fibrotic lung disease and malignancies.
Measurement. It is necessary to determine the number of airborne respirable fibres by sampling onto a cellulose acetate filter for subsequent microscopic analysis and counting. A respirable fibre is defined as one that is greater than 5 µm in length, has a length to breadth ratio of at least 3 : 1 and a diameter of less than 3 µm. Sampling should be carried out in accordance with HSE Guidance Note EH10 and MDHS 39/4.
Occupational exposure limits. HSE control limits:
(a) for asbestos consisting of or containing any crocidolite or amosite:
　(i) 0.2 fibres per millilitre of air averaged over any continuous period of 4 h;
　(ii) 0.6 fibres per millilitre of air averaged over any continuous period of 10 min;
(b) for asbestos consisting of or containing other types of asbestos, but not crocidolite or amosite:

(i) 0.5 fibres per millilitre of air averaged over any continuous period of 4 h;

(ii) 1.5 fibres per millilitre of air averaged over any continuous period of 10 min.

Legal requirements and HSE guidance. The Control of Asbestos at Work Regulations 1987 (SI 1987 No. 2115 as amended by SI 1988 No. 712). The Asbestos (Licensing) Regulations 1983 (SI 1983 No. 1649). The Asbestos (Prohibitions) Regulations 1985 (SI 1985 No. 910). Asbestos (Vol. 1) Final Report of the Advisory Committee (Simpson), HMSO, 1980. Work with Asbestos Insulation and Asbestos Coating: Approved Code of Practice and Guidance Note, revised edition, HSC, 1983. A Guide to the Asbestos (Licensing) Regulations MS(R) 19. EH10 (Rev) Asbestos — Control Limits, Measurement of Airborne Dust Concentrations and the Assessment of Control Measures (revised 1990). EH51 Enclosures Provided for Work with Asbestos Insulation and Coating 1989. EH52 Removal Techniques for Asbestos Insulation Coatings and Insulation 1989. EH57 The Problems of Asbestos Removal at High Temperatures 1993. EH71 Working with Asbestos Cement and Asbestos Insulating Board 1996. MDHS 39/4. MS 13.

Coal dust (see also section on lung diseases, p. 43)
Occurrence. Mainly underground and world-wide. Formed due to the prehistoric accumulation of rotting vegetation.
Properties. Vary with the type and rank of coal.
Uses. Combustion, petrochemicals.
Metabolism. None.
Health effects. Acute: none. Chronic: pulmonary fibrosis ranging from simple pneumoconiosis to progressive, massive fibrosis, which is a frequent precursor of death from respiratory failure.
Health surveillance. Lung function tests, especially spirometry. Serial chest radiography.
Treatment. Removal from exposure. Management of chronic respiratory disease.
Measurement. Sampled for airborne respirable fraction by drawing a known volume of air through a pre-weighed filter for reweighing and analysis. Respirable size selection for personal exposure is undertaken by means of a cyclone separator at an air flow rate of 2.2 l min^{-1} (SIMPEDS) or, for static sampling, by means of a horizontal parallel plate elutriator, as in the MRE 113A sampler, at an air flow rate of 2.5 l min^{-1}. As quartz dust is often found with coal, it may be necessary to determine the respirable quartz content. Therefore, the following filters may be

required: for gravimetric analysis alone, glass fibre; for X-ray diffraction analysis for silica, silver membrane; for infrared analysis for silica, PVC.

Occupational exposure limits. Permitted levels of respirable dust in coal mines are laid down in the Regulations given below. Exposure limits for workplaces other than coal mines: coal dust containing less than 5% quartz: TWA, 2 mg m^{-3} respirable dust; coal dust containing more than 5% quartz: see silica below.

Legal requirements. Coal Mines (Respirable Dust) Regulations 1975 (SI 1975). Coal Mines (Respirable Dust Amendment) Regulations 1978 (SI 1978).

Cotton dust (see also section on lung diseases, p. 43)

Occurrence. Cotton occurs on the plant as a 'boll', which is picked either by hand or by machine, and usually contains some stem and leaves. The bolls pass through a 'ginning' process, that separates the seeds and other materials from the raw cotton, which is then baled for transportation. The ginning process usually occurs close to the cotton fields. At the mills, the bales are opened and the cotton is mechanically cleaned by blowing. It is then combed or 'carded' before being spun, dyed and woven. The dustiest areas are the blowing, blending and carding rooms, where the dust consists of 'fly', i.e. large fibres of cotton (up to 3 cm in length) which are too large to be inhaled, 'trash', which is a mixture of plant debris and soil, and fine, inhalable, cotton dust.

Health effects. The health hazard is from byssinosis, with its characteristic cough, chest tightness and difficulty in breathing, particularly prevalent on the first day back to work after a break, e.g. Monday mornings. Schilling has graded the symptoms of byssinosis into five grades (0,1/2,1,2,3).

Measurement and standards. Many studies have shown a direct relationship between total airborne dust measured in milligrams per cubic metre and the prevalence of byssinosis. The standard is therefore gravimetric. The HSE OES for cotton dust is 0.5 mg m^{-3} TWA of collected dust less fly. Sampling is therefore based on gravimetric techniques using a specially designed apparatus unique to the cotton industry. It draws air at about 10 l min^{-1} through a glass fibre filter paper, which is screened by a gauze of 2-mm mesh, using 0.2-mm wire, to eliminate the fly. During the sampling period, the screen has to be cleared of fly from time to time to prevent it from becoming a pre-filter reducing the collected fibre amounts.

Legal requirements and HSE guidance. The Cotton Cloth Factories

Regulations 1929 (S, R and O 1929 No. 300). Cotton Cloth Factories Regulation Hygrometers Order 1926 (S, R and O 1926 No. 1582). EH 25 Cotton Dust Sampling. MS9 Byssinosis.

Silica dust (see also section on lung diseases, p. 43)
Occurrence. World-wide, as Earth's crust contains 28% silicon.
Properties. Silica (SiO_2) is a hard, rock-like compound capable of fragmentation into fine particles. It is a constituent of many ore-bearing rocks, coal seams, granites, china clay, sandstones and sand.
Uses. Abrasives, building materials, ceramics, foundry work, road stone.
Health effects. Inhalation into the lungs triggers a florid fibrotic reaction from the pulmonary tissues. Acute: none. Chronic: severe nodular pulmonary fibrosis, mainly in the upper lung zone, with surface calcification of lymph nodes and a predisposition to tuberculosis. The possibility of a carcinogenic effect of silica on the lungs is discussed on p. 49.
Health surveillance. Pulmonary function tests, particularly spirometry. Serial chest radiography.
Treatment. Removal from exposure. Management of chronic pulmonary fibrosis.
Measurement. Airborne dusts that may contain silica require to be analysed for crystalline silica. It is usual to collect the respirable fraction by drawing a known volume of air through a pre-weighed filter for reweighing and analysis. Respirable size selection for personal exposure is undertaken by means of a cyclone separator (Higgins and Dewell, SIMPEDS) at an air flow rate of 2.2 l min^{-1} or, for static sampling, by means of a horizontal parallel plate elutriator, as in the MRE 113A sampler, at an air flow rate of 2.5 l min^{-1}. The nature of the crystalline silica is determined by sampling onto a silver membrane filter for subsequent analysis using X-ray diffraction.
Occupational exposure limits. Silica, respirable (all forms) MEL: 8-h TWA, 0.3 mg m^{-3} (under review).
HSE guidance. MDHS 51/2.

Synthetic mineral fibres (man-made mineral fibres, MMMFs)
Occurrence and uses. Manufactured by drawing, blowing, centrifuging and flame attenuation at very high temperature, using various raw materials, and producing a range of fibres with differing diameters and properties.
  Continuous filament: glass-drawn material, molten at 1000–1500°C,

3–15 mm in diameter; product forms — yarn, roving, woven fabrics; uses — industrial textiles, glass-reinforced plastics.

Insulation wools: rockwool, slagwool, glass wool; basalt or dolerite rock, blast furnace slag, glass-blown or centrifuged material at 1000–1500°C, 4–9 μm in diameter; product forms — bulk fibre, blanket, slab, board, mattress; uses — acoustic and thermal insulation.

Refractory fibres: ceramic materials or alumina drawn or blown at 1000–1500°C, 2–3 μm in diameter; product forms — bulk fibre, needled blanket, board, paper, woven cloth, rope, specially moulded shapes; uses — high-temperature insulation for turbines, boilers, heat exchangers, fire protection, hot face linings in furnaces and kilns, seals, gaskets, expansion joints, high-temperature gas and liquid filters. Have a low thermal mass, and thus furnaces can be lighter and respond more quickly.

Special purpose fibres: lime-free borosilicate glass flame attenuated; 0.1–3 μm in diameter; product forms — bulk fibre, felt mat, blanket; uses — aeroengine and rocket insulation, jet engine pipes and fuel systems.

Health effects. Fibres are not crystalline; they break transversely rather than longitudinally. Therefore, crushing and attrition do not yield smaller fibres. The larger fibres cause skin irritation, but there is no evidence of lung disease. Implantation and some inhalational studies on animals show that fibres below 0.25 μm in diameter produce tumours. The production of fibres below 1 μm in diameter is a recent development, and thus the effects on humans will not become apparent for many years. Recent international studies of MMMF workers have failed to resolve the question of whether MMMFs are human carcinogens. At present, there remains a serious suspicion of carcinogenicity — particularly for the ceramic fibres and, perhaps, the rockwool/slagwool fibres. Glass fibres appear to be less implicated.

Measurements and standards. The HSE has published a gravimetric standard, i.e. an MEL of 5 mg m^{-3}, for fibres that are not respirable. Sampling is by drawing a known volume of air through a pre-weighed glass fibre filter mounted in a modified UKAEA or IOM sampling head; the weight gain in milligrams is divided by the volume of air sampled in cubic metres. For respirable fibres, the method is similar to that of asbestos sampling and is explained in MDHS 59. A respirable fibre is defined as one that is greater than 5 μm in length, with a length to breadth ratio of at least 3 : 1 and a diameter of less than 3 μm. See also MDHS 59.

HSE guidance. MDHS 59 Man Made Mineral Fibres 1988.

Wood dust

Wood dust causes irritation of the eyes, nose and throat. The particles generated by the machining and processing of timber are usually large particles which affect mucosal surfaces and the upper respiratory tract. Glues and wood preservatives can be used for timber products, and dust from such sources may release formaldehyde and organic solvents. Western red cedar wood dust has been associated with the development of occupational asthma. Iroko and pine have been known to cause irritant and allergic contact dermatitis. Chronic exposure to hardwood dusts in the furniture trade has been linked to the development of adenocarcinoma of the nasal sinuses. The exact chemical agent in hardwood dust responsible for this effect has not been identified.

Health surveillance. Advice to wood workers on the early recognition of relevant symptoms, and clinical evaluation and follow-up of those with symptoms. Lung function tests indicated for those who are exposed to dusts and woods known to cause asthma.

Management. Reduction of exposure for those who develop occupational asthma or dermatitis. Medications may provide symptomatic relief. Job change to be considered for those with severe health effects.

Measurement. Sampled by drawing a known volume of air through a pre-weighed glass fibre mounted in a modified UKAEA or IOM sampling head; the weight gain in milligrams is obtained by dividing by the total flow volume in cubic metres.

Occupational exposure limits. HSE MEL: 5.0 mg m^{-3}.

HSE guidance. MDHS 14/2.

Dusts (other than those mentioned separately)

We are cautioned by the HSE that, although not all dusts have been assigned occupational exposure limits, the lack of such limits should not be taken to imply an absence of hazard, and that exposure should be controlled to the minimum that is reasonably practicable. However, where there is no indication of the need for a more stringent standard, personal exposure should not exceed 10 mg m^{-3} total dust and 4 mg m^{-3} respirable (alveoli fraction) dust. Any airborne dust concentrations above these values should be regarded as 'substantial concentrations' for the purposes of Regulation 2 of COSHH and, as such, are substances hazardous to health.

HSE guidance. EH44 Dust in the Workplace: General Principles of Protection. MDHS 14/2.

Fume

This is regarded as solid particles generated by chemical reactions or condensation from the gaseous state, usually from the volatilisation of molten metal. Often the particles are in the region of 1 μm in diameter, unless oxidisation has taken place, as with zinc fume, and then the diameters will be larger.

Some welding processes generate fume that contains components which have specific MELs or OESs: these limits should be applied to control exposure if these substances are present in the fume. In any other case, HSE OES: welding fume, 5 mg m^{-3}.

5 Light, Heat, Noise, Vibration, Pressure and Radiation

5.1) Light

Regulation 8 of the Workplace (Health, Safety and Welfare) Regulations 1992 requires that every workplace shall have suitable and sufficient lighting and the lighting shall, so far as is reasonably practicable, be by natural light.

Lighting levels at work can affect health and safety in a number of ways, notably the following.

- When people move about, they must be able to see obstacles that could lead to accidents from tripping, falling or by just walking into them.
- The tasks must be adequately lit to enable workers to see sufficient detail so that these jobs can be carried out correctly.
- Operators of machinery must be able to see the controls, information dials and screens.
- Colours should be correctly rendered if that forms part of the work.
- Stroboscopic effects on rotating machinery must be minimised to prevent the moving part from appearing stationary.
- Items being worked on must have a three-dimensional shape and not appear flat.
- Glare must be minimised.

The above points imply that:

- the lighting levels falling on a work surface must be of the correct intensity;
- the light must be positioned to provide good modelling;
- the colour output of any artificial light source must not distort the colour of the item being worked on if that is important;
- the background levels of light sources or the reflections from surfaces must not be too great to cause glare;
- where rotating machinery is concerned, the source of illumination must not oscillate in time with the frequency of the electrical supply.

5.1.1 Units used in lighting

Luminous intensity. Unit, candela (cd); a measure of brilliance or brightness, which is the power of a source to emit light.

Luminous flux. Unit, lumen (lm), which is the luminous flux emitted within unit solid angle (1 steradian (sr)) by a point source having a uniform luminous intensity of 1 cd. A lamp of 1 cd emits 4π lm.

Luminance. Unit, cd m^{-2}; the flow of light in a given direction.

Illuminance. Unit, lux (lx or lm m^{-2}); this is the unit that expresses the amount of light falling on a surface.

5.1.2 Recommended lighting standards

A comprehensive guide to the most suitable lighting levels (illuminance) for many workplaces is given in the 'Code for Interior Lighting', published by the Chartered Institute of Building Services Engineers, but some typical levels are given below:

Area	Recommended lighting level (lx)
Circulation areas, e.g. corridors, stairs, lifts	100–150
Entrances, lobbies, waiting areas	150
Enquiry desks	500
Factories	300–500 (dependent on the degree of detail to be viewed)
Offices, general at desk	500
Offices, drawing boards	750
Typical outdoor levels	10 000

5.1.3 Glare

As a result of the illumination of a task, it will reflect light to the eye at a certain level of luminance. Surrounding the task will be an immediate field and, in the background, will be yet another field, both of which emit light at a certain luminance. If any of these fields emit too much light into the eye, glare will occur. Where there is a direct interference with vision, as with an undipped car headlamp at night, the condition is known as *disability glare*. If there is no direct impairment of vision, but there is discomfort or annoyance, it is known as *discomfort glare*. Where the task is satisfactorily illuminated, but the surroundings are too bright, a distraction is caused that may lead to visual fatigue. Such a situation is often found in open-plan offices, where lines of lamps hanging below a ceiling appear to merge into the distance, creating one distracting source. This is prevented by recessing the light fittings into a false ceiling, or by turning the worker's desk through 90°. Another example is where a computer screen is placed with a window as a background; the intensity of daylight seen around the screen is far greater than the intensity received from the screen, and discomfort glare occurs.

To minimise glare, the ratio of task to immediate surround to background surround emission should be 10 : 3 : 1. For example, if the task emits 500 cd m^{-2}, the immediate surround should emit no more than 150 cd m^{-2} and the far background no more than 50 cd m^{-2}.

5.1.4 Colour effects

No artificial lamp reproduces exactly the combination of light wavelengths that is found with daylight, and therefore colours seen under artificial light may appear to be different from those illuminated naturally.

Where the matching of colours is important, as with electronic assembly work, the fabric trade and interior decorating, it is essential that any artificial light uses lamps that are as close to the daylight frequencies as possible.

5.1.5 Stroboscopic effects

Lamps that operate from the mains electrical supply, which is at a frequency of 50 Hz, turn on and off 100 times per second. With certain fluorescent lamps, the light output, in effect, ceases at that frequency. If a piece of machinery rotates as an exact function of the mains supply frequency and is illuminated by such a lamp, it may appear to be stationary, which could lead to an accident. Filament lamps glow even when the supply is off and thus their light output is continuous.

5.1.6 Lighting surveys

A full lighting survey will provide details of any defects in the lighting system, but also any potentially acute or chronic occupational health problems. However, some basic information, collected on the report sheet shown in Fig. 5.1, will probably highlight the more obvious problems; where detailed measurements are required, it is suggested that an occupational hygienist with comprehensive knowledge of this field is contacted.

5.2 Heat

5.2.1 Health effects

Body temperature is maintained within close limits by an efficient homeostatic mechanism, although diurnal variation is observed over a range of 0.5–1°C. Physical exercise will increase body temperature in proportion to oxygen consumption, the range being 0.5°C for moderate exercise up to 4°C for marathon running. In normal conditions, however, the body temperature stays within the range 36–39°C as a balance is struck between the following:
* metabolic heat (M);

Lighting survey sheet

Date .... Time ....

Location Address ....
Survey Person ....
Reason for Survey ....

> Room Dimensions: L = ... W = ... H = ...
> Window Dimensions: H = ... W = ...

Daylight Availability: Side Glazing .... Roof Glazing ....

Artificial Lighting: Luminaires/Lamps ....
Luminaire Type ....
Lamp Type ....
Lamp Rating ....
Date of Lamp Change ....

Condition of Equipment and Room Fabrics:
Ceiling ....
Walls ....
Floor ....
Windows ....
Luminaires ....

Principal Visual Tasks ....

Principal Planes of Interest ....

CIBSE Recommended Illuminance Values ....

Fig. 5.1 Typical lighting preliminary report sheet.

- evaporation (E);
- convection (C);
- conduction (K);
- radiation (R);
- storage (S).

Traditionally, this is expressed as:

$$M = E \pm C \pm K \pm R \pm S$$

Diving in a full suit or working in hot, humid conditions can greatly alter this homeostasis. For example, sweating ceases to be an effective means of heat loss at ambient temperatures above 37°C, at a relative humidity of 80% or greater. Against this is the fact that acclimatisation to heat is possible over a period of 10 days, and is facilitated by a greatly increased sweating rate. Furthermore, physical fitness improves an individual's ability to cope with the stresses of heat.

The severity of health effects from heat increases with the temperature, humidity and duration of exposure. In order of increasing seriousness, these effects are:

- lassitude, irritability, discomfort;
- lowered work performance and lack of concentration;
- heat rashes;
- heat cramps;
- heat exhaustion;
- heat stroke.

Any effect up to heat cramps is readily amenable to cooling and the administration of salt and water supplements. Heat exhaustion and heat stroke signify the onset of the failure of the thermoregulatory mechanism, and this demands rapid and effective cooling, with fluid and electrolyte replacement by parenteral routes if necessary. Complete recovery of homeostasis may take a further week.

5.2.2 Environmental monitoring

The four means of heat exchange are: conduction, convection, radiation and evaporation; however, these are not measured directly. The thermal environment around the body, which affects the rate of heat flow, is instead expressed by the following four parameters:

- the dry bulb temperature of the air;
- the moisture content or water vapour pressure of the air;
- the air velocity;
- the radiant heat exchange between the skin and surrounding surfaces.

The relationship between the dry bulb temperature and the moisture content is shown in the psychrometric chart given in Fig. 5.2. The two conditions which can be measured and plotted on this chart are the ventilated wet bulb and dry bulb temperatures, as measured by the sling or aspirated psychrometer. Other factors, such as the moisture content, percentage saturation (approximately the same as the relative humidity), specific enthalpy and specific volume, can be read from the appropriate scales from the point of intersection of the wet and dry bulb temperatures, as shown in Fig. 5.3.

The air velocity is measured by an air flow meter (such as a cup anemometer or rotating vane anemometer), unless the value is low, in

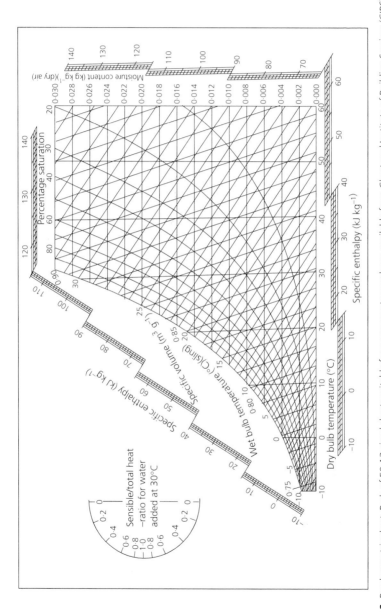

Fig. 5.2 Psychrometric chart. Pads of 50 A3-sized charts suitable for permanent records are available from Chartered Institute of Building Services (CIBS), 222 Balham High Road, London SW12 9BS.

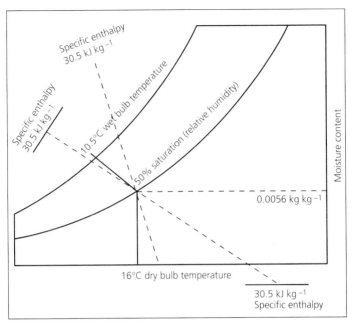

Fig. 5.3 The use of the psychrometric chart. (From Ashton and Gill, 1991.)

which case a kata thermometer is used. The air velocity is obtained from the cooling time of the kata thermometer, using the nomograms given in Figs 5.4 and 5.5.

The radiant heat exchange is obtained from the globe thermometer, which integrates the radiant heat flux from all the surfaces which surround it. As the instrument is affected by the air temperature and velocity, a correction is made, using the nomograms given in Fig. 5.6(a–d), to provide the mean temperature of the surroundings (mean radiant temperature).

Other factors which affect body heat gains and losses are:

- the metabolic rate of the subject due to the degree of activity;
- the type of clothing worn;
- the duration of exposure to the heat or cold.

Typical metabolic rates for different activities are shown in Table 5.1.

Work rates tend to be self-regulating, because a worker will voluntarily reduce their rate if they feel overheated, except in fire fighting and rescue work, where psychological pressures may overcome normal scruples.

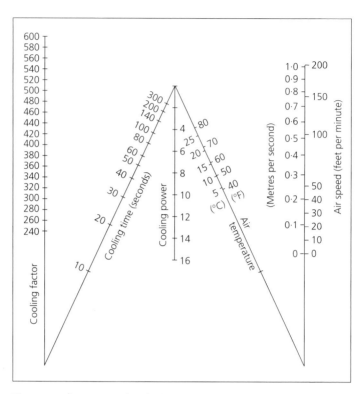

Fig. 5.4 Kata thermometer chart for the temperature range 38–35°C. (After a withdrawn British Standard, BS 3276, 1960.)

Clothing assemblies have varying resistances to heat flow, expressed by the unit 'Clo' (1 Clo = 0.155°C m² W⁻¹). Typical Clo values for various clothing assemblies are given in Table 5.2.

External factors, such as moisture content and wind, will influence the resistance of clothing to heat flow. Moist clothing will have a lower resistance. Higher air velocities tend to collapse clothing, reducing its thickness and hence its resistance, whilst with open weave clothing wind can remove the inner layers of warm air. Except when used as a protection against chemicals or other hazards, personal insulation tends to be self-regulating, people adding or removing layers of clothing according to their feelings of comfort.

The *duration of exposure* can be varied by work/rest regimes, preferably with the rest period being taken in a less extreme

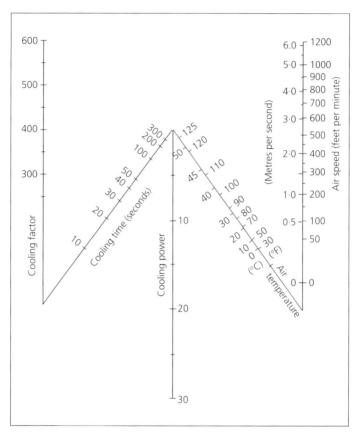

Fig. 5.5 Kata thermometer chart for the temperature range 54.5–51.5°C. (After a withdrawn British Standard, BS 3276, 1960.)

environment. In certain circumstances, such as in hot mines and places of extreme climate, it may not be possible to remove the worker from the environment. This also occurs with rescue work, where the motive to continue the work at all costs is uppermost in the worker's mind.

It is usually either ill advised or not possible to assess hazards/risks in a thermal environment by the use of just one of the parameters mentioned previously, and therefore attempts have been made to bring together these parameters into a single index representing a thermal environment, from which the degree of hazard can be assessed. Some indices are given below.

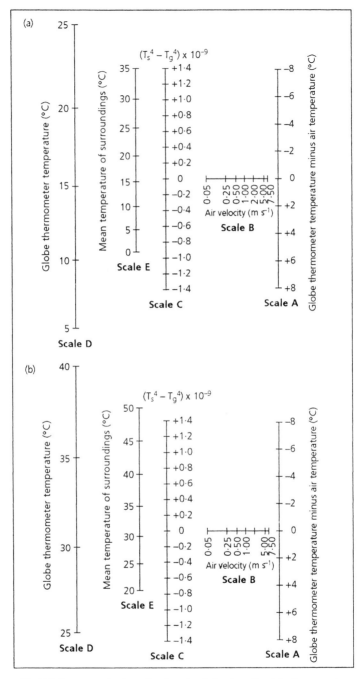

Fig. 5.6 Nomogram for the estimation of radiation from the globe thermometer. (a) Range 5–25°C; (b) range 25–30°C *Continued.*

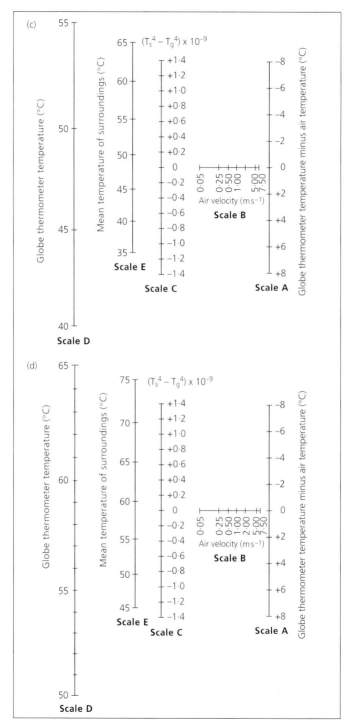

Fig. 5.6 *Continued.* (c) Range 40–55°C; (d) range 50–65°C.

Table 5.1 Typical metabolic rates.

Activity	Metabolic rate (W)
Sitting	95
Standing	115
Walking at 4 km h^{-1}	260
Standing: light hand work	160–210
Standing: heavy hand work	210–260
Standing: light arm work	315
Standing: heavy arm work (e.g. sawing)	420–675
Work with whole body: light	315
Work with whole body: moderate	420
Work with whole body: heavy	560

Table 5.2 Typical Clo values.

Clothing assembly	Clo
Naked	0
Shorts	0.1
Light summer clothing	0.5
Typical indoor clothing	1.0
Heavy suit and underclothes	1.5
Polar clothing	3–4
Practical maximum	5

Wet bulb globe temperature (WBGT)

For indoor use:

WBGT (°C) = $0.7t'_n + 0.3t_g$

For outdoor use:

WBGT (°C) = $0.7t'_n + 0.2t_g + 0.1t$

where t'_n is the natural or unventilated wet bulb temperature, t_g is the globe temperature and t is the dry bulb temperature.

Note that the ventilated wet bulb can be used instead of the natural wet bulb according to the following rules:
- if the relative humidity of the air is below 25%, add 1°C to the ventilated wet bulb temperature;
- if the relative humidity of the air is between 25 and 50%, add 0.5°C to the ventilated wet bulb temperature;
- if the relative humidity of the air is above 50%, use the ventilated wet bulb temperature.

Recommended work/rest regimes for various WBGTs are given in Table 5.3.

Clothing correction for WBGT

Corrections should be made to Table 5.3 to allow for the type of clothing worn as follows:

- light summer clothing, 0;
- cotton overalls, –2;
- winter clothing, –4;
- water barrier (permeable), –6.

Hence, Table 5.3 is suitable only for persons wearing light summer clothing; a new table would have to be drawn up for each clothing type by applying the correction given above to all values in the table.

Table 5.3 WBGTs and recommended work/rest regimes (°C).

	Workload (total)		
	Light	Moderate	Heavy
Continuous	30.0	26.7	25.0
75% work, 25% rest each hour	30.6	28.0	25.9
50% work, 50% rest each hour	31.4	29.4	27.9
25% work, 75% rest each hour	32.2	31.1	30.0

Workload: light, 230 W; moderate, 230–400 W; heavy, 400–580 W. For example, at a WBGT of 30°C, a person could undertake continuous light work, but, if heavy work was involved, he/she could only maintain it for 25% of the time in any hour.

Effective and corrected effective temperatures (ET and CET)

The three charts in Fig. 5.7(a–c) give the 'basic', 'normal' and 'adjusted' scales of the (corrected) effective temperature. The 'basic' scale refers to a worker stripped to the waist, the 'normal' scale refers to a worker lightly clothed and the 'adjusted' scale takes into account the work rate.

To use the charts, it is necessary to join the globe or dry bulb temperature reading to the wet bulb temperature with a straight line. The ET or CET can be read from the nomogram at the point of intersection of the line with the air velocity line. If the dry bulb temperature is used, it will provide the answer as ET, whereas, if the globe temperature is used, the answer will be CET.

Heat stress index (HSI)

This index is calculated as follows:

$$HSI = (E_{req}/E_{max}) \times 100\%$$

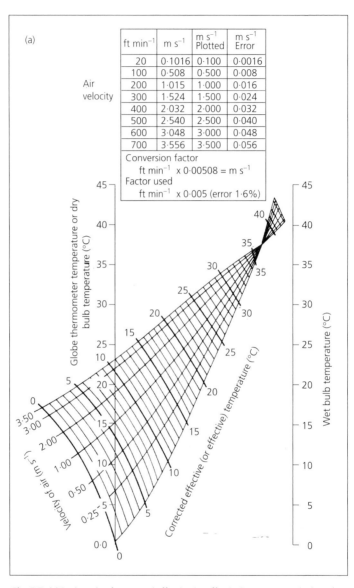

Fig. 5.7 (a) Basic scale of corrected effective (or effective) temperature (stripped to the waist). *Continued.*

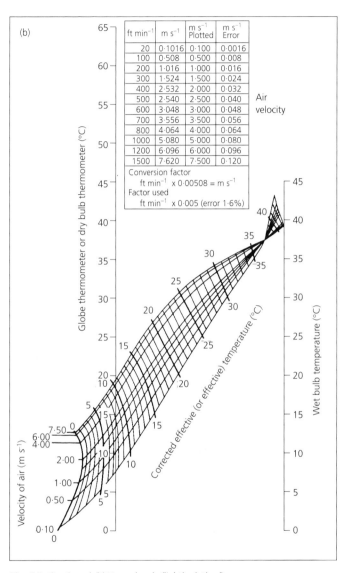

Fig. 5.7 *Continued.* (b) Normal scale (lightly clothed).

(c)

ft min^{-1}	m s^{-1}	m s^{-1} Plotted	m s^{-1} Error
20	0·1016	0·100	0·0016
100	0·508	0·500	0·008
200	1·016	1·000	0·016
300	1·524	1·500	0·024
400	2·032	2·000	0·032
500	2·540	2·500	0·040
600	3·048	3·000	0·048
700	3·556	3·500	0·056
800	4·064	4·000	0·064
1000	5·080	5·000	0·080
1200	6·096	6·000	0·096
1500	7·620	7·500	0·120

Conversion factor
ft min^{-1} × 0·00508 = m s^{-1}
Factor used
ft min^{-1} × 0·005 (error 1·6%)

Air velocity

Sweat rate = 2·5 l

Fig. 5.7 *Continued.* (c) Normal scale with additional nomogram including work rates.

....

where E_{req} (W) $= M + R + C$. For lightly clothed persons:

E_{max} (W) $= 12.5v^{0.6}(56 - \rho_s)$

M (W) $=$ metabolic rate of the worker

R (W) $= 7.93(t_r - 35)$

C (W) $= 8.1v^{0.6}(t - 35)$

For persons stripped to the waist:

E_{max} (W) $= 21v^{0.6}(56 - \rho_s)$

R (W) $= 13.2(t_r - 35)$

C (W) $= 13.6v^{0.6}(t - 35)$

where ρ_s is the water vapour pressure in millibars, an approximate value of which can be found by reading across horizontally from the dry bulb/wet bulb intersection (on the psychrometric chart) until it meets the air moisture content in kg kg^{-1} and multiplying that value by 1560, t_r is the mean radiant temperature (°C), t is the dry bulb temperature (°C) and v is the air velocity (m s^{-1}). A work/rest regime can be calculated from:

$$\text{Exposure time (min)} = \frac{4400}{E_{req} - E_{max}}$$

$$\text{Rest time (min)} = \frac{4400}{E_{max} - E_{req}}$$

Note that, for the rest time, E_{max} and E_{req} refer to the thermal environment in the rest room, if one is used, and normally the work rate will be less.

The upper limit for safety is if the HSI reaches 100%. Any value above this will result in an increase in the deep body temperature, which, if allowed to continue for any length of time, may lead to stress. A negative value indicates cold stress.

One very useful aspect of the HSI is that, if an environment has been found to be unacceptable, potential values to control the environment can be tried in the equation; for example, if the real work environment has a wind velocity of 0.5 m s^{-1}, a value of 1 m s^{-1} can be tried in the equation. If this is still not satisfactory, and 1 m s^{-1} is the maximum value that can be used, but the water vapour pressure can be changed, the combined effect of these can be tried until a satisfactory outcome is achieved.

The *required sweat rate*, the most comprehensive HSI published to date, is given in detail in ISO 7933. It takes into account potential heat stress from the acclimatised and non-acclimatised worker. However, the equations are complex and are best suited to computer solutions; ISO 7933 provides a computer program for their solution.

Wind chill index

In a cold environment, the effect of wind is important. Figure 5.8 shows the equivalent still-air temperatures of various wind velocities. The curves are labelled with a heat loss value in kilocalories per hour per square metre. At a heat loss of 1750 kcal h^{-1} m^{-2}, exposed flesh freezes in approximately 20 min, but, at 2800 kcal h^{-1} m^{-2}, it freezes in 1 min.

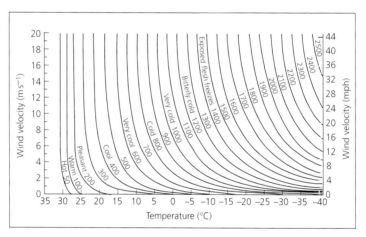

Fig. 5.8 The wind chill index (WCI). Values marked against the curves are the rates of cooling in kcal h^{-1} m^{-2} (multiply by 1.16 to convert to W m^{-2}) at different combinations of wind velocity (m s^{-1}) and temperature (°C).

5.3 Noise

Sound involves pressure changes in the air which are picked up by the eardrum and transmitted to the brain. Pressure is measured in pascals (Pa). The threshold of human hearing is at approximately 0.00002 Pa, but, at 25 m from a jet aircraft taking off, the pressure is 10^7 times greater, at 200 Pa. The expression of such a wide range of sound is simplified with the decibel scale, which compares the actual sound with the reference value of 0.00002 Pa, using a logarithmic scale (to base 10) as follows:

Decibel (dB), $20 \log_{10} \dfrac{P_a}{P_r}$

where P_a is the pressure of the actual sound and P_r is the reference sound pressure at the threshold of hearing.

Typical sound intensities are given in Table 5.4.

Table 5.4 Typical noise levels.

	Pressure (Pa)	Decibel (dB)
Threshold of hearing	0.00002	0
Quiet office	0.002	40
Ringing alarm clock at 1 m	0.2	80
Ship's engine room	20	120
Turbojet engine at 25 m	200	140

5.3.1 Addition of sounds

If two sounds are being emitted at the same time, their total combined intensity is not the numerical sum of the decibel levels of each separate intensity. Because of the logarithmic nature of the decibel scale, they must be added according to the graph given in Fig. 5.9.

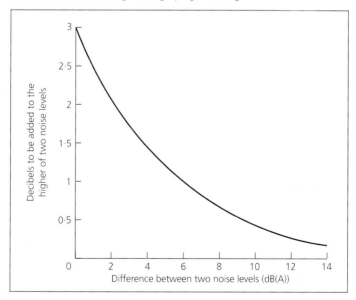

Fig. 5.9 Graph for adding two unequal noise levels.

5.3.2 Sound spectrum

The lowest frequency sound that can be detected by the human ear is about 20 Hz, and the highest, for a young person, is up to 18 kHz. With age, the ear becomes less sensitive to the higher frequencies. A doubling of the frequency raises the pitch of the note by one octave. The ear is most receptive to sounds between 500 Hz and 4 kHz; indeed, 500 Hz to 2 kHz is the frequency range of speech. Unless a sound is a pure tone, which is unusual, most noises are made up of sounds of many frequencies and intensities; when assessing the intensity, it may be necessary to discover the intensity values over the whole range of frequency, i.e. to measure the sound spectrum. This is especially useful for controlling noise. For convenience, it is usual to divide the sounds into octave bands, and to use a measuring instrument which assesses the intensity of all notes between the octaves and expresses it as a mid-octave intensity. The mid-octave frequencies chosen for this analysis are: 62.5 Hz, 125 Hz, 250 Hz, 500 Hz, 1 kHz, 2 kHz, 4 kHz, 8 kHz and, sometimes, 16 kHz. Thus, a spectrum of noise will quote the intensities at each of these mid-octave band frequencies.

5.3.3 Noise rating

Because of the sensitivity range of the ear, it can tolerate louder sounds at lower frequencies than at higher ones. A range of octave band curves, known as 'noise rating (NR) curves', has been produced, which indicates the recommended octave band analyses for various situations. The curve lying immediately above the measured octave band analysis of the noise in question represents the NR of that noise. A range of NR curves is given in Fig. 5.10, and the recommended rating for various situations is given alongside it.

5.3.4 Decibel weightings

As noise is a combination of sounds at various frequencies and intensities, the noise intensity can either be expressed as a spectrum, mentioned previously, or as a combination of all frequencies summed together in one value. As the human ear is more sensitive to certain frequencies than others, it is possible to make allowances for this in the electronic circuitry of a sound level meter, i.e. certain frequencies are suppressed as others are boosted, in order to approximate to the response of the ear.

This technique is known as weighting, and there are A, B, C and D weightings available for various purposes. Figure 5.11 shows the A, B and C weighting networks. That which is most usually quoted is the A

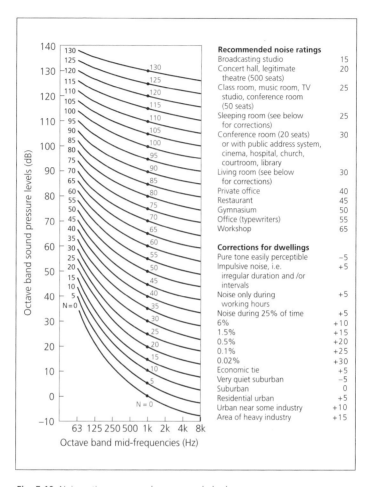

Fig. 5.10 Noise rating curves and recommended values.

weighting, and instruments measuring sound intensity with that weighting give readings in dB(A). The weightings given to the mid-octave band frequencies for the dB(A) scale are shown in Table 5.5.

5.3.5 Noise dose and L_{eq}

Exposure to noise normally varies in intensity over a working period and, in order to estimate an equivalent noise level that would give the same total amount of sound energy as the fluctuating noise, the unit L_{eq} has been devised. In order to measure the L_{eq}, personal noise dosemeters are

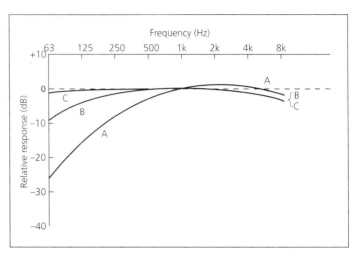

Fig. 5.11 Relative responses of the weighting networks.

Table 5.5 Mid-octave band frequency corrections for dB(A) weighting.

Frequency (Hz)	62.5	125	250	500	1000	2000	4000	8000
Correction (dB)	−26	−16	−9	−3	0	+1	+ 1	−1

used; these are convenient, as they fit into the worker's pocket and the readout (depending on type) is directly in percentage dose, L_{eq}, maximum peak, Pa^2 h, etc.

Guidance for the UK Noise at Work Regulations 1989 recommends that measurement should be made in the 'undisturbed field'; however, results are unlikely to be significantly affected by reflections if the microphone is kept at least 4 cm away from the operator (it should also be placed on the side of the subject likely to receive most noise) (see Fig. 5.12); therefore, most dosemeter microphones are provided with a clip to hold them onto the brim of a safety helmet or overall lapel. Thus, the microphone receives the same sound pressure as the worker's ear, which the dosemeter 'A' weights, and then, after squaring, totals over the measurement period and displays as the noise dose.

The recommended maximum noise doses for the unprotected ear are given in Table 5.6. Each of the doses shown represents the same amount of sound energy and is regarded as 100% noise dose. Noise dosemeters sold on the British market are set to indicate a percentage dose based on this value. For example, if a dosemeter were placed on an unprotected

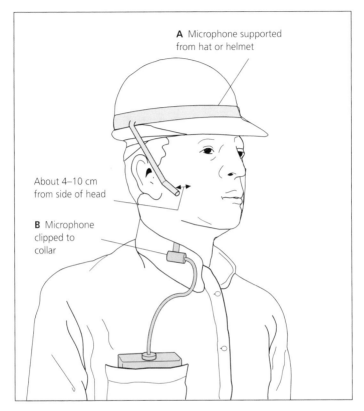

A Microphone supported from hat or helmet

About 4–10 cm from side of head

B Microphone clipped to collar

Fig. 5.12 Location of microphone for dosemeters: A, head-mounted microphone; B, collar- or shoulder-mounted microphone. (From Health and Safety Executive (HSE), 1990.) Crown copyright is reproduced with the permission of the Controller of The Stationery Office.

worker for a period of time and the reading showed 150%, the recommended dose would have been exceeded, but, if it showed 30%, it would not.

This degree of energy does not fully protect some people from suffering noise-induced hearing loss if exposed day after day; a more suitable dose is 85 dB(A) for 8 h. A slightly modified version of these two noise doses is now written into the Noise at Work Regulations 1989 as the 'first action level' (85 dB(A) $L_{EP,d}$) and the 'second action level' (90 dB(A) $L_{EP,d}$). The term $L_{EP,d}$ refers to a daily dose rather than one of 8 h. The Noise at Work Regulations 1989 are summarised in Section 5.3.7. These Regulations are published together with two Health and

Table 5.6 Noise exposures equivalent to 90 dB(A) for 8 h.

Limiting dB(A) (L_{eq})	Maximum duration of exposure
90	8 h
93	4 h
96	2 h
99	1 h
102	30 min
105	15 min
108	7 min
111	4 min
114	2 min
117	1 min
120	30 s

Safety Executive (HSE) Noise Guides, and a further five Noise Guides are published separately. All are available from The Stationery Office (formerly HMSO) (see Chapter 13).

The noise dose for workers exposed to reasonably steady sources of sound can be estimated from the chart in Fig. 5.13, taken from HSE Noise Guide 3. By drawing a line joining the duration of exposure on the right-hand side of the chart to the intensity of steady noise on the left-hand side, the $L_{EP,d}$ can be read from the centre line of the chart. Also shown on the centre line are numbers marked f, which represents the fraction of 100% dose mentioned above. If a worker moves into other noisy areas, f numbers can be added from each to give a total fractional dose for the day.

Example.

An unprotected worker works in a steady 105 dB(A) for 10 min, 95 dB(A) for 4 h and 88 dB(A) for 3 h. What is the noise dose?

Answer.

105 dB(A) for 10 min: $f = 0.7$.

95 dB(A) for 4 h: $f = 1.5$.

88 dB(A) for 3 h: $f = 0.25$.

Total: $f = 2.45$ or 245% dose.

This level of noise is equivalent to a daily exposure of 94 dB(A), which is in excess of the 'second action level' as defined in the Noise at Work Regulations 1989.

5.3.6 Control of noise exposure levels

As with the control of all situations in the working environment, one must attempt to prevent rather than control exposure and, if prevention/elimination is not possible, to descend the hierarchy of

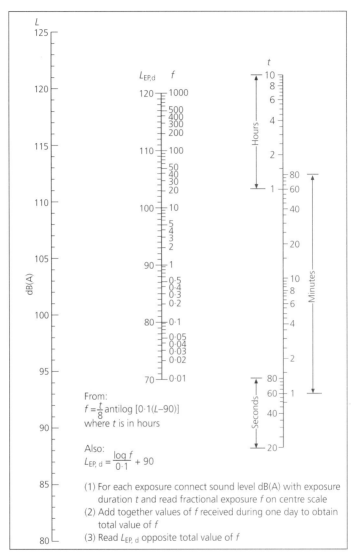

Fig. 5.13 Nomogram for the calculation of $L_{EP,d}$. (After HSE Noise Guide 3, 1990.) Crown copyright is reproduced with the permission of the Controller of The Stationery Office.

acceptable/effective control measures (see Chapter 8). The control of noise exposure provides the classic example of viewing the work environment in three distinct sections: source, transmission path and receiver (Fig. 5.14).

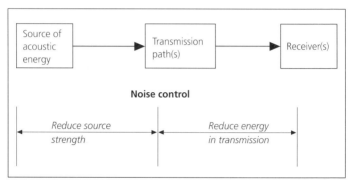

Fig. 5.14 Energy flow diagram.

Noise reduction at source

Because movement causes vibration, which is passed on to air particles and perceived as sound, minimisation of movement in any process will achieve a measure of noise control at source. A number of methods of preventing noise generation are given below:

- substitution for a quieter process, i.e. welding not riveting;
- avoid or cushion impacts;
- introduce or increase the amount of damping;
- reduce turbulence of air exhausts and jets by silencers, either of the 'absorption' type, where the attenuation (insertion loss) is achieved by a lining of absorbent material, or the 'expansion chamber' type, where the insertion loss is achieved by acoustic mismatch between the volume of the chamber and inlet/outlet pipe (a number are now a hybrid of these two types);
- use of low-noise air nozzles and pneumatic ejectors;
- match the pressure of the supplied air to the needs of the air-powered equipment;
- avoid 'chopping' air streams by rotating components;
- improved design of fans, fan casings, compressors, etc.;
- dynamic balancing of rotating parts;
- use of better quality control in design and manufacturing procedures to obviate the need for *post hoc* rectification;
- better machine maintenance;

• limit the duration for which a noisy machine or part of a machine is used.

Control of the transmission path

Having made every effort to control the noise exposure at the source, the next most appropriate course of action is to minimise the progress of the energy from the source to the receiver. A number of examples are given below:

• use of correctly chosen reflecting and absorbent barriers for the direct component;
• use of correctly chosen absorbent material on surrounding surfaces to minimise the reflected component;
• use of anti-vibration mountings under machines;
• enclosure of the source;
• provision of a noise refuge;
• increase the distance between the source and receiver:
    • segregation of noisy processes;
    • use of remote control;
    • use of flexible exhaust hoses to ensure that the exhaust is discharged away from the operator(s);
• active noise control, where the addition of a second source with the same amplitude, but with reversed phase, causes destructive superposition.

Control of noise exposure for the receiver

Other than a reduction in the time for which a worker is exposed, ear protection is the main means of control, and this is discussed in much more detail in Chapter 9.

5.3.7 The Noise at Work Regulations 1989 (SI 1989 No. 1790)

The following is a summary of the Regulations — the wording is that of the authors, not the Health and Safety Commission (HSC). They came into force on January 1, 1990.

Regulation 2 — interpretation

'First action level': daily personal noise exposure of 85 dB(A).
'Second action level': daily personal noise exposure of 90 dB(A).
'Peak action level': sound pressure 200 Pa (140 dB).

Employer includes self-employed persons in respect of themselves. Employee includes self-employed persons.

Regulation 3 — exceptions

On board ship under the direction of the master.
On board an aircraft or hovercraft under power.

Regulation 4 — assessment of exposure

Where any employees are above the first action level, the employer shall have an assessment made by a competent person to:

- identify which employees are so exposed;
- obtain sufficient information to enable him or her to comply with Regulations 7, 8, 9 and 11.

Review the assessment if:

- it is no longer valid;
- there is a significant change in the work.

Regulation 5 — assessment records

A record of that assessment or reviewed assessment shall be kept until a further noise assessment is made.

Regulation 6 — reduction of risk of hearing damage

Every employer shall reduce the risk of damage to the hearing of his/her employees from exposure to noise to the lowest level reasonably practicable.

Regulation 7 — reduction of noise exposure

When any employees are exposed to noise levels above the second action level or the peak action level, the employer shall reduce the exposure so far as is reasonably practicable by means other than personal ear protectors.

Regulation 8 — ear protection

- When employees are exposed to levels between the first and second action levels, the employer shall provide the employee, on request, with suitable and efficient ear protectors.
- When employees are exposed to levels above the second action level or the peak action level, the employer shall take all reasonable steps to provide suitable ear protectors, which, when properly worn, can reasonably be expected to keep the risks to hearing to below that level.

Regulation 9 — protection zones

Every employer shall ensure that:

- ear protection zones are demarcated and identified by means of signs specified in British Standard BS 5378, which show that it is an ear protection zone and that hearing defenders must be worn in that zone;
- people who enter the zone must be wearing hearing defenders;
- ear protection zone means wherever the employees are likely to be exposed to levels above the second action level.

Regulation 10 — maintenance and use of equipment

- The employer must take reasonable steps to ensure that the equipment provided is (a) properly used and (b) maintained in an efficient state, in efficient working order and in good repair.
- Every employee shall take all reasonable steps to make full and proper use of the equipment provided.

Regulation 11 — provision of information to employees

Every employer shall make adequate arrangements to provide each of his/her employees, who is likely to be exposed to levels above the first action level or peak action level, with adequate information, instruction and training on:

- the risk of damage that such exposure may cause;
- what steps the employee can take to minimise that risk;
- how to obtain personal ear protectors;
- the employee's obligations under these Regulations.

Regulation 12 — modification of Section 6 of Health and Safety at Work, etc. Act (HASAWA) 1974 regarding articles for use at work

Section 6 of HASAWA is modified to include a duty to ensure that articles used at work, that are likely to result in an employee being exposed to the first action level or the peak action level, are supplied with adequate information concerning the noise likely to be generated by them.

This Regulation also applies to fairground equipment.

Regulation 13 — exemptions

Subject to a time limit and the power to revoke at any time, the HSE may exempt any employer from the following.

- Regulations 7 and 8(2), where the daily personal dose averaged over a week does not exceed 90 dB(A) and arrangements are made to ensure this.
- Regulation 8(2), if compliance is likely to cause a risk to the health or safety of 8(2) and if it is not reasonably practicable to wear the ear

defenders affording the highest degree of protection in the circumstances.

Such exemptions will not be granted if the HSE is of the opinion that the health and safety of persons are likely to be affected.

Regulation 14 — for the Ministry of Defence

In the interests of national security, the Secretary of State for Defence may exempt (subject to a time limit and powers to revoke) the following:

- Her Majesty's Forces;
- visiting forces;
- any member of a visiting force working in or attached to any headquarters or defence organisation.

However, he/she must be satisfied that suitable arrangements have been made to assess and control the exposure to noise of these people.

Regulation 15 — revocation

Regulation 44 of the Woodworking Machines Regulations 1974(a) is revoked.

5.3.8 Auditory health effects

The ear is not well equipped to protect itself from the deleterious effects of noise. Admittedly, a sudden loud sound is rapidly followed by a reflex contraction of muscles in the middle ear, which can limit the amount of sound energy transmitted to the inner ear. Nevertheless, in the occupational setting, such circumstances are relatively rare. Most workers exposed to noise suffer prolonged exposure, which may be intermittent or continuous. Such energy transmission, if sufficiently prolonged and intense, will damage the organ of Corti and eventually can lead to permanent deafness.

Noise-induced hearing loss differs from presbycusis in being primarily centred on the ear's ability to hear sound at around 4 Hz — the upper level of speech appreciation. With time, this loss extends over the range 3–6 kHz, and this has the effect of removing the sibilant consonants and, thereby, diminishing the hearer's appreciation of the spoken word. Unlike presbycusis, noise-induced hearing loss is not improved by the use of a hearing aid. The degree of hearing loss is related to the level of noise and the duration of exposure. Hence, the attempt to establish a maximum permissible exposure level for dB(A), L_{eq}, with time, outlined above. Figure 5.15 shows the progressive stages of noise-induced hearing loss.

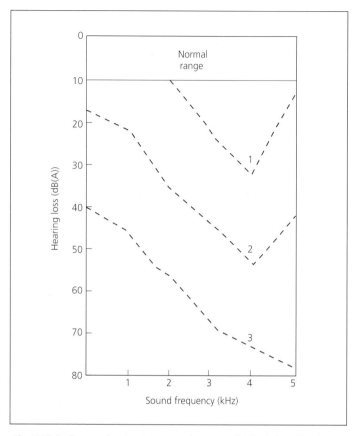

Fig. 5.15 Audiogram showing the progressive stages of noise-induced hearing loss.

5.4 Vibration

5.4.1 Introduction

Vibration is oscillatory motion about a point. In occupational health, workers may be exposed to two types.

1 *Hand-transmitted vibration* is the vibration that enters the body through the hands. It is caused by various processes in industry, agriculture, mining and construction, where vibrating tools or workpieces are grasped or pushed by the hands or fingers.

2 *Whole-body vibration* occurs when the body is supported on a surface which is vibrating (e.g. sitting on a seat which vibrates, standing on a vibrating floor or lying on a vibrating surface). Whole-body vibration occurs in all forms of transport and when working near some industrial machinery.

5.4.2 Characteristics of vibration

Vibration magnitude
During the oscillatory displacements of an object, it has alternately a velocity in one direction and then a velocity in the opposite direction. This change in velocity means that the object is constantly accelerating, first in one direction and then in the opposite direction. Figure 5.16 shows the displacement waveform, the velocity waveform and acceleration waveform for a movement occurring at a single frequency (i.e. a sinusoidal oscillation). A vibration can be quantified by its displacement, its velocity or its acceleration, but now the magnitude of vibration is usually expressed in terms of the acceleration and measured using accelerometers. The units of acceleration are metres per second per second (i.e. $m\,s^{-2}$). The acceleration due to gravity on Earth is approximately $9.81\,m\,s^{-2}$.

The magnitude of vibration is expressed in terms of an average measure of the acceleration of the oscillatory motion, usually the root-

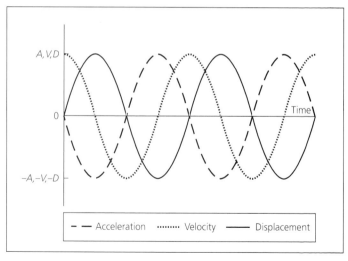

Fig. 5.16 Displacement, velocity and acceleration waveforms for a sinusoidal vibration. If the vibration is of frequency f and peak displacement D, the peak velocity $V = 2\pi f D$ and the peak acceleration $A = (2\pi f)^2 D$.

mean-square value (i.e. m s^{-2} r.m.s.). (For a sinusoidal motion, the r.m.s. value is the peak value divided by √2.)

Vibration frequency

The frequency of vibration is expressed in cycles per second using the SI unit, hertz (Hz). The frequency of vibration determines the extent to which vibration is transmitted to the surface of the body (e.g. through seating), the extent to which it is transmitted through the body and the response to vibration within the body. Oscillations at frequencies below about 0.5 Hz can cause motion sickness. The frequencies of greatest significance to whole-body vibration are usually at the lower end of the range from 0.5 to 100 Hz. For hand-transmitted vibration, frequencies as high as 1000 Hz or more may have detrimental effects.

Vibration direction

The responses of the body differ according to the direction of the motion. Vibration is usually measured at the interfaces between the body and the vibrating surfaces in three orthogonal directions. Figure 5.17 shows a coordinate system used when measuring vibration in contact with a hand holding a tool.

The three principal directions for seated and standing persons are: fore and aft (x axis), lateral (y axis) and vertical (z axis). Figure 5.18 illustrates the translational and rotational axes for an origin at the ischial tuberosities of a seated person. A similar set of axes is used to describe

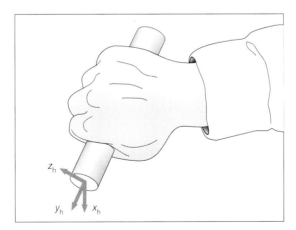

Fig. 5.17 Axes of vibration used to measure hand-transmitted vibration.

the directions of vibration at the back and feet of seated persons. The vibration of a control held in the hand or a display viewed by the eyes can also be important.

Vibration duration

Some effects of vibration depend on the total duration of vibration exposure. Additionally, the duration of measurement may affect the measured magnitude of the vibration. The r.m.s. acceleration may not provide a good indication of vibration severity if the vibration is intermittent, contains shocks or otherwise varies in magnitude from time to time.

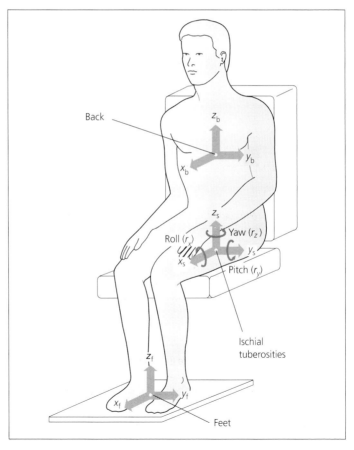

Fig. 5.18 Axes of vibration used to measure whole-body vibration.

Hand-transmitted vibration

Prolonged and regular exposure of the fingers or the hands to vibration or repeated shock can give rise to various signs and symptoms of disorder. The precise extent and interrelation between the signs and symptoms are not fully understood, but five types of disorder may be identified (see Table 5.7). The various disorders may be interconnected: more than one disorder can affect a person at the same time, and it is possible that the presence of one disorder facilitates the appearance of another. The onset of each disorder is dependent on several variables, such as the vibration characteristics, the dynamic response of the fingers or hand, individual susceptibility to damage and other aspects of the environment.

There are two types of effect: vascular and neurological.

Table 5.7 Five types of disorder associated with hand-transmitted vibratiion exposures. Some combination of these disorders is sometimes referred to as the 'hand–arm vibration syndrome' (HAVS). (From Griffin, 1990.)

Type	Disorder
Type A	Circulatory disorders
Type B	Bone and joint disorders
Type C	Neurological disorders
Type D	Muscle disorders
Type E	Other general disorders (e.g. of the central nervous system)

Vascular — vibration white finger (VWF)

Vibration white finger (VWF) is characterised by intermittent blanching of the fingers, with the tips usually being the first to blanch. Attacks of blanching are precipitated by cold (i.e. cold weather or objects) and continue until the fingers are rewarmed.

Once other conditions that cause similar signs and symptoms (e.g. primary Raynaud's disease) have been excluded, a number of diagnostic tests are available:

- cold provocation;
- photoplethysmography;
- digital systolic blood pressure (Doppler);
- dermal sensitivity (aesthesiometry).

The specificity and sensitivity of these tests have not yet been fully evaluated.

The severity of the effects of vibration is sometimes recorded by reference to the stage of the disorder (Stockholm classification) (see Table 5.8).

Table 5.8 Stockholm Workshop scale for the classification of vibration white finger. (From Gemne *et al.*, 1987.)

Stage	Grade	Description
0		No attacks
1	Mild	Occasional attacks affecting only the tips of one or more fingers
2	Moderate	Occasional attacks affecting distal and middle (rarely also proximal) phalanges of one or more fingers
3	Severe	Frequent attacks affecting all phalanges of most fingers
4	Very severe	As in stage 3, with trophic skin changes in the fingertips

If a person has stage 2 in two fingers of the left hand and stage 1 in a finger on the right hand, the condition may be reported as 2L(2)/1R(1). There is no defined means of reporting the condition of digits when this varies between digits on the same hand. The scoring system is more helpful when the extent of blanching is to be recorded.

A numerical procedure for recording the areas of the digits affected by blanching is known as the 'scoring system' (see Fig. 5.19). The blanching scores for the hands shown in Fig. 5.19 are 01300_{right} 01366_{left}. The scores correspond to areas of blanching on the digits commencing with the thumb. On the fingers, a score of 1 is given for blanching on the distal phalanx, a score of 2 for blanching on the middle phalanx and a score of 3 for blanching on the proximal phalanx. On the thumbs, the scores are 4 for the distal phalanx and 5 for the proximal phalanx.

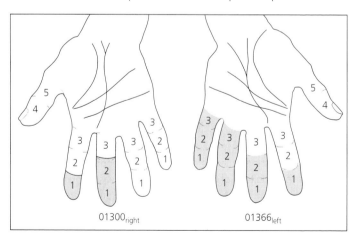

Fig. 5.19 Method of scoring the areas of the digits affected by blanching. (From Griffin, 1990.)

Neurological effects

Neurological effects of hand-transmitted vibration (e.g. numbness, tingling, elevated sensory thresholds for touch, vibration, temperature and pain and reduced nerve conduction velocity) are now recognised as separate effects of vibration, and not merely symptoms of VWF (see Griffin, 1990). A method of reporting the extent of vibration-induced neurological effects has been proposed (see Table 5.9). This staging is not currently related to the results of any specific objective test: the 'sensorineural stage' is a subjective impression of a physician based on the statements of the affected person or the results of any available clinical or scientific testing.

Table 5.9 Proposed 'sensorineural stages' of the effects of hand-transmitted vibration. (From Brammer *et al.*, 1987.)

Stage	Symptoms
0_{SN}	Exposed to vibration, but no symptoms
1_{SN}	Intermittent numbness with or without tingling
2_{SN}	Intermittent or persistent numbness, reduced sensory perception
3_{SN}	Intermittent or persistent numbness, reduced tactile discrimination and/or manipulative dexterity

Tools and processes causing hand-transmitted vibration

Table 5.10 lists the processes and tools which are often associated with vibration injuries, with Table 5.11 providing some techniques of preventive action.

Whole-body vibration

Various industrial machines and all forms of transport cause whole-body vibration.

Effects of vibration magnitude

The absolute threshold for the perception of vertical whole-body vibration in the frequency range 1–100 Hz is approximately 0.01 m s^{-2} r.m.s.; a magnitude of 0.1 m s^{-2} r.m.s. will be easily noticeable, magnitudes around 1 m s^{-2} r.m.s. are usually considered to be uncomfortable and magnitudes of 10 m s^{-2} r.m.s. are usually dangerous. The precise values depend on the vibration frequency and exposure duration, and are different for other axes of vibration (see British Standard BS 6841, 1987; Griffin, 1990).

Table 5.10 Tools and processes potentially associated with vibration injuries. (After Griffin, 1990.)

Type of tool	Examples of tool type
Percussive metalworking tools	Riveting tools
	Caulking tools
	Chipping tools
	Chipping hammers
	Fettling tools
	Hammer drills
	Clinching and flanging tools
	Impact wrenches
	Swaging
	Needle guns
Grinders and other rotary tools	Pedestal grinders
	Hand-held grinders
	Hand-held sanders
	Hand-held polishers
	Flex-driven grinders/polishers
	Rotary burring tools
Percussive hammers and drills used in mining, demolition and road construction	Hammers
	Rock drills
	Road drills, etc.
Forest and garden machinery	Chainsaws
	Anti-vibration chainsaws
	Brush saws
	Mowers and shears
	Barking machines
Other processes and tools	Nut runners
	Shoe-pounding-up machines
	Concrete vibro-thickeners
	Concrete levelling vibro-tables
	Motorcycle handlebars

A doubling of the vibration magnitude (expressed in m s^{-2}) produces an approximate doubling of discomfort. A halving of the vibration magnitude can therefore produce a considerable improvement in comfort.

Effects of vibration frequency and direction
The dynamic responses of the body and the relevant physiological and psychological processes dictate that subjective reactions to vibration depend on the vibration frequency and vibration direction.

Table 5.11 Some preventive measures to consider when persons are exposed to hand-transmitted vibration. (After Griffin, 1990.)

Group	Action
Management	Seek technical advice
	Seek medical advice
	Warn exposed persons
	Train exposed persons
	Review exposure times
	Policy on removal from work
Tool manufacturers	Measure tool vibration
	Design tools to minimise vibration
	Ergonomic design to reduce grip force, etc.
	Design to keep hands warm
	Provide guidance on tool maintenance
	Provide warning of dangerous vibration
Technical at workplace	Measure vibration exposure
	Provide appropriate tools
	Maintain tools
	Inform management
Medical	Pre-employment screening
	Routine medical checks
	Record all signs and reported symptoms
	Warn workers with predisposition
	Advise on consequences of exposure
	Inform management
Tool user	Use tool properly
	Avoid unnecessary vibration exposure
	Minimise grip and push forces
	Check condition of tool
	Inform supervisor of tool problems
	Keep warm
	Wear gloves when safe to do so
	Minimise smoking
	Seek medical advice if symptoms appear
	Inform employer of relevant disorders

Effects of vibration duration

Vibration discomfort tends to increase with increasing duration of exposure to vibration. The precise rate of increase may depend on many factors, but a simple 'fourth power' time dependence is sometimes used to approximate how discomfort varies with exposure duration from the shortest possible shock to a full day of vibration exposure (i.e. $(\text{acceleration})^4 \times \text{duration} = \text{constant}$).

Control of whole-body vibration

Wherever possible, the reduction of vibration at source is preferred. Methods of reducing the transmission of vibration to operators require an understanding of the characteristics of the vibration environment and the route for the transmission of vibration to the body. Table 5.12 lists some preventive measures which may be considered.

Table 5.12 Summary of preventive measures to consider when persons are exposed to whole-body vibration (After Griffin, 1990.)

Group	Action
Management	Seek technical advice
	Seek medical advice
	Warn exposed persons
	Train exposed persons
	Review exposure times
	Policy on removal from work
Machine manufacturers	Measure vibration
	Design to minimise whole-body vibration
	Optimise suspension design
	Optimise seating dynamics
	Ergonomic design to provide good posture, etc.
	Provide guidance on machine maintenance
	Provide guidance on seat maintenance
	Provide warning of dangerous vibration
Technical at workplace	Measure vibration exposure
	Provide appropriate machines
	Select seats with good attenuation
	Maintain machines
	Inform management
Medical	Pre-employment screening
	Routine medical checks
	Record all signs and reported symptoms
	Warn workers with predisposition
	Advise on consequences of exposure
	Inform management
Exposed persons	Use machine properly
	Avoid unnecessary vibration exposure
	Check seat is properly adjusted
	Adopt good sitting posture
	Check condition of machine
	Inform supervisor of vibration problems
	Seek medical advice if symptoms appear
	Inform employer of relevant disorders

5.5) Pressure

In normal circumstances, humans are exposed to atmospheric pressure — variously defined in pounds per square inch, millimetres of mercury or in SI units: newtons per square metre (pascals). Conveniently, the pressure at sea level is 1 atm, 1 bar, 14.2 lb in^{-2} or 10^5 Pa (N m^{-2}). Rapid changes in pressure can be rapidly fatal, but, in occupational health, the main occupational groups are:

• deep-sea divers;
• caisson (tunnel) workers;
• high-flying aviators.

The first two groups experience *increased* pressures, the last *decreased* pressures. Most of the ill effects of pressure in working environments result from decompression. These are as follows:

• direct effects (barotrauma): ruptured tympanic membrane, ruptured alveoli, sinus pain, dental cavity pain, etc.;
• indirect effects due to nitrogen dissolved in the blood at increased pressure being released as bubbles on rapid decompression (Henry's law); this myriad of potential pathologies that occurs as nitrogen bubbles block blood vessels and damage tissues is called *decompression sickness*.

The symptoms of decompression sickness can be acute or chronic:

Acute	
Type I	Mild to severe limb pain
	Skin mottling
Type II	Sensory or motor nerve effects to the limbs
	Dizziness
	Headaches
	Breathlessness
	Chest pains
	Convulsions
	Coma
Chronic	Permanent neurological or cerebral effects
	Aseptic bone necrosis

The effects depend on the rate and degree of decompression, and can range from minor discomfort to death. Treatment involves recompression in a special chamber, and a measured decompression using the standard decompression tables (in the UK, called the 'Blackpool tables'; in the USA, called the 'State of Washington's tables').

The selection of workers for diving requires careful medical surveillance, which must be carried out by approved medical practitioners. Particular attention is paid to dental and aural health, with the obese or those with previous cardiovascular or respiratory disease likely to be excluded from such work. Radiography of the chest and major joints is regularly undertaken. A previous history of Type II decompression sickness is also likely to preclude further hyperbaric work.

5.6 Radiation

Radiation is energy which is transmitted, emitted or absorbed in the form of particles or waves. The effect of such radiation on living tissue is variable, but the ability of this energy to ionise the target tissue distinguishes the two main sections of the electromagnetic spectrum, i.e. ionising radiation and non-ionising radiation. The range of the whole spectrum is enormous (see Fig. 5.20).

5.6.1 Ionising radiation

Ionising radiation is of two main types: electromagnetic and particulate. The electromagnetic group includes X-rays and gamma (γ) rays, and the particulate group includes electrons (beta (β) particles), protons, neutrons and alpha (α) particles. The degree of activity is measured in units of disintegration per second (becquerels, Bq), whilst the effects of radiation, such as the absorbed radiation dose, are measured in grays (Gy). To compare the effects of different radiations with a reference standard, the absorbed dose is multiplied by a weighting factor. The product is called the equivalent dose and is measured in sieverts (Sv).

The health effects of ionising radiation can be divided into non-stochastic and stochastic, i.e. effects for which there is a threshold (and thus a progression of severity of effect with dose) and effects for which there is no threshold. These are as follows.

Non-stochastic:
- acute radiation syndrome — gut, blood, central nervous system (CNS);
- delayed — cataracts, dermatitis.

Stochastic:
- cancer, genetic damage.

The major consequence of radiation exposure is a shortening of life, acutely so for doses in excess of 5–10 Gy, whereas lower doses will produce late effects, such as cancer 1–40 years after exposure. There are three clinically important radiation syndromes following acute exposure:
- 30–100 Gy — CNS damage leading to death from cerebral oedema within hours;

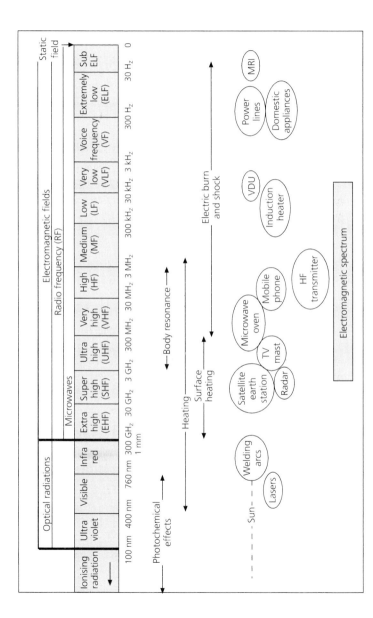

Fig. 5.20 The electromagnetic spectrum. (By convention, wavelength (nanometres to millimetres) is used for optical radiation and frequency (gigahertz to hertz) for electromagnetic fields.)

- 10–30 Gy — gastrointestinal syndrome with nausea, vomiting and diarrhoea; dehydration and overwhelming infection lead to death within days;
- 1–10 Gy — haemopoietic damage, with loss of peripheral cellular components and destruction of stem cells; death occurs within a few weeks from bleeding and overwhelming infection.

Occupational exposures are at lower levels, but are more prolonged. Thus, it is the neoplastic risk which is uppermost in most people's minds. The tumour site will depend on whether the source of radiation 'seeks' out a particular organ (e.g. ^{131}I and the thyroid, ^{90}Sr and bone) and on the site irradiated. Rapidly dividing cells are particularly radiosensitive; hence, the bone marrow, gonads and gastrointestinal mucosa are at particular risk. Additionally, care must be taken to protect target organs incapable or only slowly capable of repair (e.g. the ocular lens and nerve tissue).

Safe dose limits are recommended by the International Commission on Radiation Protection (ICRP), and have been adopted by the HSC as published in the Ionising Radiation Regulations 1985. The current dose limits are given in Table 5.13.

Table 5.13 Annual dose limits for ionising radiation.

	General public	Radiation workers
Whole body	1 mSv*	20 mSv*
Lens of the eye	15 mSv	150 mSv
Skin	50 mSv	500 mSv

*Averaged over 5 years maximum. In any one year, 5 mSv (general public) and 50 mSv (radiation worker).

To put this in perspective, let us consider the average person's dose in the UK (which is probably less than 2 mSv). This is made up of the following radiation components:

Cosmic 13%
Gamma (γ) 16% ⎫
Radon 33% ⎬ Mainly building materials
Medical 20.7%
Fall-out 0.4%
Occupational 0.4%
Discharges 0.1%
Miscellaneous 0.4%

Occupational exposure is not therefore a major factor in normal radiation dosage, but it is a potential danger for a large number of workers (estimated to be in excess of 7 million workers in the USA).

Controlling human exposure to radiation hazards is based on three principles.

• *Justification*. No practice shall be undertaken involving radiation unless it is likely to bring net benefit.

• *Optimisation*. Radiation doses and risks should be kept 'as low as reasonably achievable' (ALARA).

• *Dose limits*. No individual shall be exposed to radiation in excess of that recommended by the ICRP.

Various instruments are available for radiological protection. They include:

• ionisation chambers;
• Geiger–Müller tubes;
• scintillation counters;
• proportional counters;
• film badges;
• thermoluminescent dosemeters (TLDs).

All the above are capable of being portable. Whereas the first four are electronic, measure current radiation levels and are capable of giving audible and visible warning signals, the last two are measures of cumulative exposure and are the usual devices worn by radiation workers. No one instrument is capable of detecting or measuring all forms of radiation — α, β, γ and X-rays. Most are usually designed to monitor the most penetrating radiations, such as γ or X-rays.

Control can be summarised in three words:

• time;
• distance;
• shielding.

The first is obvious; the second is important because, for radiation, the inverse square law applies, i.e. trebling the distance from the source reduces the radiation dose to one-tenth. Shielding will vary with the type of radiation source. Paper or water may be effective enough for α and β rays, but thicker, denser materials, such as lead or concrete, may be required for X-rays.

All that has gone before relates mainly to external sources of radiation. 'Internal' radiation must also be considered; thus it is important to make sure that the radiation source cannot penetrate the skin, be inhaled or be swallowed. Once inside, so to speak, removal of the source of radiation is a complicated and frequently incomplete procedure. Thus prevention of absorption is of paramount importance.

The legal requirements are listed below.

• Radioactive Substances (Carriage by Road) (Great Britain) Regulations 1974 (SI 1974/1 No. 735).

• Ionising Radiations Regulations 1985 (SI 1985 No. 1333).

• The protection of persons against ionising radiations arising from any work activity — Approved Code of Practice.

5.6.2 Non-ionising radiation

For practical purposes, the two most important sources are lasers and microwaves. Both are capable of producing localised heating of tissues, which may be intense and dangerous, and both may be either continuous wave (CW) or pulsed.

The instrumentation required for the measurement of *laser radiation* is complex due to the wide range of wavelengths and energies exhibited by commercial laser systems. Control measures largely revolve around instrument shielding and/or personal protective clothing, such as goggles. Measurement criteria for estimating maximum permissible exposure levels are given in the British Standards Institution Guide, BS 4803 (1983).

Microwave exposure limits vary in different countries. Table 5.14 provides a summary of those which have set standards. The devices used to monitor such radiations are usually small dipoles consisting of a diode or thermocouple device for converting microwave energy into electrical energy, which can then be measured by a voltmeter. Control measures to limit exposure consist of effective containment of the microwaves within the apparatus concerned. Mesh screens or even concrete may occasionally be used, but personal protective clothing is rarely involved.

Table 5.14 Exposure (W m^{-2}).

Country	Continuous	Intermittent	Maximum
UK	100	10 (0.1 h^{-1})	500
USA	100	10 (0.1 h^{-1})	250
Poland	2	32	100
Sweden, Czech Republic and Canada		$\text{Time} = \dfrac{32}{(\text{power surface density})^2}$	
Russia	0.1	—	10

Power surface density levels are set in units of watts per square metre.

During the past few years, great interest has been created over the possible health effects of radiowaves and electric power lines. The frequency ranges from 30 Hz to 30 GHz, an enormous spectrum. For electric power lines, the range is 50–300 Hz and, because of the increasing exposure of the general public and occupational groups alike, recent epidemiological studies provide some cause for concern. The putative health risks are leukaemia and brain cancer. However, the most recent studies of electricity generation and transmission workers have failed to resolve the issue. Some suggest modest rises in risk for brain cancer, others for acute myeloid leukaemia, but pooling the data does not lead to any clear-cut excess risk (similar conclusions are obtained for studies of children and adults living near overhead power lines).

One of the problems is the poor quality of retrospective exposure assessments. The other relates to the immense complexity of finding a valid exposure measure — or even an instrument which will accurately assess exposures. Indeed, it is not clear whether the relevant exposure is the electric field or the magnetic field, or a combination of the two. There is no doubt that occupational exposures can be higher in certain industrial processes — such as electric arc furnaces, welding or induction heating processes.

Exposures to radiowaves were, in the past, largely restricted to radiomast maintenance personnel, but the explosion in the growth of cellular telephone communication has highlighted the risk of exposure. The risk to mobile phone users is unquantified at present, but the dose is clearly concentrated close to the brain — and, indeed, the salivary glands.

6 Occupational Infections

6.1 Introduction

Certain work activities are associated with an increased risk of contracting infections. This may be because the work brings an individual into contact with large numbers of people with infections, e.g. health-care workers, or materials that contain infectious agents, e.g. pathological or laboratory samples, or infected animals, as in zoonotic infections. Others affected include those who have to travel to endemic areas during the course of their work. Occupationally acquired infections can be caused by a variety of infectious agents — from viruses and bacteria to rickettsiae and parasites. In addition to considering the risk of acquiring infections from work activities, there is also a need to ensure that infected individuals do not transmit infection to others during their work, e.g. health-care workers to patients.

6.2 Blood-borne infections

The main occupational blood-borne infections of concern are hepatitis B and acquired immune deficiency syndrome (AIDS). This is despite the fact that non-occupational methods of transmission for these diseases, e.g. from unprotected sexual activity involving multiple partners, are far more common than occupational factors. Some of the general concerns are a result of media publicity, public reaction, the nature of the illness and the lack of effective treatment for these infections. Health-care workers have been infected through work activities — usually inadvertent contact with large amounts of blood, and often involving needlestick injuries or through skin lesions or abrasions. Needlestick injuries involving hollow-bore used needles pose a considerable risk of transmission. Prevention includes care in the use of sharp instruments, the use of gloves for surgical, obstetric and dental procedures and phlebotomy, the safe disposal of sharp instruments in well-designed strong containers that are not overfilled and attention to safe systems of work, especially during the performance of exposure-prone procedures.

6.2.1 Hepatitis B

Causative organism: hepatitis B virus.

Hepatitis B infection can be sexually transmitted, and there can also be vertical transmission from mother to child. The disease is prevalent in countries in the Far East. Some of these countries, e.g. Taiwan, Singapore and Hong Kong, have an active programme of hepatitis B immunisation for the population. In occupational settings, the most common cause is from contact with infected blood and body fluids. Occupational groups at risk include nurses, doctors, laboratory and research staff and other categories of health-care workers.

Infection will lead to full recovery, a chronic carrier state or liver failure and death. Carrier status is indicated by the presence of antigens: hepatitis B surface antigen (HBs) and/or e-antigen (HBe). Those with these antigen markers have an increased risk of chronic liver disease and liver malignancy. HBe carriers are infectious carriers, and the majority of cases of hepatitis B transmitted from health-care workers to patients have involved such carriers. HBs-positive but HBe-negative carriers were thought to be of low infective risk, but recent cases have indicated the potential for passing the infection to patients. Core antibody (anti-HBc) is a marker in carriers and also those who are naturally immune. It indicates previous infection, and does not appear as a result of vaccination.

Immunoglobulins have been administered to prevent infection soon after a needlestick injury or substantial contact with blood from a known hepatitis B carrier or case. The use of interferon to reverse carrier status has been attempted with variable success.

The protection of individuals at risk can be achieved by the use of a serum-derived or yeast-derived genetically engineered vaccine (hepatitis B immunisation). Newer vaccines are being developed that appear to be even more effective in achieving sero-conversion. A full course of vaccination consists of three intramuscular (deltoid) injections of 0.5 ml of vaccine, with 1 month between the first and second doses and 5 months between the second and third doses. Checking for sero-conversion is recommended 2 months after the full course. A booster dose is suggested after 5 years. Poor antibody response requires a second course of vaccine. Some individuals do not produce antibodies in spite of several doses of vaccine. These individuals may be true non-responders or may be carriers of the disease.

Counselling and advice are necessary before checking for antigen status to determine if non-response is due to carrier state. Implications for continuing or changing occupation or job activities in a known carrier should be considered by clinicians, nurses or occupational health staff providing advice to the individual. The current advice is that HBe carriers should not carry out exposure-prone procedures, as this poses a risk to the patients. Exposure-prone procedures include those where the worker's gloved hands may be in contact with sharp instruments, needle tips and sharp tissues (spicules of bone or teeth) inside a patient's open body cavity, wound or confined anatomical space, where the hands or fingertips may not be completely visible at all times. The UK Department of Health have excluded the taking of blood, setting up and maintaining intravenous lines, minor surface suturing, incision of abscesses, uncomplicated endoscopies and normal vaginal delivery from that definition.

6.2.2 Other hepatitis viruses

These include hepatitis A, hepatitis C, hepatitis D (delta agent) and other newly identified viruses capable of causing liver disease. Hepatitis A is food borne and a vaccine is available for conferring protection. Sewage workers are a group at risk. The other hepatitis viruses are blood-borne infections, with no effective vaccines yet available. The occupational measures for preventing hepatitis B (and human immunodeficiency virus (HIV)) also apply in preventing these hepatitis infections. Unfortunately, some individuals who have been immunised against hepatitis B are often under the mistaken impression that they are then protected against all blood-borne infections. Considerable effort is therefore required from occupational health departments in providing information, instruction and training to reduce the likelihood of occupationally acquired hepatitis infections.

6.2.3 Acquired immune deficiency syndrome (AIDS)

Causative organism: human immunodeficiency virus (HIV).

HIV is a retrovirus, which can remain as a dormant infection with no overt clinical features, or may progress to a clinical syndrome, AIDS, which is manifested as an increased susceptibility to infection, e.g. *Pneumocystis carinii* lung infection. There is also an increased risk of a skin malignancy — Kaposi's sarcoma. There have been over 40 published cases of occupationally acquired HIV sero-conversion. The majority of these cases resulted from needlestick injuries or splashes involving samples of infected blood. Although there are public concerns about the transmission of HIV from an infected health-care worker to patients, the number of documented instances of transmission in this direction is limited to only two cases in the world-wide literature. The first case described was that of an HIV-positive dentist in Florida infecting several of his patients, and the second reported case was that of an orthopaedic surgeon in France transmitting the infection to a patient during surgery.

6.3 Vector-borne infections

6.3.1 Malaria

Causative organism: *Plasmodium falciparum* and other species.

This is an infection transmitted by mosquitoes (*Anopheles* sp.), and is endemic in tropical and subtropical areas, such as parts of Africa and Asia. The organism enters red blood cells and causes haemolysis and anaemia. It also affects liver cells and the spleen, leading to hepatosplenomegaly. With infection by *Plasmodium falciparum*, cerebral malaria can result in delirium, coma and death. The presence of sickle-cell trait confers some protection against *falciparum* malaria.

Occupational groups at risk include forestry workers, agricultural advisers and temperate zone expatriates and travellers. Anti-malarial tablets, such as chloroquine or proguanil, are recommended for areas without drug resistance. Where there is drug resistance, alternative medications include mefloquine, doxycycline or a combination of pyrimethamine–dapsone or proguanil with chloroquine. Various drug regimens have been recommended for different countries. These regimens for prophylaxis are revised periodically in the light of data on emerging drug resistance, and, in the UK, the latest advice on malaria prevention should be obtained from the Malaria Reference Laboratory. Chemoprophylaxis should be started 1 week before leaving for malarious areas, and should continue for 4 weeks after return. Drug prophylaxis is not 100% effective, and all febrile illnesses occurring within a year of return from an endemic area should be investigated, with malaria being a possible diagnosis.

Advice should also be given on the possible side-effects of medication, e.g. mefloquine and neuropsychiatric side-effects, photosensitisation with doxycycline and retinal effects from chloroquine. Occupational health departments should be aware of the contraindications to the use of such medication, e.g. mefloquine should not be used in the first trimester of pregnancy, and proguanil affects the efficacy of anticoagulants. Other important measures are those aimed at preventing mosquito bites. These include the use of mosquito nets, long-sleeved shirts, skin lotions, ointments and insecticides. Although there have been attempts to produce a vaccine for malaria, there is currently no effective vaccine widely available for general use.

6.3.2 Lyme disease

Causative organism: Borrelia burgdorferi.

This is a tick-borne disease that affects deer and rodents and can be transmitted to humans. Occupational groups at risk are farmers and forestry workers. The disease is manifested as skin lesions with possible neurological or cardiac complications.

6.4 Food- and water-borne infections

These include cholera, shigellosis, typhoid and paratyphoid fever and *Escherichia coli* infection. Occupational health departments may be involved in dealing with such infections: (i) if they occur in a food handler; and (ii) when members of the workforce have to travel abroad during the course of their work.

Where a food handler is diagnosed as having enteric fever (includes typhoid and paratyphoid), six consecutive negative stool samples, taken at 2-weekly intervals, are recommended before return to work. If the infection involves verocytotoxin-producing *Escherichia coli* (VTEC), of which the commonest strain is *E. coli* 0157:H7, two consecutive negative stool samples taken 48 h apart are required.

If a food handler has non-specific diarrhoea and vomiting, a 48-h asymptomatic period without medication is advised before review and return to work duties. Re-emphasising the necessity for good hygiene practice is important before return to work.

For travellers abroad, immunisations for food-borne infections can be arranged based on an awareness of outbreaks of diarrhoeal diseases in the countries to which they travel. Typhoid vaccine may be administered parenterally (heat-killed organism or phenol-preserved antigen) or orally (live, attenuated vaccine) for travel to areas with a recognised risk of exposure to *Salmonella typhi*. For cholera, the vaccine available is less than 60% effective. There is no effective vaccine against *E. coli* or shigellosis. Travellers abroad should exercise care in the consumption of food and water.

6.5 Infections spread by droplets and close contact

6.5.1 Tuberculosis (TB)

Causative organism: *Mycobacterium tuberculosis*.

Pulmonary TB manifests as persistent chronic cough, with loss of weight, night sweats and possibly haemoptysis. TB can also affect the bones, meninges and other parts of the body. Diagnosis is by the detection of pulmonary infiltration, cavitation or fibrosis, often in the upper lung zones on a chest X-ray. Mantoux or Heaf test can be strongly positive, and Gram-negative, acid-fast bacilli may be detectable on sputum culture.

Tuberculosis is of higher prevalence in developing countries than in the West. However, it generally tends to affect those in poor socioeconomic situations. There is an increased risk in AIDS patients due to their

199

compromised immune status. Occupational groups at risk include mortuary staff, pathologists and post-mortem room personnel. Agricultural workers and veterinary staff occasionally acquire a related infection due to *Mycobacterium bovis*. There is also a concern regarding TB-infected health-care personnel transmitting the infection to their patients. Hence, procedures, such as the determination of TB immune status by checking the history of BCG (bacillus Calmette–Guérin) immunisation, confirming the presence of a BCG scar and the use of a Heaf test or Mantoux test where necessary, have been included in the pre-employment screening of groups of health-care staff. Treatment can be by the use of drug regimes including streptomycin, isoniazid, *p*-aminosalicylic acid and rifampicin.

6.5.2 Meningococcal meningitis

Causative organism: *Neisseria meningitidis*.

Close occupational contact, e.g. mouth-to-mouth resuscitation of an infected patient, poses a possible risk to the health-care worker, e.g. ambulance crew. Avoiding direct mouth-to-mouth resuscitation will reduce the likelihood of this occurring. However, if there is close contact, prompt administration of a course of ciprofloxacin or rifampicin is appropriate prophylaxis. Rifampicin can interfere with the efficacy of the oral contraceptive pill, and suitable advice should be provided to female health-care workers who have to be given this medication prophylactically.

6.6) Zoonotic infections

6.6.1 Anthrax

Causative organism: *Bacillus anthracis*.

Historically, this Gram-positive, spore-forming bacillus was responsible for 'woolsorter's disease' — where spores of the organism present in animal hides, hair, bone, fur, wool or horns were inhaled causing pneumonic anthrax. Skin contact with spores leads to the formation of a characteristic ulcerative lesion, termed an 'eschar'. The eschar appears as a pustule with a ring of blisters and marked oedema. Anthrax can also present as a septicaemia. Antibiotic treatment of anthrax is by the use of penicillin. The incidence of occupationally acquired anthrax in developed countries has been reduced through the treatment of animal hides and horns at the country of origin, before they are exported for further processing. Immunisation is also available for workers at risk.

6.6.2 Orf

Causative organism: orf (parapox) virus.

The disease affects sheep, young lambs and goats. It is transmitted to farmers and shepherds via contact with contaminated wool and carcasses. It presents as a pus- and fluid-filled circumscribed lesion usually on the hands. There may be associated lymphadenitis, and the disease is self-limiting.

6.6.3 Psittacosis (ornithosis)

Causative organism: *Chlamydia psittaci*.

The disease affects mainly birds and poultry, and the organism is present in dusts from desiccated bird droppings and feathers. Occupational groups at risk are pet-shop keepers, poultry workers, taxidermists and zoo workers. Those who keep birds as pets are also at risk. The disease manifests as a 'flu-like illness', often developing into a patchy pneumonia, with fever, headache and chest symptoms. It can be severe, but is rarely fatal. Diagnosis is by the detection of an increase in antibody titres in serum. Tetracyclines are effective for treatment.

6.6.4 Q fever

Causative organism: *Coxiella burnetii*.

The disease affects sheep, goats and cattle, and can be transmitted to humans by droplet infection or through direct contact with infected meat, birth fluids from animals or contaminated wool, straw and milk. Occupational groups at risk are abattoir workers, laboratory personnel, wool processors, vets and farmers. The disease may present as a mild influenza-like illness, although severe sequelae, such as carditis, meningitis, hepatitis, renal failure and pneumonia, have been reported. Diagnosis is by the detection of a serial increase in specific antibodies. Tetracyclines are effective for treatment. Prevention includes separate enclosures for calving and lambing, use of gloves and aprons in abattoirs and vaccination of groups at risk. Vaccination of animal herds is of doubtful efficacy.

 ## Other infections

6.7.1 Legionnaires' disease

Causative organism: *Legionella pneumophila*.

This organism was described after an outbreak of severe pneumonia that resulted in the death of several ex-American Legion members following attendance at a function at the Bellevue Stratford Hotel in Philadelphia in 1976. The cause of the pneumonia was traced to a Gram-negative flagellate bacillus, which is present in nature in soil, pools of water and in water samples from cooling towers. It grows optimally at 35°C (20–45°C). The organism is transmitted by airborne particulates, rather than from person to person.

Legionnaires' disease tends to affect susceptible individuals, such as immunocompromised patients in hospitals, or the aged, especially those with chronic pulmonary disease. Affected patients present with fever, non-productive cough, headache and malaise. Other features can include respiratory, gastrointestinal, cardiovascular and central nervous system symptoms. Chest X-rays show patchy consolidation. Diagnosis is on the basis of a fourfold or greater increase in antibody titre. Erythromycin is the treatment of choice.

(Pontiac fever is a limited, non-pneumonic form of infection by *Legionella*, with a shorter incubation period.)

Occupational health perspective

Staff exposed to the organism may develop antibodies without clinical disease. Workplace exposures include buildings where the bacilli proliferate in the water and spread through the ventilation or water supply system. Outbreaks have been reported from hospital cooling towers and in hotels, office blocks and large commercial buildings. Hospital inpatients, visitors and outpatients are amongst the groups affected.

Control measures include cleaning up the ventilation, water supply and water humidification systems, keeping the water supply below 20°C or above 45°C and the hyperchlorination of water. Biocides can be used, although with care as they can affect some exposed individuals. Looking for the organism in the water supply or ventilation systems in the absence of an outbreak is not recommended, as the bacillus is widespread in nature.

6.7.2 Methicillin-resistant *Staphylococcus aureus* (MRSA)

This is a commensal present on the skin, nose and throat of a large proportion of the general population, and does not usually pose a risk to healthy individuals. However, in immunocompromised or debilitated patients, and those with open surgical or traumatic wounds, the organism can cause an infection which is difficult to treat. Some hospitals screen staff who are to work in surgical, renal, accident and emergency and other clinical wards for MRSA carrier state, and then eradicate the organism using topical applications, such as chlorhexidine or bacitracin cream, before allowing the individual to start work in these areas. There are practical difficulties with this, in that MRSA has a tendency to recolonise the skin after eradication. The transport of MRSA-colonised patients by ambulance does not pose a risk to the ambulance crew. Measures such as washing hands with soap and water or the use of an alcohol-based wipe between the handling of patients will minimise the risk of transmission of MRSA between patients.

7 Risk Assessment

7.1) 7.1 Introduction to risk assessment

In the Health and Safety at Work, etc. Act 1974, the concept of risk assessment was introduced (but, unfortunately, only by implication) by the phrase '*so far as is reasonably practicable*'. A number of subsequent pieces of legislation, such as the Control of Lead at Work Regulations 1980 and the Ionising Radiation Regulations 1985, required the risks to health from specific hazards to be assessed. However, it was probably the Control of Substances Hazardous to Health Regulations 1989 that formalised the need for risk assessments in environments other than those for which specific legislation existed.

The approach of risk assessment is now much more common due to the 'framework' directive (89/391/EEC), which the UK has implemented in the Management of Health and Safety at Work Regulations (MHSWR) 1992 and other related Regulations. The fundamentals of all of these Regulations are the three tenets of occupational health:

- recognise;
- evaluate;
- control.

Since these various pieces of legislation have come into force, there has been some confusion about the terms used in risk assessment, specifically 'hazard' and 'risk'. These terms are defined elsewhere in this book (see Chapter 3), but also here for the purpose of emphasis and clarity.

A *hazard* is something with the potential to cause harm, such as a substance, a piece of equipment, a form of energy, a way of working or a feature of the environment. *Harm* (in terms of occupational health) includes death and major injury and any form of physical or mental ill health. *Risk* is a measure of the likelihood that the hazard (defined previously) will manifest some degree of harm. It follows, therefore, that the highest risk is where something very hazardous is almost certainly going to result in severe harm.

Other than for simple legislative compliance, the only real reason for determining risk is to decide what to do with the level of risk ascertained (see Fig. 7.1). Therefore, it is now common for risk assessment and risk management to be integrated together; clearly, the latter follows from information gained from the former. The steps below include elements of both, but only those for risk assessment will be expanded upon in this chapter.

- Consider all activities and situations, both routine and non-routine, including foreseeable emergencies and loss of control.

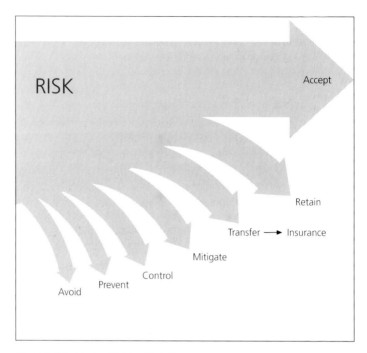

Fig. 7.1 What to do with identified risk.

- Identify the hazards, both intrinsic and those generated by all of the activities discussed above.
- Identify which individuals or groups of workers may be exposed to the hazards (include non-employees, and those identified to be at extra risk by virtue of susceptibility, illness and other medical conditions).
- Determine and assess the risks to health from the hazards.
- Determine the degree of control of these risks, and whether this is adequate.
- Can this (these) risk(s) be eliminated or reduced?
- Implement new or improved risk control measures.
- Monitor the effectiveness of these controls and, if necessary or appropriate, the health of those at risk.
- Review and, if necessary, implement any appropriate corrective action.

The purpose of the structure of this chapter is to lead the reader through the basic elements of risk assessment, from the perspective both of an occupational hygienist (i.e. the environment) and of an occupational physician (i.e. the individual). This chapter does not attempt to describe the more sophisticated probabilistic risk assessment or epidemiological modelling techniques (e.g. Failure Modes and Effects Analysis and Fault Tree Analysis).

7.2 Walk-through surveys

One of the most important and most simple acts, generally as an occupational health professional, but critically in the context of this chapter, is to actually venture into the workplace and 'see for oneself' what people do and how they do it. In order to maximise the benefit of the visit, it is common for people to use a walk-through check-list, both as an *aide-mémoire* and to try to ensure objectivity.

The suggested pro forma below will contain elements which are not always necessary and may even be difficult to complete (technically or politically). However, it is our attempt at being comprehensive, in order that the reader can extract the relevant aspects for his/her needs. It is also acknowledged that most workplaces contain a multitude of processes, all with their own hazards; it will therefore be necessary for the person undertaking the walk-through survey to determine whether separate sheets need to be completed for each process or section.

....

General Site Information

Name of Company/Factory
Address of Site
Site Contact (Name/Tel. No.)
- Managing Director
- Human Resources Manager
- Union Representative
- Site Engineer

Site Details
- Past Activities (brief)
- Current Activities
- Employee Details
  - No. of employees
    - Management
    - Workforce
    - Maintenance/cleaners
  - Subcontracted activities
  - Age profile
  - Sex ratio
  - Race
  - Shift patterns
  - Staff turnover
- Shower/Changing Rooms
- Canteen

Occupational Health Dept. (no. + qualifications)
Staff
- Occupational hygienist
- Occupational physician
- Occupational health nurse
- Safety officer
- Ergonomist/acoustician/etc.

Facilities
- Equipment
  - Type
  - Quantity/quality/appropriateness
  - Deficiencies

Activities
- Executive or advisory role
- Pre-purchase review of substances/equipment
- Statutory measurements
- Non-statutory measurements
- Specification/design of control measures
- Pre-employment
- Periodic health surveillance
- Post sickness review/rehabilitation
- Disability employment procedure
- Immunisation
- Health promotion
- Counselling
- Training
- Disaster planning

Hazard	Comment	Type and adequacy of control	Action required	Person at risk				Harm					Likelihood					Risk ranking
				EMP	CON	VIS	PUB	NO	MIN	MOD	MAJ	FAT	IMP	REM	POS	PROB	DEF	
Use of equipment																		
Rotating/moving parts																		
Free movement																		
Machine/vehicle movement																		
Fire explosion																		
Work practices and premises layout																		
Hazardous surfaces																		
Working at height																		
Awkward posture/ movement																		
Confined space																		
Slips/trips																		
Electrical																		
Electrical switchgear																		
Electrical installations																		
Electrically operated equipment																		
Portable electric tools																		
Physical agents																		
Electromagnetic radiation																		
Noise																		
Vibration																		
Heat																		
Light																		
Ionising radiation																		
Non-ionising radiation																		

Continued on p. 212

Continued

Hazard	Comment	Type and adequacy of control	Action required	Person at risk				Harm					Likelihood					Risk ranking
				EMP	CON	VIS	PUB	NO	MIN	MOD	MAJ	FAT	IMP	REM	POS	PROB	DEF	
Biological agents																		
Viruses																		
Bacteria																		
Fungi																		
Protozoa																		
Algae																		
Parasites																		
Naked genetic material																		
Agents of transmissible spongiform encephalopathy																		
Cell lines																		
Genetically modified organisms																		
Chemical agents																		
Dust																		
Fibre																		
Smoke																		
Fume																		
Mist																		
Liquid																		
Gas																		
Vapour																		

Person at risk. EMP, employee; CON, contractor; VIS, visitor; PUB, public.

Harm. NO, no injury; MIN, minimal (cuts, bruises, etc.); MOD, moderate (prolonged but not permanent damage or effect); MAJ, major (permanent ill health or disability); FAT, fatality.

Likelihood. IMP, improbable; REM, remote (possible, but highly unlikely); POS, possible; PROB, probably (is likely to occur); DEF, definite (will occur at some point in time).

	Comments	Action required

Psychological factors
Intensity/monotony of work
Role ambiguity and/or conflict
High demand/low control
Workplace dimensions
Contribution to decision making

General
Safety policy (adequacy)
Written work procedures (followed?)
Housekeeping
Suitability of personal protection
    equipment (PPE)
Supervision of PPE usage
Interaction of workplace and human
    factors
• Dependence of safety systems, a
  need to receive and process
  information accurately
• Dependence on knowledge and capabilities
  of staff
• Dependence on norms of behaviour
• Dependence on good communication
• Impact of reasonably foreseeable departures
  from safe working procedures
Preception of company commitment to health
  and safety
Perception of local site commitment to health
  and safety
Perception of workforce motivation to work
  safely
Dangers caused by other people
    Public (violence)
    Workforce (bullying)
Proximity, suitability and speed of access for
  emergency services

Comments

It is worth drawing the reader's attention to a number of points before this walk-through survey pro forma is used. Despite the fact that a crude means of assessing risk has been included, the primary function will always remain the *identification* of hazards. Therefore, the most important part of the form is the 'comments' section, furnished by the reviewer's senses (sight, smell, sound, taste and touch). So much can be achieved without the need for the formal measurement of contaminants (i.e. many organic chemicals have distinctive smells, with some having their odour threshold around their occupational exposure limit (OEL) (perchloroethylene, 50 ppm), fine particles are made visible by shafts of light (Tyndall beam) and the ear can determine the intensity and frequency of industrial sounds).

In order to be systematic about reviewing all parts of a process, it is often best to observe the process from beginning to end, with, for example, chemicals being looked at from raw materials through to the final product. Included along the way should be an evaluation of the intermediates, by-products and waste/excess material.

For most of the hazard types listed above, it is also important to be aware of the route of entry into the body. For example, a volatile liquid can be ingested, inoculated, absorbed via the skin or, most commonly, inhaled (vapour).

On the pro forma, the means of separating harm and likelihood into one of the five groups is crude, but is designed to assist in the process of assessing risk and ranking risk. There may be some situations in which anomalous risk rankings arise, but the individual is advised to review these with care.

7.3 Sampling strategies

The previous section on walk-through surveys provided some information on the questions to be asked and the observations made to make a qualified judgement about the risks to health in an environment. When decisions cannot be reached by these means, or when an estimate of the level of exposure is required (e.g. design of ventilation system or litigation), measurements taken as part of a coherent sampling strategy are necessary.

Most occupational measurements are taken for comparison with OELs or relevant standards (i.e. noise, ionising radiation, etc.). Occasionally, more enlightened companies are taking measurements for epidemiological purposes. For some time, the perception has been that the sampling strategies for the two are markedly different, but current thinking is suggesting that a well-constructed strategy should provide adequate data for both. However, regardless of this, all sampling strategies should contain the same basic elements, having answered the following simple questions.

- Why sample?
  - Level of approach?
- What to measure?
- How to sample?
- Whose exposure should be measured?

- Where to collect the sample?
- When to measure?
- How long to sample for?
- How many measurements?
- How often to sample?
- What to do with the data?
- What to record?

7.3.1 Why sample?

A number of reasons for taking measurements have been alluded to above, but it is critical that the individual undertaking any sampling is very clear exactly what the purpose is for the collection of such data and what they are going to do with the results. The reason why more than one sample needs to be taken is that real-world exposure varies massively — from moment to moment, person to person, etc. This variability is dependent upon factors such as the nature, density and intensity of activity/process/people, the contaminant(s) of interest and environmental components including temperature, wind speed and direction, humidity, etc. Examples of the influence of these factors are shown in Fig. 7.2(a–f).

7.3.2 Level of approach?

Having determined the reason for sampling, it is then necessary to determine the need or importance of the answer, thereby prioritising which contaminants and/or processes are associated with the highest degree of risk. Some risk determinants include: the number of potentially exposed individuals; the toxicity of the substance(s); the quantities used over some arbitrary reference period; the likely duration and concentration of exposure (plus exposure via routes other than inhalation), i.e. dose; the existence of and confidence in control measures; the likelihood and magnitude of change to the process and its control; and the presence of substances which may be potentiators or act synergistically or antagonistically with contaminants.

Occupational hygiene surveys can be broken down into four levels relative to the level of priority assigned: an initial assessment, a preliminary survey, a detailed survey and routine monitoring. The level of survey is obviously related to the importance associated with the answer (as described above), and the magnitude of the survey is related to the factors involved (numbers of people, variability, etc.). Figure 7.3 shows a self-explanatory flow diagram to aid in the visualisation and understanding of this process.

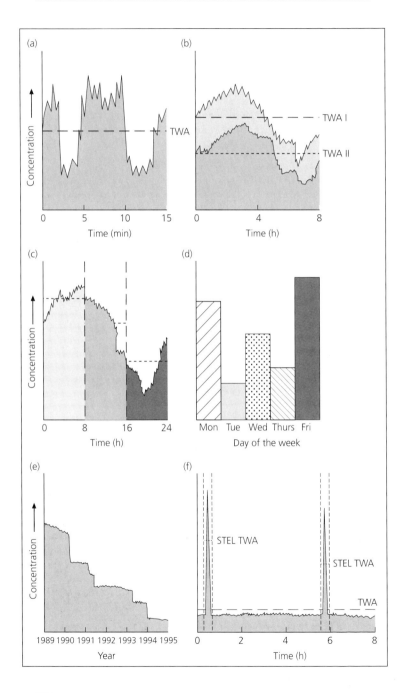

....

7.3.3 What to measure?

Rarely, in industrial situations, is only one substance used (usually this is not a problem for other contaminants, such as ionising radiation, noise, etc., where the sampling instrumentation is designed to be contaminant specific), and therefore a decision must be made as to which, of potentially many substances, should be measured. Reference to the original aim of sampling will assist (i.e. compliance or health risk). There are three main options, which involve the assessment of: (i) all, or many, of the contaminants; (ii) the 'mixture' as a whole; or (iii) reference/surrogate substance(s).

1 The increasing availability of techniques able to identify and quantify large numbers of contaminants has improved the possibility of measuring multicontaminant mixtures; however, this process will certainly be expensive. For compliance purposes, there may be a number of substances in the mixture with OELs and with the same site of action, thereby necessitating this approach, together with the use of the additive equation:

$$C_1/L_1 + C_2/L_2 + C_3/L_3 \ldots < 1$$

This approach may also be necessary when the components in the mixture and their relative ratios are constantly changing.

2 Instead of breaking down a mixture into its component parts (as in (i) above), the contaminant of interest is, by definition, a mixture (e.g. rubber, foundry or welding fume). The OEL is therefore set and assessed on this basis. Again, this approach may satisfy the needs of compliance testing, but not those of health risk assessment; for example, with welding, issues such as the proportion of hexavalent chromium may be important for both compliance and health risk assessment. Another example is the measurement of non-specific dusts (either respirable or

---

Fig. 7.2 (*opposite*) Examples of the variability of exposure. (a) Hypothetical personal exposure as measured by continuous monitoring and the integrated 15-min time-weighted average (TWA) exposure. (b) Hypothetical continuous trace and integrated TWA personal exposure for two individuals undertaking the same work over an 8-h period. (c) Hypothetical continuous trace and integrated TWA personal exposure for three individuals undertaking the same work on different shifts over a 24-h period. (d) Hypothetical 8-h TWA personal exposures for an individual undertaking the same work over a period of 1 week. (e) Hypothetical trace of weekly TWA personal exposures for an individual undertaking the same work over a number of years. (f) Hypothetical trace of personal exposure and 8-h and 15-min TWAs of a contained process with occasional fugitive omissions.

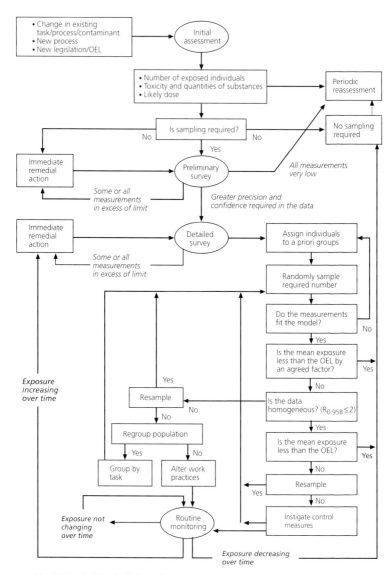

Fig. 7.3 A decision logic flow diagram.

total inhalable), whose values are compared with the respirable and total dust standards of 4 and 10 mg m^{-3}, respectively.

3 Where a mixture has been well characterised in terms of constituents and relative ratios throughout a process, it is possible to measure one or a limited number of these as a surrogate for the whole. The choice of which one(s) may be dictated by the difficulty/ease of measurement/analysis and/or the state of toxicological knowledge and existence of OELs.

If approach (**3**) is to be undertaken, issues such as the types of standard (occupational exposure standard (OES) or maximum exposure limit (MEL)) and the basis on which they have been set, the toxicity of the various components (i.e. carcinogen), the proportion of each component in the bulk material and the volatility (and, thereby, the likely airborne concentrations of each component) should be addressed. It is believed that, using method (**3**), if the concentration of the most volatile and/or toxic substance is under control, then, by default, so should everything else be.

A useful means of combining both the OEL (ppm) and the volatility of a substance (which is temperature dependent) is the 'vapour hazard index or ratio (VHR)':

$$VHR = \frac{\text{concentration of saturated vapour (SC)}}{OEL}$$

where OEL is the relevant occupational exposure limit for the material in question (in parts per million by volume, ppm) and SC is the saturation concentration (also in ppm), given by:

$$SC = \frac{VP_{STP} \times 10^6}{BP}$$

in which the barometric pressure (BP) is 760 mmHg and VP_{STP} is the vapour pressure in millimetres of mercury at standard temperature (20°C) and pressure (760 mmHg).

Applying the above to the examples of hydrazine and hexane, we obtain the following:

Hydrazine	SC = 13 158 ppm
	OEL = 1 ppm
	VHR = 13 158
Hexane	SC = 163 158 ppm
	OEL = 500 ppm
	VHR = 326

From which we can see that hydrazine is potentially much more hazardous to health, despite its lower vapour pressure and, hence, lower magnitude of exposure.

In some cases, it is also important to consider the extent to which a material, when it is airborne, can exist as a vapour or an aerosol. To quantify this, SC — as defined above — is first converted into a mass concentration (mg m^{-3}). This is then compared with the OEL (also expressed in mg m^{-3}). Thus, we have the following possible scenarios.

1 If SC/OEL < 1, the airborne material will appear mostly as an aerosol.

2 If 1 < SC/OEL < 100, the airborne material will contain some aerosol.

3 If SC/OEL > 100, the airborne material will appear as vapour.

For example, mercury has an OES listed as 0.025 mg m^{-3} under the assumption that the material is present as vapour and that there is no aerosol exposure. Mercury has a vapour pressure of 1.8×10^{-3} mmHg, leading to SC = 19.6 mg m^{-3}. Therefore, SC/OEL = 19.6/0.025 = 784. This therefore confirms that the setting of an OEL for mercury based on the assumption of a vapour is correct.

7.3.4 How to sample?

Depending on the question being addressed and the level of approach required, it is not always necessary to use the technique with the greatest accuracy, precision, sensitivity and specificity. Not forsaking practical issues, such as the intrinsic safety, user acceptability (i.e. weight and size) and performance (i.e. flow rate range and battery longevity) of the equipment, the sampling and analytical methods chosen should meet the requirements of the sampling strategy and not vice versa.

All measuring techniques are subject to error, certainly random and perhaps systematic. A knowledge of the error for all parts of the sampling train and subsequent analyses is necessary to ensure that it is minimised and that comparability is maximised, and may include the contaminant stability, sampling device (i.e. dust head), sampling medium and its stability (i.e. absorber/adsorber or filter), tubing, pump (i.e. flow rate fluctuations) and analytical technique. The potential and magnitude of the error vary within a sampling train and between the sampling trains required for different contaminants. For example, the flow rate can easily be set incorrectly relative to the requirements of the instrument (i.e. cyclones) or in absolute terms (i.e. the rotameter may read 2.2 l min^{-1}, but, in reality, it is 1.8 l min^{-1}).

7.3.5 Whose exposure should be measured?

In all sampling strategies, the decision of who to sample is vital. In the past, compliance testing strategies have focused on 'worst case scenarios', whereby people undertaking the jobs likely to give rise to the highest exposure, or intrinsically 'dirty workers', are sampled. The philosophy behind this was that, if the exposure was less than the OEL, then, by default, so would the exposure be in all other situations. Unfortunately, this biased selection process was driven by legislative requirements to ascertain the probability that a person would exceed the OEL on a particular day; however, these data are profoundly limited for other purposes.

The current promulgated technique is for groups of workers with common exposure to be formed either prospectively or retrospectively, and for a subset of these to be sampled randomly. Common exposure means that the group should be exposed to the same substances, and that each of the exposure distributions for the individual workers should have the same means and standard deviations. This is often referred to as homogeneity.

Prospective grouping

The grouping of prospective employees relies on the ability of the occupational hygienist to assign individual workers to a group on the basis of observations, such as the similarity of tasks, contaminants and environment (process equipment and controls). A proportion of workers from within each group should be selected randomly and sampled, with the data assessed for homogeneity. Environments in which populations generate data that meet this definition of homogeneity are almost unheard of, and therefore a more 'workable' definition is required. The Health and Safety Executive (HSE) have suggested a crude but useful rule, i.e. if a worker's exposure is less than half, or greater than twice, the group mean, he or she should be reassigned to another group. Another definition of a homogeneous or monomorphic group is described below in the retrospective grouping of employees.

Retrospective grouping of employees

As it is not always possible to assign workers to the correct groups simply on the basis of observation, especially those involved in maintenance or non-routine tasks, it may be preferable to sample everyone randomly. This procedure gains in significance if it is possible to undertake at least two sets of repeat measurements on those sampled, and helps to identify the components of variability of exposure, i.e. total distribution and distributions within and between workers. The groups of workers can then be calculated on the basis of the exposure data (concentration and variability). A grouping is deemed to be monomorphic if 95% of the individual mean exposures lie within a factor of two. This implies that the ratio of the 97.5 percentile to the 2.5 percentile ($R_{0.95B}$) is not greater than two, which equates to a between-worker geometric standard deviation (GSD) ($\sigma g \beta$) of 1.2 or less. If the groups used in an epidemiological study are not homogeneous, then the distribution of each group's may overlap (i.e. lack contrast) and hence non-differential misclassification exposure may occur. This tends to attenuate the exposure–response relation — although it is more important for the hygienist to ensure that, even if the groups are not homogeneous, they do not overlap — wherein the estimate of the relative risk at certain exposure level will be unbiased but lacking precision.

7.3.6 Where to collect the sample?

The occupational hygienist has two main choices with regard to the location of the sampling device: to place the equipment on the individual (personal) or to fix it to a tripod, in which case it will be static over the duration of sampling (static or area). If an assessment of compliance or health risk is being undertaken, the preferred location is personal, as this is most likely to reflect the individual's exposure. In fact, for all but a few substances (e.g. cotton dust, the annual MEL for vinyl chloride monomer and subtilisins (proteolytic enzymes)), the OELs are specific to personal exposure.

It is conventional to call the micro-environment to which an individual will be exposed the 'breathing zone', and this is defined as approximately 20–30 cm from the nose/mouth (Fig. 7.4a). However, marked spatial variation between the two lapels is possible. It is also known that substances with a high degree of thermal buoyancy, such as welding fume and colophony, generate a reasonably well-defined plume which rises sharply. A significant proportion of this may miss the lapel-located sampler, but, as a result of the nature of the work and therefore the required body position, will generate significant exposure. The welding head sampler is therefore mounted on a cranial cap or on the inside of air stream welding helmets (Fig. 7.4b). Clearly, consideration of the work activity must be given before placement of the equipment, and discussion with the worker with regard to wearability may be fruitful.

As there is a poor relationship between static samples and real personal exposure, their use is less prevalent; however, they do have specific roles. The main one is in the assessment of the requirements and performance of control measures. The fixed location of the sampler strengthens the validity of comparing concentrations pre- and post-control intervention, without the additional variability inherent with an individual moving around the workplace. Some measuring devices are large and barely portable. This is especially true for continuous

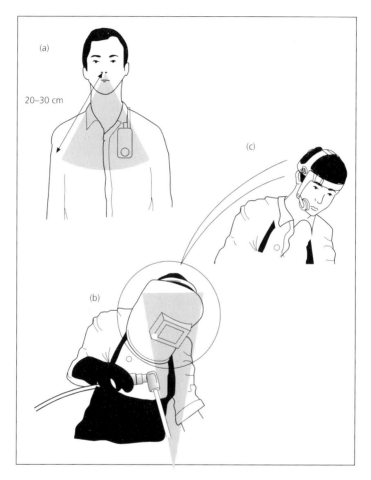

Fig. 7.4 Location of sampler. (a) Breathing zone highlighted with sampler located in its normal 'lapel' position. (b) Well-defined plume missing the normal 'lapel' position (a), and sampler located underneath welding helmet next to nose/mouth (b). (From HSE, 1989, 1990.)

monitoring devices, or where very large volumes of air need to be sampled due to the low ambient concentrations. Occasionally, static samples can be used as a surrogate for personal exposure, especially where the nature of the work may make the wearing of additional sampling equipment more hazardous, or where a clear relationship between static measurements and personal exposure has been defined (e.g. on return roadways in coal mines).

7.3.7 When to measure?

Processes can be split into three main types, continuous, cyclic or random, with most major processes being made up of different proportions of all three — for example, in a chemical factory, the production is continuous, the packaging is cyclic and the reactive maintenance is random. If a worker's job involves just one of these types of process, both cyclic and random exposures will vary considerably, but will be more stable for a continuous process. This exposure variability will be even greater if a worker is involved in two or more types of process. Clearly, there is a need to be aware of this variability, and to sample at such times as to reflect this most accurately. If a random sampling programme is used, care must be taken to ensure that sufficient samples are obtained so that rare tasks are likely to be included.

7.3.8 How long to sample for?

This is an area of great potential divergence between the requirements of compliance and epidemiology. Compliance testing requires the comparison of exposure with legislative airborne standards of which there are, in the main, two time-weighted average (TWA) reference periods — 8 h and 15 min. However, it is not necessary to sample for these exact durations because, within the reference time, there may be periods of known exposure (zero or some other value). This thereby facilitates greater precision and accuracy to be gained for the periods that are evaluated. It is then possible to calculate the TWA exposure relative to the control periods.

Epidemiological evaluation poses greater problems because it is necessary to have some knowledge of the rate at which the contaminant causes a biological effect. Thus if the substances have an acute effect (seconds to hours), the duration of sampling must be able to reflect this variability within a shift, whereas, if the effect is chronic, a more appropriate duration may be a weekly, monthly, annual, average or lifetime dose.

For substances known to cause an immediate effect on, for example, mucous membranes, such as sulphur dioxide, ceiling values are quoted in some countries. The instantaneous measurement of these contaminants is difficult as instrumentation only exists for a small number of substances, and the accuracy, precision and specificity are often limited. Epidemiologically, the problem may be compounded further by issues of the exposure profile. It has been postulated that it is in some way the 'peakiness' of the exposure (profile) to sensitisers that causes the sensitisation rather than the dose.

Periods of work greater than 8 h

The ever-changing requirements of employers, in terms of the duration of work or shifts, may mean that potential difficulties arise when comparing exposures with OELs devised for five 8-h days per week. Clearly, the longer the day over which the contaminant is absorbed, the shorter the period of recovery before the next insult. For substances with very short half-lives, this may not be a problem, but, for those whose half-lives approach or exceed 16 h (the period of recovery for an 8-h working day), the body burden may rise over the week/shift period. A number of sophisticated models utilising pharmacokinetics have been put forward, but, unfortunately, they require a great deal of substance-specific information, which is very rarely available. A more simplistic model by which OELs can be adjusted was postulated by Brief and Scala (1975) for longer working periods:

$$\text{OEL multiplication factor} = \frac{8}{H} \times \left(\frac{24 - H}{16}\right)$$

where H is the number of hours worked per day.

7.3.9 How many measurements?

The only way to ensure that an absolute measure of an individual's exposure has been achieved is to measure them on every day of their working life for every contaminant. Clearly, this is not possible, but equally foolish is the perception that one can take a few measurements and, by so doing, characterise an individual's exposure. Therefore, it is usually a balance between the scientific (statistical) needs of multiple samples and the logistical/political/financial aspects of reality. Obviously, the further towards the scientific needs one is able to go the better. Fortunately, there are some crude guides that assist us in the process of selecting the number of samples.

The National Institute for Occupational Safety and Health (NIOSH) promulgated a method by which one could decide that one wanted at least one measurement from the sampled population to be in the top $T\%$ with $C\%$ confidence. This was designed specifically as a compliance tool, but has been used in epidemiological studies. Tables exist wherein one specifies the upper fraction of exposure (i.e. top 10%) and the confidence with which one wants to find an exposure measurement in that fraction (i.e. 95% confidence). The total number of individuals in the defined homogeneous group is determined (group size), and the required number of samples to be taken in that day is read off (Table

Table 7.1 Sample size selection (NIOSH).

Top 20% with 90% confidence (use $n = N$ if $N \leq 5$)		Top 20% with 95% confidence (use $n = N$ if $N \leq 6$)		Top 10% with 90% confidence (use $n = N$ if $N \leq 7$)		Top 10% with 95% confidence (use $n = N$ if $N \leq 11$)	
Size of group (N)	No. of samples required (n)	Size of group (N)	No. of samples required (n)	Size of group (N)	No. of samples required (n)	Size of group (N)	No. of samples required (n)
6	5	7–8	6	8	7	12	11
7–9	6	9–11	7	9	8	13–14	12
10–14	7	12–14	8	10	9	15–16	13
15–26	8	15–18	9	11–12	10	17–18	14
27–50	9	19–26	10	13–14	11	19–21	15
51–∞	11	27–43	11	15–17	12	22–24	16
		44–50	12	18–20	13	25–27	17
		51–∞	14	21–24	14	28–31	18
				25–29	15	32–35	19
				30–37	16	36–41	20
				38–49	17	42–50	21
				50	18	∞	29
				∞	22		

7.1). These values are not dependent upon a knowledge of the distributional form.

A knowledge of the geometric mean and geometric standard deviation from previous surveys can be used to calculate the required number of samples. If no data are available, mean exposures and their standard deviations can be either estimated or extracted from published data for comparable industries. It is preferable to overestimate rather than underestimate the geometric standard deviation, as this will maximise the sample size (i.e. $n > 2$). Therefore, the number of samples required (n) can be calculated from these data using the formula:

$$n = \left(\frac{t\,CV}{E}\right)^2$$

where CV is the coefficient of variation (standard deviation divided by mean), E is the acceptable or chosen level of error and t is the t-distribution value for the chosen confidence level ($n_0 - 1$) degrees of freedom.

For example, for normally distributed amorphous silica data, with an arithmetic mean of 6.0 mg m^{-3}, standard deviation of 2.0 mg m^{-3}, chosen error limit of 5%, 95% confidence level and $t = 1.960$ (degrees of freedom):

$$n = \left(\frac{1.960 \times 2.0/6.0}{0.05}\right)^2$$

$n = 171$ samples

Therefore, to estimate the mean concentration of the population within 5% of the 'true' mean with 95% confidence, 171 samples from the same group would be needed! Clearly, the greater the homogeneity and acceptable/allowable error and the less the confidence required, the smaller the number of samples needed.

Much more sophisticated techniques exist for the calculation of the required number of samples, especially for epidemiological use, but it is suggested that the reader refers elsewhere for these.

7.3.10 How often to sample?

As with the number of samples, the answer to this question is reliant upon the variability — specifically the day-to-day variance. The greater the day-to-day variance, the greater the frequency of sampling. In addition, if certain events happen on an infrequent basis, and a random sampling schedule is being used, it is necessary to sample often in order that at least one estimate will include this rare occurrence. Again, esoteric techniques exist to calculate accurately the frequency, but are outside the remit of this text.

7.3.11 What to do with the data?

It is prudent to know exactly what you are going to do with whatever data are collected; this is the least the individuals who supplied the data deserve. Unfortunately, this is not always the case, and one is reminded of the adage, 'Don't ask a question if you don't know what to do with the answer'. A number of statistical packages are now available, but care needs to be taken because most of these are significantly more sophisticated than the user's ability to interpret the plethora of inappropriate analyses performed.

The belief exists that almost all personal exposure data are log-normally distributed; however, this assumption is rarely tested. It is possible to test the skewness and kurtosis of a distribution, but this is complex and not always informative. More readily interpretable and certainly less complex is the cumulative probability plot. This is a plot of the individual data points as a cumulative frequency curve, where the percentage scale has been adjusted so that log-normally distributed exposure data will produce a straight line. The drawn line will summarise the characteristics of the population from which the samples were taken, and enables generalisations and predictions to be made (Fig. 7.5).

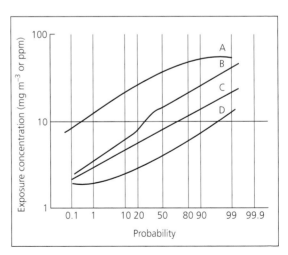

Fig. 7.5 Four hypothetical probability plots: A, probability plot of a right-truncated distribution; B, probability plot of a mixture of two distributions; C, probability plot of a log-normal distribution; D, probability plot of a left-truncated distribution.

Table 7.2 Log-probability plotting points.

Rank order	Sample size (n)																Rank order
	5	6	7	8	9	10	11	12	13	14	15	16	17	18	19	20	
1	12.9	10.9	9.4	8.3	7.4	6.7	6.1	5.6	5.2	4.8	4.5	4.2	4.0	3.8	3.6	3.4	1
2	31.5	26.6	23.0	20.2	18.1	16.3	14.9	13.7	12.7	11.8	11.0	10.3	9.8	9.2	8.7	8.3	2
3	50.0	42.2	36.5	32.1	28.7	25.9	23.7	21.8	20.1	18.7	17.5	16.4	15.5	14.7	13.9	13.2	3
4	68.5	57.8	50.0	44.0	39.4	35.6	32.4	29.8	27.6	25.7	24.0	22.5	21.3	20.1	19.1	18.1	4
5	87.1	73.5	63.5	56.0	50.0	45.2	41.2	37.8	35.1	32.6	30.5	28.7	27.0	25.5	24.2	23.0	5
6		89.1	77.1	67.9	60.7	54.8	50.0	46.0	42.5	39.6	37.0	34.8	32.8	31.0	29.4	27.9	6
7			90.6	79.8	71.3	64.4	58.8	54.0	50.0	46.5	43.5	40.9	38.5	36.4	34.5	32.8	7
8				91.7	81.9	74.1	67.6	62.1	57.5	53.4	50.0	47.0	44.3	41.8	39.7	37.7	8
9					92.6	83.7	76.3	70.2	64.9	60.4	56.5	53.1	50.0	47.3	44.8	42.6	9
10						93.3	85.1	78.3	72.4	67.4	63.0	59.2	55.8	52.7	50.0	47.6	10
11							93.9	86.3	79.9	74.3	69.5	65.3	61.5	58.2	55.2	52.5	11
12								94.4	87.3	81.3	76.0	71.4	67.3	63.6	60.3	57.4	12
13									94.8	88.2	82.5	77.5	73.0	69.1	65.0	62.3	13
14										95.2	89.0	83.6	78.8	74.5	70.6	67.2	14
15											95.5	89.7	84.5	79.9	75.8	72.1	15
16												95.8	90.3	85.4	81.0	77.0	16
17													96.0	90.8	86.1	81.9	17
18														96.2	91.3	86.8	18
19															96.4	91.7	19
20																96.6	20

For sample size > 20: plotting point = $\dfrac{\text{rank order} - 0.3}{\text{sample size} + 0.4} \times 100$.

To draw a log-probability plot, the data should be ranked in ascending order, the number of results counted, the appropriate plotting points taken from Table 7.2 and the results plotted against the corresponding point on log-probability paper (Chartwell 5575). If it is possible to draw a straight line 'by eye', then this can be done, but it is preferable to calculate the correct line. One method by which this can be carried out is by taking logarithms of the data, calculating the geometric mean (GM) and geometric standard deviation (GSD) and then plotting $GM \times GSD^{1.65}$ against the 95th percentile and $GM/GSD^{1.65}$ against the 5th percentile. A straight line is drawn between the two points and, as a check, it is seen whether the line passes through the geometric mean at the 50th percentile. Care needs to be taken as this is not a 'goodness of fit' test.

A number of useful measures, such as the GM and GSD, can be estimated from the plot (provided that this has not already been undertaken to calculate the line itself): the GM by reading up from the 50th percentile until intersection of the line, and then reading off the concentration from the y axis, and the GSD by dividing the value gained from the 84th percentile by that gained from the 50th percentile. The gradient or slope of the line is therefore indicative of the variability of the results: the steeper the gradient, the greater the variability.

Other valuable information which is readily obtainable from these plots includes a simple guide to the proportion of the population above/below a certain level of exposure. For example, the proportion of exposure measurements likely to be above 10 (arbitrary units) in Fig. 7.5 (line C) is about 30%. In addition, if the line is right truncated (i.e. flattened to horizontal at the top), it is suggestive of the measuring device reaching the point of saturation (Fig. 7.5, line A), whereas if it is left truncated (i.e. flattened to horizontal at the base), it is suggestive that the exposure is low and therefore the measuring device has reached its limit of detection due to insufficient sensitivity (Fig. 7.5, line D). If there appear to be potentially two distinct line segments, this is suggestive that in fact two separate populations have been measured (Fig. 7.5, line B). Lastly, two or more lines can be drawn on the same plot, perhaps to compare different systems of work or control techniques.

7.3.12 What to record?

It is always necessary to record observations both at the time of sampling and in any subsequent reports. It is also advisable to record more information than one would have thought to be necessary at first as, on enquiry, the memory may have rapidly faded and, if someone else is attempting to read and interpret the report, additional qualifying

Monitoring Record Sheet

Author and Any Assistants	Tel. No.	Date of Sampling
Name of Occupier		
Address of Premises/Location/Identity		
Total No. of People on Site		
Total No. of People in Area/Process of Interest		

	1	2	3
Contaminant			
CAS No.			
Product/Trade Name			
Sampling/Analysis Details			
MDHS/NIOSH/ OSHA Ref.			

	Ref. No.	Male/ Female (M/F)	Personal Identifier	Sample Type Personal/ Static(P/S)	Sample Description (e.g. name/task /process /equipment)	Reason for Sampling (Compliance/ Random/Ratio etc.)	Exposure Modifier (e.g. other routes of absorption, confounding factors etc.)	Work Period (i.e. shift)	Start/ Stop Times	Duration (min)	Result	TWA ppm or mg m^{-3}	Result	TWA ppm or mg m^{-3}	Result	TWA ppm or mg m^{-3}
1																
2																
3																
4																
5																
							Current Occupational Exposure Limits	8 hour								
								15 min								

Fig. 7.6 Sample record sheet.

information is always of benefit. Figure 7.6 shows an example of a sample record sheet which is useful for both on-site recordings and for formalising the information provided in a report.

The Control of Substances Hazardous to Health (COSHH) Regulations 1994

This section provides a synopsis of the requirements of the COSHH Regulations 1994. These Regulations provide an excellent example of the need to review the workplace to identify hazards (as highlighted in Section 7.2) and, if necessary, to collect exposure data in a rigorous and reliable way, and reveal the structure and style of modern risk assessment legislation. They came into force on October 1, 1989 and were revised in 1994.

The following is a summary of the essential sections of the COSHH Regulations 1994. It should be noted that the wording below is that of the authors and not that of the Regulations as published. The following abbreviations are used:

COSHH	Control of Substances Hazardous to Health
MEL	maximum exposure limit
OES	occupational exposure standard
EMA	Employment Medical Adviser
CHIP	Chemicals (Hazard Information and Packaging for Supply)
HSE	Health and Safety Executive
AFARP	as far as reasonably practicable
ARP	as reasonably practicable

Regulation 2 — interpretation
'Substance hazardous to health' means any substance that creates a hazard to the health of any person arising out of or in connection with work which is under the control of the employer and includes:
- any substance listed in the CHIP 2 Regulations 1994 and for which the classification is specified as: very toxic, toxic, harmful, corrosive, irritant;
- any substance that has an MEL or OES;
- a micro-organism which creates a hazard to health;
- dust of any kind when present in substantial concentrations in air.

Regulation 5 — application of Regulations 6–12
Exceptions are where other Regulations apply, namely the Control of Asbestos at Work Regulations 1987, Mines (Respirable Dust) Regulations 1980 and Control of Lead at Work Regulations 1980. Other exceptions

include hazardous substances due to radioactive, explosive or flammable properties, work at high or low pressures and the administration of a substance during the course of medical treatment.

Regulation 6 — assessment of health risks created by work involving substances hazardous to health

An employer shall make a suitable and sufficient assessment of the risks to the health of workers exposed to substances hazardous to health with a view to controlling those hazards.

Regulation 7 — control of exposure to substances hazardous to health

Every employer shall ensure that the exposure of employees is prevented or adequately controlled. Where an MEL exists, exposure should be reduced AFARP below that limit. Where an OES exists, exposure should be: (i) not exceeded; or (ii) if exceeded, the reasons identified and appropriate action taken to remedy the situation as soon ARP. Control should not be achieved by resorting to respiratory protective equipment, but, if it has to be used, it shall be suitable for the purpose and HSE approved.

Regulation 8 — use of control measures

Every employer shall ensure that the control measures or protective equipment is properly used, and every employee shall make full and proper use of the control measures and equipment provided and report any defects.

Regulation 9 — maintenance of control measures, etc.

Every employer shall ensure that the control measures provided are maintained in an efficient state and working order and in good repair.

Where local exhaust ventilation is provided, its performance shall be examined and tested at least every 14 months, except for certain specified processes, as indicated in Schedule 3 of the Regulations, and for any other process at suitable intervals. Where respiratory protective equipment is provided, it shall be examined and tested at suitable intervals. Records shall be kept for 5 years of any test made under this Regulation.

Regulation 10 — monitoring exposure at the workplace

Whenever necessary to maintain adequate control of exposure, to protect the health of employees or for substances listed in Schedule 4, regular monitoring is required, the records shall be kept for at least 5 years or, if required to be kept with medical records as described in Section 11, records shall be kept for 30 years.

Regulation 11 — health surveillance

• Where appropriate for their protection, employees exposed to substances hazardous to health shall have regular and suitable health surveillance if exposed to a substance or if engaged in a process listed in Schedule 5, or if an identifiable disease or ill effect may occur, or if there are valid techniques for the early detection of disease or ill effect.

• The employer is to keep an approved health record of those employees for 40 years.

• Where an employee is exposed to a substance listed in Schedule 5, Part II, health surveillance shall include medical surveillance by an Employment Medical Adviser (EMA) or appointed doctor.

• The frequency of medical surveillance is specified in Schedule 5, Part II, and can continue for a specified period after exposure has ceased.

• An EMA or appointed doctor may inspect any workplace in order to carry out his/her functions under this Regulation.

• An EMA or appointed doctor can prevent an employee from working with that substance or he/she can lay down conditions under which that employee shall work.

• An employee shall present himself/herself for medical examinations which shall be during working hours and at the employer's expense and, if on the employer's premises, shall be in suitable accommodation.

• An employee may see his/her own medical record and if aggrieved by what it contains may apply for a review.

• Medical records shall be made available to an EMA or appointed doctor as he/she may reasonably require.

Regulation 12 — information, instruction and training for employees who may be exposed to substances hazardous to health

• An employer who undertakes work which may expose an employee to substances hazardous to health shall provide such information, instruction and training as is adequate for him or her to know: the nature of the substance and the risks to health created; the precautions which should be taken; the results of any monitoring and whether the MEL has been exceeded; and the collective results of any health surveillance undertaken under Section 11.

• Every employer shall ensure that any person who carries out work in connection with duties under these Regulations is given such information, instruction and training as will enable him or her to carry out that work effectively.

The Approved Code of Practice explains in some detail how the

Process	Minimum frequency
Processes in which there is blasting in or incidental to metal castings, in connection with their manufacture	Monthly
Processes, other than wet processes, in which metal articles (other than of gold, platinum or iridium) are ground, abraded or polished, using mechanical power in any room for more than 12 h in any week	Six monthly
Processes giving off dust or fume in which non-ferrous metal castings are produced	Six monthly
Jute cloth manufacture	Monthly

COSHH Regulations 1994 should be complied with.

Summary of schedules referred to above

Schedule 3. Frequency of thorough examination and test of local exhaust ventilation plant used for certain processes.

Schedule 4. Specific substances and processes for which monitoring is required.

Substances or processes	Minimum frequency
Vinyl chloride monomer	Continuous or in accordance with a procedure approved by the Health and Safety Commission
Vapour or spray given off from vessels at which an electrolytic chromium process is carried on, except trivalent chromium	Every 14 days

Schedule 5. Medical surveillance.

Substances for which medical surveillance is appropriate	Processes
Vinyl chloride monomer	In manufacture, production, reclamation, storage, discharge, transport, use or polymerisation
Nitro or amino derivatives of phenol and of benzene or its homologues	In the manufacture of nitro or amino derivatives of phenol and of benzene or its homologues and the making of explosives with the use of any of these substances
Potassium or sodium chlorate or dichromate	In manufacture
1-Naphthylamine and its salts. *ortho*-Tolidine and its salts. Dianisidine and its salts. Dichlorobenzidine and its salts	In manufacture, formation or use of these substances
Auramine Magenta	In manufacture
Carbon disulphide Disulphur dichloride Benzene, including benzol Carbon tetrachloride Trichloroethylene	Processes in which these substances are used, or given off as vapour, in the manufacture of india-rubber or of articles or goods made wholly or partially of india-rubber
Pitch	In manufacture of blocks of fuel consisting of coal, coal dust, coke or slurry with pitch as a binding substance

COSHH assessments

It could be suggested that the section on chemical/biological agents of the walk-through survey, described in Section 7.2, could be supplemented by the assessment required under these Regulations. A pro forma approach is again necessary for these assessments, and that developed by The Institute of Occupational Health, University of Birmingham is given below.

....

ASSESSMENT FORM

Company name
Works address
Location of workplace

Single workstation/process assessment   One substance/more than one
Number of workers exposed
List of substances used
Name (trade and IUPAC)
Physical state (dust, fibre, gas, etc.)
Mode of exposure (inhalation, skin)
Toxicity class (very toxic, etc.)
OEL
Known occupational exposure
Toxic effects of each substance (brief description of chronic and acute effects on target organs)

Sketch and/or flow chart of process if relevant (use separate sheet if necessary)

SOURCE OF EXPOSURE
(In the descriptions below outline how the substance(s) come into contact with the worker(s))

Storage (description to include type of container, location, method of opening, also how stores issues are controlled) ....
....
Are leaks possible?   Yes/No   If yes, give method of prevention if any
....

Packaging and labelling
Is suitable packaging and labelling provided?   Yes/No
If no, state what improvements should be made ....
....

Transport and transfer (describe how substances are moved from store to point of use) ....
....
Is inhalation or skin contact possible?   Yes/No
If yes, state which and describe the method of control if any ....
....
Are spills possible?   Yes/No
If yes, state how and the method of control if any ....
....

Use (describe how substance is used; refer to the sketch where necessary)
....
....
Is inhalation or skin contact possible?   Yes/No
If yes, state how and method of control if any ....
....

Continued on p. 238

ASSESSMENT FORM *Continued*

Disposal of excess material (describe how disposal is achieved) ....
....

Is inhalation or skin contact possible?   Yes/No
If yes, state how and method of control if any ....
....

Emissions to atmosphere (describe what is likely to be present in any emission to
outside atmosphere from within the building) ....
....

Are these emissions likely to cause any environmental problems?   Yes/No
If yes, state how they can be minimised ....
....

Waste products (describe what products and how they are disposed of; include
these products in the list of substances above) ....
....

Is inhalation or skin contact possible?   Yes/No
If yes, state how and method of control if any ....
....

Intermediate products (list any intermediate products that might occur and state
where they could be inadvertently emitted into the workroom; also include these
products in the list of substances above) ....
....

Is inhalation or skin contact possible from these fugitive emissions?   Yes/No
If yes, state how their effects could be minimised ....
....

Monitoring

Workplace monitoring
Are airborne concentrations monitored?   Yes/No   If yes, state frequency
....

If no, state whether measurements should be taken; give details ....
....

Give results with dates; if frequently or routinely, give the results of the last three
surveys (where appropriate with summary results) and state reference number of
the appropriate reports or result sheets (append extra sheets if necessary)
....
....

Do the results above show that a hazard to health exists? Yes/No If yes, give details
....

Are surface contamination measurements necessary?   Yes/No
If yes, give details ....
....

Health/medical surveillance
Is health/medical surveillance undertaken?   Yes/No
If yes, give or append collective results ....
....

Continued

ASSESSMENT FORM *Continued*

If no, state whether surveillance should be undertaken and give details ....
....

Biological monitoring
Are biological measurements taken?   Yes/No
If yes, state what and give reference numbers of records and summary of results;
do not mention individuals
....

Do results of health/medical surveillance or biological monitoring show any risk
to health?   Yes/No   If yes, give details
....

CONTROL

Ventilation methods of control
If ventilation methods of control are used, state frequency of routine measurement and give reference number of record sheet ....
....

Do the results show any malfunctioning of the ventilation systems?   Yes/No
If yes, give details ....
....

Protective equipment
If protective equipment is used, describe the type used and method of selection,
inspection and maintenance ....
....

Is protective equipment suitable and in good order?   Yes/No   If no, give details
....

Is decontamination of protective equipment necessary?   Yes/No
If yes, is it undertaken?   Yes/No   If yes, give details ....
....

If no, what is required?...
....

Other methods of control not mentioned above
Give details of any methods of control ....
....

Are these methods operating satisfactorily? Yes/No   If no, state what
improvements could be made ....
....

Training
Do any of the work methods described involve special training?   Yes/No
If yes, give details ....
....

Is any training given with regard to the health and safety aspects of the
work?   Yes/No
If yes, give further details ....
....

Continued on p. 240

ASSESSMENT FORM *Continued*

Is this training adequate to minimise the health risk?   Yes/No
If no, give details of extra training required ....
....

Welfare and personal hygiene
List the provisions for welfare and personal hygiene ....
....
Are these provisions satisfactory?   Yes/No   If no, state what
improvements are required ....
....

Health and safety work sheets
Are any health and safety work sheets issued?   Yes/No
If yes, append a copy
If no, give details of what should appear on such a sheet; append a draft if possible
....
....

THE ASSESSMENT
Having considered the information provided on the previous pages, I am/we are
of the opinion that (tick as appropriate):
- risks to health are unlikely
- risk is significant but adequate controls are in operation
- risk is significant and controls need to be applied as follows ....
....
- risk is unknown; the following actions are recommended ....
....
This assessment should be reviewed (tick as appropriate):
- when the above actions are implemented
- when circumstances change
- .... months from the date given below
Assessor(s)

Name .... Qualifications ....
Position ....
Signature .... Date ....

Initial assessment procedures

In order to make a start on the assessment, it is useful to have a sequence
of actions to follow.

1 *List the substances in the area to be assessed*. This important first stage
helps to define the size of the task. If the list becomes very large, the
areas to be assessed should be reduced and subdivided into manageable
packages. A decision is required on whether a complete production
process is to be assessed or whether a subprocess within it is more
manageable. The number of individual substances appearing in any one
operation will probably be the deciding factor.

It is also important to determine the volume of storage and use of the substances under review.

2 *Determine which of those substances are actually used.* This important consideration has proved to be a useful economic exercise in itself, as many companies are finding their storerooms and cupboards well stocked with chemicals no longer used but not yet discarded. They are also finding that different sections of the plant are using different chemicals for the same or similar processes, and that some rationalisation of their purchasing policy is required which will benefit the company financially. The COSHH assessment has provided the ideal opportunity to remove all the old substances from the site, some of which may be in an unstable condition, and others in containers that are deteriorating rapidly and may soon become an occupational or environmental danger.

3 *Determine the true chemical names and/or Chemical Abstracts Series (CAS) numbers.* Most substances appear in the workplace under a trade name or code number. If the toxic nature of the substance is to be determined from the standard texts, a precise identification is required. All chemicals are issued with a unique name by the International Union of Pure and Applied Chemistry (IUPAC) and a unique number known as the CAS number.

4 *Obtain suppliers' data sheets.* There is a duty under Section 6 of the Health and Safety at Work, etc. Act 1974 for suppliers to provide adequate information on substances supplied, and this is reinforced by the Consumer Protection Act 1987. This information is usually provided by the supplier in the form of a data sheet (see 'Hazard data sheets', p. 243). The quality of the information supplied is very variable, the best giving all the information required to appraise the toxicity of the substance, the worst giving information that is misleading and sometimes dangerous.

It is advisable to have standard letters available to request this information and more strongly worded back-up letters in the event of default.

5 *Evaluate data sheets.* It is wise to check the validity of the information supplied on the data sheets. For example, the IUPAC name of the substance or substances may not be given, making it difficult to check the toxicity information provided. Alternatively, if the substance is a mixture of chemicals, such as a proprietary solvent, not all the ingredients may be shown. It is understandable if the exact formulation of a mixture is not given, because the supplier has 'trade secrets' to protect, but a list of substances present without the exact proportions can be given without running the risk of industrial espionage!

6 *Check the toxicological data given and rewrite data sheet.* Once the name of the substance is known, a simple check on the accuracy of the toxicological data given should be made before writing the data sheet to suit the way the substance is used in the situation being assessed. The data sheet will need to be rewritten or supplemented to take into account the way in which the substance is to be used. The suppliers cannot be expected to anticipate the way their substance is to be stored, transported or handled in the workplace under review, but the employees will require some guidance. This is a requirement of Regulation 12 of the COSHH Regulations 1994 (see 'Hazard data sheets', p. 243).

7 *Inspect the places where the substances are handled.* Now is the moment to inspect the way the substance is being handled to establish the modes of exposure and the possible risk to those employed. The ways in which the material is stored, transferred to the point of use, dispensed into the process and disposed of after use all pose a potential risk to those involved. It is in this way that it is possible to establish whether the exposure is to the skin or via inhalation, the two most common modes. At the same time, on-site observations can be made of the eating, drinking and smoking activities in the workplace, all of which can be a potential means of causing systemic absorption.

8 *Inhalation route — check airborne monitoring.* If the substances are dusty or volatile, and there are open containers providing surfaces for evaporation, there is a likelihood of inhalation being the main route of entry. If it is not possible by other means, it may be necessary to measure the airborne concentration of the substances in the 'breathing zone' of the worker and to compare the results with published standards. Occupational hygiene surveys may need to be arranged.

9 *Skin contact route.* Observations on the method of handling will reveal whether skin contact is likely. When liquids are being transferred from one receptacle to another, even if mechanically handled, splashing could occur, and, with any open surface of liquid, accidental contact is possible. In addition, the handling of wet materials with unprotected hands is an obvious source of exposure. Measurements of airborne exposure may not be adequate to establish the degree of exposure, but the wary eye, backed up with a knowledge of the material's potential dangers, may be what is needed to assess this hazard. If not, biological monitoring should be considered.

10 *Look at the method of control.* The performance of control methods (Chapter 8) needs to be assessed. In some cases, this can be performed by observation, whereas, for others, it will involve some technical measurements. If airborne substances are being controlled, the ultimate test is the airborne concentration in the breathing zone of the workers involved. If the levels are substantially below an applicable MEL, or below the OES, usually it is not unreasonable to assume that control has been achieved.

More subtle methods of control involving working procedures and good supervision will have to be checked and seen to be working satisfactorily before accepting that the process is free from risk.

11 *Implement improvements before the final assessment.* If, as a result of this initial assessment procedure, some obvious faults are seen, they should be rectified speedily before completion of the final assessment. If the improvements appear to require time to implement, an interim assessment should be made with a view to reassessment later.

Hazard data sheets

The purpose of the data sheet is twofold:
- the receipt of product information from the supplier;
- the provision of information to users within the company.

The latter is necessary in order to fulfil the company's obligations under Regulation 12 of the COSHH Regulations 1994. The sheets should not be the same for the reasons given below.

A good supplier's hazard data sheet should contain the following information.

- *Identification.* Product name, physical form, e.g. powder, liquid, etc., colour, odour.
- *Supplier.* Name, address, emergency telephone number, contact person.
- *Composition.* chemical names of constituents, CAS numbers, synonyms, proportions, formulae, occupational exposure limits, impurities.
- *Physical data.* Boiling point, vapour pressure, specific gravity, melting point.
- *Health hazards.* Short- and long-term effects of inhalation, skin contact, ingestion, injection, eye contact, first detectable signs of overexposure.
- Emergency and first aid procedures.
- Spillage procedures.
- Fire precautions and likely products of combustion.
- Recommended control measures other than personal protective equipment (PPE).
- Recommended PPE.

- Storage, packaging and labelling advice.
- Reactivity data: stability, decomposition products, known interactions.
- Special precautions.
- Legal requirements.
- Sources of information.

Very few will be as comprehensive as this (or will need to be) if the substance poses a low risk. Users who are heavy consumers of a particular product may ask their suppliers to complete a company standard data sheet for circulation within the company and to be kept on an 'in-house' database.

For 'shop floor' purposes, the supplier's data sheet may contain too much information or be couched in unintelligible scientific terms. In addition, the sheet for shop floor use must contain details of safe systems of use and details of the local methods of control. For example, the solvent 1,1,1-trichloroethane is used in large quantities on the shop floor for degreasing and in small quantities in the office as a correcting fluid; the methods of exposure and control will be different in each situation. A separate data sheet should be provided for the two types of user. Data sheets should also be written in language that the shop-floor worker can understand and, where necessary, may have to be issued in several languages.

7.5 Health assessment

7.5.1 Introduction

In occupational health practice, health assessment refers to the evaluation of the health status of an individual or group of workers. The reasons for assessment include the following.

- Obtaining baseline data on the state of health before occupational exposure to enable comparisons to be made in the future.
- Early detection of effects from occupational exposure (health surveillance). This allows removal from further exposure before chronic or permanent ill health results. It also signals the need for the review of control measures.
- Diagnosis of occupational disease.
- Determination of the extent of disability from non-occupational diseases, and assessment of compatibility with current job duties. A consequence of health assessment for this reason may be a recommendation for adjustments to the current job, relocation to a new job or retirement on grounds of ill health.

Health assessment uses some combination of symptom review, clinical examination, differential diagnosis (i.e. considering various clinical conditions that can cause similar health effects) and laboratory or physiological tests. It is normally a task for occupational health nurses or physicians. Perhaps the most important piece of information to be checked at the pre-employment assessment is the occupational history.

7.5.2 The occupational history

This is a full description of the individual's previous jobs and occupational exposures from the time of leaving school. It is a crucial part of any medical examination and, indeed, every medical student and occupational health student should be taught to take a full occupational history. If the occupational history is incomplete or not taken, an important aspect of a patient's history will be omitted. This could lead to an error in diagnosis, or a delay in diagnosis and management.

Some stated occupations, such as 'civil servant', 'maintenance man' or 'retired', need further clarification, as these vague terms do not give much indication of occupational exposures. Ramazzini emphasised this point over 200 years ago, when he noted in the introduction to his book, *De Morbis Artificium*, how important it was to ask the patient the nature of his work. It is, he says, 'concerned with exciting causes and should be particularly kept in mind when the patient belongs to the common people. In medical practice, attention is hardly ever paid to this matter though, for effective treatment, evidence of this sort has the utmost weight'.

The occupational history should contain information on the following items for each job:

- job title;
- description of tasks/duties within the job title;
- employer and nature of the company/industry;
- duration of employment in each job;
- hours of work, including overtime and shift work;
- exposure to occupational hazards;
- provision and use of personal protective equipment;
- sickness absence, especially for work-related ill health or injury.

Information about past occupations can be as relevant as that about the present job. Previous occupations may be the cause of the patient's current health problems, particularly for diseases of long latent period, such as cancer or asbestosis. For these cases, a detailed past history is vital, and an example of a format for obtaining the full occupational history is given in Table 7.3. The authors have found this useful for clinical occupational medicine practice. It is important to remember that the

Table 7.3 Format for obtaining full occupational history.

Please fill in the table below, listing all the jobs at which you have worked for more than 6 months. Start with your present job and go back to the first. Use additional paper if necessary:

Workplace (employer's name and address)	Dates worked from	Dates worked to	Full/part time	Describe type of industry	Describe job duties	Known health hazards in workplace (dusts, solvents, etc.)	Protective equipment used	Were you ever off work for a health problem or injury?

patient's pastime or hobbies may, in addition, cause diseases often attributed to occupation, e.g. the amateur boat builder who becomes sensitised to isocyanates, or the bird fancier who develops extrinsic allergic alveolitis. The occupational history is thus not only an essential part of pre-placement assessment, but is indispensable in any thorough medical examination.

7.5.3 Pre-employment assessment

Pre-employment or pre-placement assessment is a function carried out by almost all occupational health departments. The main purpose is to ensure that the person has no pre-existing ill health or disability which may make the performance of the proposed job difficult or unsafe for the individual, coworkers and for third parties, e.g. visitors or customers. Pre-existing disorders not detected before commencing work can add to the liability of the employer in the event of future claims of work-related disease. The assessment is also used to see whether the workplace can be adapted to meet the needs of the disabled individual, and it provides baseline data for future assessments. However, these aims are sometimes subsumed by other procedures, which attempt to make full use of the presence of the new employee at the occupational health department. Thus, the pre-employment examination is sometimes used to introduce the facilities of the department to the new starter, to bring the individual's immunisations up to date, to reinforce advice on health promotion or to see whether the individual meets the health criteria for joining the company's pension scheme.

With the implementation of legislation on disability discrimination in some countries, e.g. the USA and UK, there is a move in these countries to review the basis for pre-employment examinations. Such examinations for prospective candidates or those on an interview short list would be better replaced by pre-placement assessment of the candidate selected after interview. This is likely to be more cost effective, as it avoids the performance of several assessments for the eventual selection of one individual. In developing countries, the rationale for the pre-employment examination may be different. Companies could be concerned about the cost implications of employing an individual with an existing health problem, especially if it is a chronic disease requiring ongoing treatment. The costs could include health-care charges for the individual met by the employer (especially in countries where health care is provided privately, rather than on a national health service basis), and lost time cost for hospital attendance for medical treatment. An important consideration is to view the possible expertise and contribution of the individual to the job, rather than just the apparent cost implications alone. An individual with a chronic ailment that is well controlled by regular treatment may indeed contribute more to a job than an equivalent 'healthy' individual with less experience or poor motivation.

Pre-employment questionnaires vary in content and length, and revised questionnaires should only ask for information that is essential to ensure no contraindication between the person's health status and the proposed job. Questions on experience of painful menstrual periods or past obstetric history may be viewed as discriminatory. If the reason for asking about 'painful periods' is a concern about whether monthly experience of pain will lead to frequent sickness absence, perhaps there should be a general question on all conditions that can cause periodic pain, including migraine, sinusitis and severe dental caries. A better alternative is to focus on the sickness absence record, regardless of cause of absence. Questions on a past history of piles, varicose veins or eating disorders may not be necessary if there is no increased risk of the conditions getting worse in the proposed job, and if they do not affect the performance of the work duties. The trend in pre-employment questionnaires is towards fewer questions which are more focused.

7.5.4 Periodic medical examinations

Health assessment by performance of periodic medical examinations has been and continues to be a major component of occupational health functions. Several reasons may explain the prominence of this activity.

• Where the occupational health team consists primarily of doctors and nurses, they will use their training, experience and clinical skills to perform activities with which they are familiar. Clinical activity is patient centred, and the clinical approach involves taking the history, examining the individual, ordering relevant investigations and formulating the diagnosis. If the diagnosis indicates an occupationally related condition, management of the case will require an evaluation of the work environment and work practices, and advice on modification and adaptation as necessary. This requires team work, and may involve the clinical team, safety engineer, occupational hygienist, managers and worker representatives.

• There is a perception, primarily amongst managers and workers, that there is merit in periodically reviewing the health status of individuals who are exposed to various noxious agents in the workplace. The analogy is often made with the legal requirements for annual inspections of motor vehicles (the 'MOT' in the UK). If individuals take care of their cars by checking their structure and functions periodically because of the ravages of wear and tear from road use, why not apply the same principle to the workforce? This is a powerful argument; however, it does not take into account the limitations of the medical examination for the early detection of preventable conditions. The range of conditions for which periodic assessments may lead to case detection and the institution of effective treatment or prevention is limited to certain communicable diseases (such as tuberculosis), diabetes, hypertension, visual defects, dental caries and some cancers (possibly colon, bladder, breast and skin). For occupational exposures to toxic chemicals, medical examinations to detect an early effect are probably of use only for a limited number of agents, e.g. examination of the nasal septum to detect early ulceration from exposure to chromic acid. What is possibly of greater benefit is to include biological monitoring as part of the periodic assessments (see p. 253). This gives some indication of exposure, which can be evaluated in conjunction with any symptoms or signs detected.

• Statutory requirements. Health and safety laws in some countries require statutory medical examinations for certain groups of workers. These are usually specified for workers with defined occupational exposures; for example, in the UK, these exist for lead, asbestos, ionising radiation, compressed air work and diving. The nature and frequency of the examinations are prescribed, and there are provisions for these to be performed by appointed doctors. In Singapore, the term used is 'designated factory doctor'. Special training requirements and/or qualifications and experience in occupational health are often required of these physicians. Annual medical examinations are the norm for a large proportion of the workforce in countries such as France and Poland. The value of these examinations is debatable. One possible secondary benefit is that the contact between occupational physician and worker is used as an occasion to review workplace practice and changes in occupational exposure or the development of symptoms of ill health that might be related to work.

• The periodic review of individuals provides an opportunity not only to advise on health and illness, but also to reinforce advice on occupational health prevention. The clinical staff will have greater credibility in discussing preventive measures if they are also seen to care for workers on a regular basis. Periodic contact facilitates the establishment of rapport and encourages discussion on all aspects of health — occupational issues as well as non-occupational. Without this, individuals may not see the clinical team as the first 'port-of-call' for raising occupational health concerns.

7.5.5 Post sickness absence review

Some occupational health departments review workers who return after a period of sickness absence. The reason for the review is to ensure that the person has no residual effects from the cause of the sickness absence, which may affect the return to work. Although hospital physicians and general practitioners (family physicians) often indicate the duration of absence required and the fitness for return to work, this may be performed without a full appreciation of the job duties or work environment. Hence, occupational health staff can consider these factors in conjunction with those providing clinical care. Close liaison between occupational health departments and physicians responsible for treatment facilitates successful return to work after sickness.

Sickness absence or absence attributed to sickness includes absence for social, family and personal reasons other than illness. Sympathetic review and assistance by occupational health staff may reduce the likelihood of recurrence of absence for these reasons. Sickness absence policies often make the distinction between frequent, short-term absences and long-term spells of absence (e.g. more than 4 weeks of continuous absence). Long-term absence results from chronic ailments, acute conditions requiring a waiting period for surgery, incomplete recovery from illness or post-surgical complications or recuperation. Frequent, short-term absences are often difficult to manage. This is especially so if the stated causes for these absences vary, suggesting that there may be factors other than a chronic underlying illness. These could include work-related factors, such as job dissatisfaction, individuals who are prone to frequent, short-term infections, non-work factors, such as illness in a family member, or drug and alcohol problems.

7.5.6 Retirement on grounds of ill health

One of the functions of occupational health departments is to assess workers wishing to retire from their jobs on health grounds. These include workers with chronic illnesses or incomplete recovery from treatment, where the continuing safe and efficient performance of their work is in doubt. Pension entitlements may be brought forward for those who are successful. The replacement of an experienced worker who retires early could be a problem for the organisation. The occupational health staff also have to consider whether the individual is capable of doing other jobs in spite of the illness. If so, redeployment of the worker to a different job within the company is a suitable alternative. Criteria for early retirement on grounds of ill health have been proposed by occupational physicians.

7.5.7 Medical surveillance for groups at risk

Medical assessments are required by law for some groups of workers exposed to specific hazards in the workplace. The term 'health surveillance' has been used for the periodic medical/physiological assessment of exposed workers, with a view to protect and prevent occupationally related diseases. This activity, when carried out by occupational health departments, requires that the medical or physiological assessments are valid, and that information is sought on the nature and extent of occupational exposures. The legal requirements vary between countries; some examples are included below.

• Lead workers. The medical assessment includes a review of exposure and symptoms which may indicate a lead effect — colic, constipation, lethargy and malaise, examination for the presence of pallor, weakness of the extensor muscles of the wrists and Burton's blue line in the gum margins (the latter being as rare as hen's teeth in the authors' opinion).

• Other statutory examinations are those for ionising radiation workers, asbestos-exposed workers, compressed-air workers and divers. These are categories specified under UK law. In Germany, the list is longer. Some countries include periodic audiometry as part of the assessment for noise-exposed workers.

• Examination of the hands and nose in workers exposed to chromic acid mist and other hexavalent chromium compounds. The rationale for periodic assessment is the early detection of 'chrome ulcers' on the skin of the hands and nasal septal ulceration or perforation, all recognised pathological effects from such exposure. Nasal examination requires experience in detecting such pathology with the aid of a nasal speculum. As for detecting skin ulceration, self-examination by individual workers with referral to occupational health is better than periodic skin examinations of all exposed workers by occupational health staff.

• Following legal action in the UK after a case of scrotal cancer from exposure to mineral oils (*Stokes* v. *GKN*), companies using such oils have implemented periodic examination of the scrotum of exposed workers by occupational health staff. It is uncertain whether the detection rate for early scrotal cancer from this activity justifies the effort involved. However, other than self-examination, which can be logistically more difficult than examination of the skin of the hands, there does not seem to be a better or less embarrassing procedure available.

• Exposure to respiratory sensitisers. The periodic review of symptoms, with lung function assessment, is recommended for workers exposed to isocyanates, platinum salts, laboratory animal dander, glutaraldehyde and other recognised respiratory sensitisers. The symptom enquiry includes wheeze, breathlessness, chest tightness and nocturnal cough. The lung function tests include spirometry and peak flow determinations. The effectiveness of occasional lung function testing in detecting asthma is questionable. Spirometry can detect obstruction of the airways during an asthmatic attack, but could well be normal in between attacks in someone with asthma.

There are other periodic medical assessments that do not fit with the description of health surveillance provided earlier. These are medical examinations of special groups, where their state of health may affect the safety of the public.

• Professional drivers. Those who drive passenger-carrying vehicles or large goods vehicles are required to have periodic medical assessments to ensure that they have not developed a disease or disability that might affect their fitness to drive and pose a danger to the public. Conditions specified under European Community Directives which will bar such drivers include uncontrolled epilepsy, severe mental handicap and liability to sudden attacks of severe giddiness or syncope (fainting spells). Further detailed advice is available in the UK Driver and Vehicle Licensing Agency's guide on the fitness to drive.

• Food handlers. The medical surveillance of this group of staff is intended primarily to protect the products from contamination by infected material. Infections of relevance for this particular occupational group include enteric fever (typhoid and paratyphoid fever), salmonellosis, verocytotoxin-producing *Escherichia coli* (VTEC) and hepatitis A. For food handlers who develop diarrhoea and vomiting, the occupational health staff should confirm that vomiting has ceased, bowel habits have returned to normal and re-emphasise advice on good hygiene practice, especially hand washing. Other than for a limited number of specific infections, such as acute enteric fever and VTEC, repeated stool testing at pre-employment or after diarrhoeal illness is not indicated.

• Psychiatric ill health. Health-care workers who have wilfully attempted to harm patients have been the subject of recent media attention. In the UK, a case of 'Munchausen syndrome by proxy', involving a nurse causing injury to infants, resulted in calls for stricter occupational health clearance. A government inquiry resulted in several recommendations, including obtaining a report from a health-care worker's personal physician if there is a declaration of mental ill health on a pre-employment questionnaire. There are also suggestions that closer scrutiny should be made of individuals who have previously been prescribed psycho-active drugs. However, these proposals have been viewed as discriminatory against those with mental illness, and the Americans with Disability Act discourages such a line of enquiry. The UK Disability Discrimination Act 1995 requires good justification for actions which may disadvantage those with mental or physical disability. Further interest in the UK on the assessment of those with psychiatric ill health was spurred by an inquiry into the case of a nurse who was thought to have caused grievous bodily harm to a patient in intensive care. One controversial recommendation was that the occupational health record should be verified by the employee's personal physician. There are limitations in the use of health assessments for detecting factors that can predict a high risk that a health-care worker might harm a patient.

7.6 Biological monitoring and biological effect monitoring

Biological monitoring refers to the analysis of biological samples for the presence of a chemical or its metabolite. The purpose of this procedure is to determine the extent of systemic absorption for a chemical encountered in the workplace. This, in turn, gives an indicator of exposure. The merit of biological monitoring is that it takes into account all routes of absorption for any chemical. The biological samples analysed are usually blood and urine. These samples are collected by occupational health staff; some essential questions that must be answered before performing biological monitoring are as follows.

- What is the chemical of interest?
- Is detection of the parent compound or the metabolite required?
- If it is the metabolite, is this unique to the compound of interest, or can it be derived from several different sources?
- When should the sampling be carried out? During or at the end of a shift, at the end of a working week, or is the time of sampling not critical?
- What biological sample should be collected? Blood, urine or other samples?
- How much of the biological sample is required?
- Are there special needles for taking blood, or special containers (with or without preservatives) for the blood or urine samples?
- Are there any special precautions for the collection of samples, packing and dispatch to the laboratory?
- Should the samples be kept at room temperature or be refrigerated before sending to the laboratory?

Approved laboratories with adequate quality control mechanisms and

Table 7.4 Biological monitoring guidance values.

Substance	Biological monitoring guidance values			
	Health guidance value*	Sampling time	Benchmark guidance value†	Sampling time
2-Butoxyethanol	240 mmol butoxyacetic acid per mole of creatinine in urine	Post-shift		
N,N-Dimethylacetamide	100 mmol N-methylacetamide per mole of creatinine in urine	Post-shift		
Lindane (γ-BHC(ISO))			35 nmol l^{-1} (10 µg l^{-1}) of lindane in whole blood (equivalent to 70 nmol l^{-1} of lindane in plasma)	Random
2,2'-Dichloro-4,4'-methylenedianiline (MbOCA)			15 µmol total MbOCA per mole of creatinine in urine	Post-shift
Mercury	20 µmol mercury per mole of creatinine in urine	Random		
4,4'-Methylenedianiline (MDA)			50 µmol total MDA per mole of creatinine in urine	Post-shift for inhalation and pre-shift next day for dermal exposure

*Health guidance values (HGVs) are set at a level at which there is no indication from the scientific evidence available that the substance being monitored is likely to be injurious to health. Values not greatly in excess of an HGV are unlikely to produce serious short- or long-term effects on health. However, regular exceeding of an HGV does indicate that exposure is not being adequately controlled. Under these circumstances, employers will need to look at current work practices to see how they can be improved to reduce exposure.

†Benchmark guidance values (BMVs) are set at a level around the 90th percentile of available validated data, collected from representative workplaces with good occupational hygiene practices. If a result is greater than a BMV, it does not necessarily mean that ill health will occur, but it does mean that exposure is not being adequately controlled. Under these circumstances, employers will need to look at current work practices to see how they can be improved to reduce exposure.

sufficient experience in such analyses should be used. For the interpretation of such results, biological exposure indices (BEIs) are published annually by the American Conference of Governmental Industrial Hygienists (ACGIH). The BEIs are reference values intended to represent equivalent exposure to the threshold limit values (TLVs). There are over 40 compounds and/or their metabolites listed in the 1997 ACGIH booklet on TLVs and BEIs. The HSE in the UK has also started publishing annual biological monitoring guidance values, with six substances listed in EH40/98. Table 7.4 gives some examples of biological monitoring guidance values.

The term 'biological effect monitoring' (BEM) was proposed for periodic assessment procedures, where the effect to be detected is a change in some biochemical parameter or physiological measure, the significance of which may still need to be determined. Like biological monitoring, this is used as an indicator of exposure. Unlike biological monitoring, it does not deal with the detection of a chemical or its metabolite. Examples of BEM are the determination of serum free erythrocyte protoporphyrin or urinary δ-aminolaevulinic acid for workers exposed to inorganic lead, and increased *N*-acetyl glucosaminidase in the urine for those exposed to cadmium. The same questions as above for biological monitoring would apply to the laboratory analysis of samples for BEM.

7.7 Medical records

Records on individual workers that are maintained by occupational health departments include the following.
• Pre-employment questionnaires.
• Occupational history information, including data on previous occupations, present job and change in job within the same organisation.
• Visits to the occupational health department, and the reason and outcome of the visits. This includes periodic attendance for statutory medical assessments, health surveillance for exposure to specific agents, emergency first aid treatment for accidents and injury, visits for advice and counselling and, in some cases, visits for the treatment of minor ailments.
• Results of physiological tests, e.g. lung function tests, audiometry or vision screening.
• Results of other laboratory investigations, e.g. antigen status and antibody levels for specific infections, biological monitoring and BEM results and blood and urine test results.

- Occupational hygiene data. These are often kept by the occupational hygiene or safety department separately from the medical records. However, if there is to be regular evaluation of occupational exposure and effect, it would be sensible for the two data sets to be brought together and compared by the relevant specialities.
- Immunisation records, including vaccination for travel and for specific protection against occupational infections in health-care workers.
- Communications and reports from family physicians, hospital doctors, physiotherapists and other health-care practitioners providing treatment for the worker.
- Consent forms, including those for access to medical reports and those allowing disclosure of certain information to management.
- Data on smoking history or alcohol consumption and current medications.

Many occupational health departments still maintain the above range of medical records in files and paper format. They can be filed in alphabetical order, by work departments or by work identification number. Increasingly, computer systems are being used for the storage of medical records. Commercial software systems are now available for such tasks as tracking immunisation status, automatic printing of reminder letters and aggregating and summarising data for groups of workers. The potential for using data kept in this format for epidemiological studies is good. However, the usefulness of the data is only as good as the completeness, consistency and accuracy of recording. There are differences, even for recording data on diagnosis. Hence, low back pain could be recorded as sciatica, lumbago, myositis or backache. Attempts have been made to develop uniform recording systems for occupational health data, with varying success. Where computer systems are used to store and retrieve occupational health records, the security of the system must be ensured. In addition to physical safeguards, such as locks and keeping the system in a locked secure room, computer software is also available to provide password protection, anti-virus mechanisms and to limit the number of individuals who have access to and can modify some or all of the records. There should also be provisions for the back-up storage of data in the event of theft or system failure. Advances in computerisation have meant the availability of equipment, such as scanners and recordable CD-ROMs, that can facilitate the storage and processing of large amounts of data. Where data about individuals are stored on computer, there are legal provisions in some countries to safeguard the accuracy and availability of that data. In the UK, the relevant legislation is the Data Protection Act (1984). In spite of computerisation, the paperless occupational health department is still far from reality. Paper copies or originals of some documents, especially those that have medico-legal implications, should still be kept.

7.8 Principles of epidemiology

7.8.1 Introduction

Occupational health may be considered to be a component part of public health. A key discipline within public health is epidemiology. Whereas clinical medicine tends to be concerned with the investigation and management of an individual patient's problem, population-based studies are an integral part of occupational health practice. There can be few workers whose job characteristics are unique to them. In this context — and misquoting John Donne — 'no worker is an island'.

It follows that, in reviewing any individual with a health-related problem or, indeed, any workplace with a hazardous environment, the investigator must ask himself/herself the question:

- who is affected/at risk?

From this follows more questions.

- Where?
- When?
- How?

To follow that with *so what*? is another way of implying that risk assessment is fundamental to the epidemiological process. This is its *raison d'être* — no problem, no question, no study.

7.8.2 Definition

Epidemiology is the study of the occurrence of human illness in populations. Occupational epidemiology is the study of the occurrence of diseases in relation to work-related determinants.

7.8.3 Types of epidemiological study

In essence, there are three types of epidemiological study — although, in practice, the third is frequently not undertaken for ethical reasons.

1 *Descriptive*. These are the questions noted above. Such descriptive procedures should lead to the development of causal hypotheses which can be tested.

2 *Analytical*. This involves the testing of hypotheses in formal epidemiological studies. If a hypothesis seems to be supported, attempts should be made to refute it in further studies and/or to undertake intervention studies.

3 *Intervention studies.* These are undertaken to see whether an alteration of exposure produces a change in the health outcome of the exposed population.

7.8.4 Databases

Although epidemiology is not just a set of number-crunching exercises, databases are crucial to the process. In this context, it is essential to remember that the fundamental question concerns the following relationship:

PUTATIVE EXPOSURE(S) → OBSERVED HEALTH EFFECT(S)

Exposure data vary greatly in quality. At worst, they may only provide information on ever/never exposed. At best, they may include a detailed record over many years of personal exposure data collected using accurate instruments and analysed by reputable techniques. As the best is rarely a reality, there has been much work recently on retrospective exposure assessment procedures in order to move the point on the exposure data spectrum closer to real-time data and away from vague statements.

   Health outcome data tend to be more accurate; however, although in most developed countries 'hard' data, such as death certificates and cancer registrations, are reasonably accurate and reliable, 'soft' data, such as sickness absence records, accident claims, hospital records and pension scheme information, are prone to inaccuracy and incompleteness. Specialist registers, such as those for mesothelioma or ionising radiation workers, have a special and useful place in studies. In the Nordic countries, where registry data are of a consistently high standard, it is possible to undertake *record linkage* studies between databases, thereby reviewing, for example, occupational registers with congenital malformation registers.

7.8.5 Cause or association?

The main thrust of an epidemiological study is to assess whether A causes B. In practice, doubt can still exist at the end of the study. If a difference is found between exposed and non-exposed groups for a given health outcome, there are four possible reasons.

1 Bias.
2 Confounding.
3 Chance.
4 Causation.

Asking a number of questions of the data can help to distinguish between these options.

- Is the disease specific to a special group of workers?
- Is it much more common than in other groups of people?
- Has the association been described by others in other relevant population-based studies?
- Does the exposure always precede effect by an appropriate time interval?
- Are there corroborative laboratory (*in vitro*) or animal (*in vivo*) data?
- Is this study result biologically plausible?
- Is this study result statistically significant?
- Is there a good dose–response relationship?

7.8.6 Survey design options
Despite the confusing terminology in many textbooks, the options are limited. They are:
- cross-sectional (prevalence) study;
- longitudinal study:
  - case control (case referent); or
  - follow-up (cohort).

Cross-sectional study
A cross-sectional study gives a snapshot view of events. It cannot relate exposure to effect. This requires a longitudinal component, which means either a case control or a follow-up study.

Case control study (Fig. 7.7)
The controls are similar to the cases, except (ideally) for the occurrence of

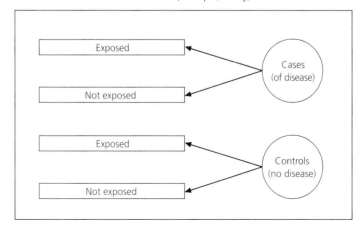

Fig. 7.7 Case control study.

the disease. The analysis consists of comparing the exposed/non-exposed ratio for the cases with that of the controls.

A case control study starts with the disease and works backwards (retrospectively) towards the exposures. Such studies, although highly suitable for rare diseases and relatively quick and easy to perform, are prone to bias of various types:

- selection of the cases or controls;
- comparability of the cases and controls (excluding the disease factor);
- recalling information on exposures;
- accuracy of diagnosis of health effects, etc.

Follow-up study (Fig. 7.8)
The analysis here allows disease rates to be calculated by exposure category.

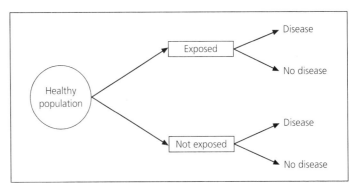

Fig. 7.8 Follow-up study. Note the direction of the arrows linking exposure with health effects.

Follow-up studies are free from many of the biases listed above for case control studies if conducted in a truly forward (prospective) manner. Whilst they are suitable for rare exposures, they are time consuming and thus expensive.

7.8.7 Shortcomings in the epidemiological method
Epidemiology is not an exact science, and some of the major flaws are listed below:

- a healthy worker effect — the comparison group has a different general health status from the cases;
- poor response rate;
- high turnover of study populations — selecting in (or out);

- latency between exposure and effect longer than study period;
- insufficient evidence of differing effects from differing exposures;
- poor quality of health effect data;
- poor quality of exposure data;
- multiple exposures;
- no effect of exposure noted — does this mean a true negative result or merely a poor/small study (non-positive result!)?

7.8.8 Appraising an epidemiological study

Even if the occupational health practitioner never intends to undertake an epidemiological study, he/she should be able to evaluate a published study and assess its worth.

The following points should be considered in any publication:

- question clearly formulated;
- appropriate study design;
- good quality health effect data;
- good quality exposure data;
- valid population choice for cases/controls;
- high response rate/good sampling strategy;
- confounders considered and allowed for;
- attempts made to reduce bias;
- population large enough to detect an effect if present;
- correct statistical techniques;
- estimates of risk include measures of variability, e.g. confidence intervals;
- cause/association issues addressed;
- non-positive/negative study result reviewed;
- effect of results on current knowledge assessed.

7.8.9 Conclusions

Despite the undoubted importance of laboratory-based studies and the skills of clinicians, the fundamental questions concerning the causation of human disease can only be answered by studying populations of humans. The fact that epidemiology proves to be an inexact science does not detract from this basic observation. However, the establishment of (or attempts to establish) causation is not the end of the story. At best, epidemiological studies will allow some estimate to be made of risk. Risk estimation should be followed by procedures to reduce that risk. Occupational health is a branch of preventive health, and epidemiological studies have a vital role to play in providing the scientific basis for preventive strategies.

8 Control of Airborne Contaminants

8.1 Introduction

The purpose of the application of workplace control techniques is to minimise worker exposure to the potential hazard, ideally so that exposure levels are below those that are considered to be hazardous. The success of the selected control will be judged by its ability to reduce personal risk. The control method should remain effective and maintain the same degree of protection over the working life of the process. Potential risk should be assessed by examining the results of failure of the control system. Where chronic hazards exist, an occasional transient failure may not be too serious, but any overexposure could have grave implications in the case of sensitisers and carcinogens, and, for asphyxiants, could be fatal. Thus, the control system must be designed to match the potential risk and, when risks are great, tolerances and safety factors should be planned accordingly. Where potential failure could have serious consequences, there will be a need to build in redundancy and back-up controls to warn of overexposure.

In accordance with good occupational hygiene practice, the control systems will take two forms — software and hardware — which can be applied together or separately.

Software consists of:
• substitution of a less hazardous material (see Fig. 8.1);
• methods of work to reduce worker exposure;
• training of workers to adopt safer methods of work;
• application of work schedules or regimes to limit the number of exposed individuals and to reduce the duration of their exposure.

Hardware consists of:
• enclosure of the process;
• suppression of emissions;
• shielding of source or worker;
• ventilation, extract at source;
• ventilation, dilution to reduce concentration;
• application of personal protective clothing to the worker.

As far as exposure to substances is concerned, there is a legal duty to *prevent* or *control* enshrined in Regulation 7 of the Control of Substances Hazardous to Health (COSHH) Regulations 1994; paragraphs 30 and 33 in the Approved Code of Practice set out the order in which the procedure should be tackled as follows.

To prevent exposure (software solutions).

1 Eliminate the use of the substance.

2 Substitute by a less hazardous substance or by the same substance in a less hazardous form (see Fig. 8.1).

To control exposure (hardware solutions).

1 Totally enclose process and handling systems.

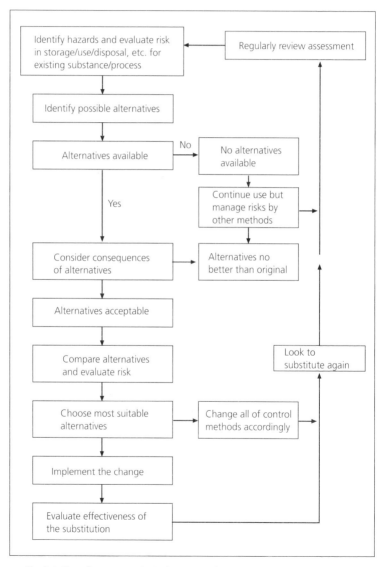

Fig. 8.1 Flow diagram to assist in the process of substitution of a contaminant.

2 Design the plant, process or systems of work to minimise the generation of the substance, or suppress or contain it.

3 If spills are likely, design the system/process to minimise the volume and area of contamination.

4 Partially enclose the source, together with local exhaust ventilation.

5 Provide local exhaust ventilation.

6 Provide sufficient general ventilation.

To control exposure (software solutions).

1 Reduce the number of employees present.

2 Exclude non-essential access.

3 Reduce the period of exposure for employees.

4 Regularly clean contamination from, or disinfect, walls, surfaces, etc.

5 Provide safe means of storage and disposal of substances hazardous to health.

6 Provide suitable personal protective equipment.

7 Prohibit eating, drinking, smoking, etc., in contaminated areas.

8 Provide adequate facilities for washing, changing and storage of clothing, including arrangements for laundering contaminated clothing.

When tackling a workplace health hazard with a view to reducing the risk, using engineering controls, the order in which the problem should be approached is as follows.

1 Deal with the *source* of emission or hazard.

2 Examine the *transmission* of the hazard between the source and the worker.

3 *Protect* the worker or the exposed population.

The hazard can be:

• an airborne pollutant, such as dust, gases and vapours, a microbiological organism or a radioactive particle, all of which enter the body via the lungs;

• a radiated emission, such as noise, heat, light or ionising and non-ionising radiation, which affects the body through the skin or other exposed organs;

• a chemical in liquid or solid form, which can affect the skin or enter the body via that organ.

8.1.1 Source

The source can be tackled, in the case of airborne pollutants, to reduce the potential for emission as follows:

• change the process so that no hazard is created;

• substitute the toxic material for one with a lower hazard potential (see Fig. 8.1);

- enclose the point of emission to minimise the area of outlet openings;
- provide extraction ventilation to capture the material at the point of release;
- suppress at source by wet methods or quenching techniques.
  The emission of radiation can be approached as follows:
- reduce the intensity of the source;
- change the wavelength of radiation to a safer one;
- enclose the point of emission;
- attenuate at the point of emission.

8.1.2 Transmission

With airborne pollutants, once the material is airborne and away from the source, control involves:

- shielding between the worker and the source;
- application of dilution ventilation;
- the use of jet ventilation to divert the contaminated air.
  In the case of radiated emissions:
- increase the distance between the worker and the source;
- attenuate the radiation;
- deflect or divert the radiation.

8.1.3 Exposed population

The workers' exposure can be minimised by examining their position in relation to the hazards.

In the case of air pollution:

- enclose the worker;
- eliminate the need for a worker using remote control of the process or automation;
- wash the worker in a stream of uncontaminated conditioned air;
- reduce the duration of exposure by means of job rotation;
- apply a safer method of work involving less contact with the pollutant;
- educate and train the worker to appreciate the hazards, so that their own behaviour will minimise the exposure.
- provide respiratory protection;
  With radiation and skin contact:
- enclose the worker in a protective cabin or behind shields;
- remove the worker by means of remote control operation of the process or by automation;
- apply a safer method of work;
- educate and train the worker in the risks involved and the application of safer methods of work.

- provide protective clothing to all vulnerable or exposed parts of the body;

This philosophy is represented diagrammatically in Fig. 8.2.

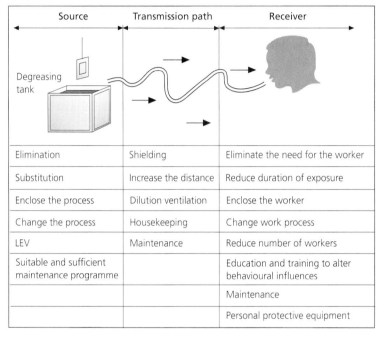

Source	Transmission path	Receiver
Elimination	Shielding	Eliminate the need for the worker
Substitution	Increase the distance	Reduce duration of exposure
Enclose the process	Dilution ventilation	Enclose the worker
Change the process	Housekeeping	Change work process
LEV	Maintenance	Reduce number of workers
Suitable and sufficient maintenance programme		Education and training to alter behavioural influences
		Maintenance
		Personal protective equipment

Fig. 8.2 Movement of a contaminant from a source to a receiver with control techniques for each component. (After Olishifski, 1988.)

8.1.4 Sources of emission

Sources of emission can be either *predictable* in time and space, being continuous or periodic, or *unpredictable* (fugitive), occurring haphazardly due to the breakdown or wear of normal engineering items. The former can be dealt with by engineering methods, some of which are outlined below, but the latter cannot, and normally involve the use of personal protective equipment (see Chapter 9).

The maintenance of plant and equipment always carries a great risk of predictable and unpredictable emissions, and maintenance workers require special attention and equipment to minimise their exposure. Software should be particularly attended to because maintenance workers work unsupervised where access is difficult and when safety and health staff are not on site.

8.1.5 Control of periodic and continuous emissions

It is necessary to examine the working process carefully to establish where the sources of emission are and how an improvement can be effected. In most cases, the emission of dust and vapours can be minimised by enclosure, or by redesigning the process so that the escape of pollutants is reduced. The openings through which pollutants escape can be fitted with doors or covers, which remain closed most of the time, and which are opened only for access. If this is impracticable, the openings for access can be fitted with extract ventilation, but it is worth remembering that, the smaller the openings, the lower the air flow rate required to capture the pollutants and, hence, the cheaper the costs.

The redesign of the process can be simple, for example:

- fitting covers on containers and openings;
- matching discharge ports to entry holes;
- using sealed transfer systems;
- using anti-splash discharge nozzles.

A more expensive solution is to enclose and automate the process completely, thus keeping the bulk of the contaminants inside; however, eventually, in most processes, the end-product has to be exposed to the atmosphere as do the raw materials at the start. With highly toxic materials, automation may be the only solution.

The provision of enclosure means that the visibility of the process is impaired, and, where it is necessary to observe the process, enclosure materials should be transparent. Closed-circuit video viewers could be adopted. Observation of the process is often necessary to judge whether a container is full or empty; thus visibility is not important if an alternative means of indication is employed. This may involve one of the following:

- placing the vessel or container on a weight indicator;
- using a float indicator;
- using a beam of light or a stream of radioactive particles to a sensor placed on the opposite side of the vessel; the intervention of the material cuts the beam, thus indicating that it has reached that level;
- using pressure switches.

Process redesign is often a cheaper expedient than the provision of extract ventilation, which requires skilful design to be successful, and is costly to build and to operate, particularly with regard to the replacement of the heat removed by the discharge of extracted air to the atmosphere. The costs of heating 'makeup' air are given later in this chapter. Many ventilation systems are unsuccessful owing to poor quality design.

8.2) **Extract ventilation design**

Where alternative solutions cannot be adopted, the pollutants can be captured before they are generally released into the working environment by means of extract ventilation. This can be achieved by some kind of hood, enclosure or slot, sufficiently negatively pressurised to ensure an inward current of air that will carry with it the airborne pollutants. The extract device will normally be connected to a fan via ducting, and thence to a point of discharge. An air cleaning system in the duct may be necessary to ensure that the discharged air is sufficiently clean, either to recirculate to the workplace or to satisfy external environmental standards if released outside.

With an unrestricted suction inlet, such as a hood, air will flow from all sides, in a zone of influence which is approximately spherical, with the inlet at the centre. Thus, with unflanged hoods, air will flow in from behind the inlet as well as in front, where there may not be any pollutants, and so this air is wasted. Flanges and screens are therefore necessary to channel the air at a sufficient velocity over the point of release of the pollutant to ensure successful capture.

The *capture velocity* is defined as that velocity which will overcome the motion of the airborne pollutant to draw it into the mouth of the extract. The following factors will influence the capture velocity:

- the velocity of release of the pollutant;
- the degree of turbulence of the air around the source;
- in the case of particulates, their aerodynamic diameter;
- the density of the materials released.

Recommended capture velocities are given in Table 8.1.

The *capture distance* is the distance between the point of release and the mouth of the inlet. The *face velocity* is the air velocity across the mouth or face of the inlet. The *aspect ratio* is the ratio of the width of the face divided by the length.

With booths, enclosures and fume cupboards, the face velocity is used rather than the capture velocity. Sufficient face velocity should be provided to prevent the pollutants released inside the enclosure from escaping back towards the worker. Recommended face velocities will depend upon the degree of toxicity of the material being handled and the amount of air turbulence found at the entrance, and will vary from 0.3 m s^{-1} for an aerodynamically shaped inlet handling low-toxicity materials up to 1.5 m s^{-1} for the opposite. It must be borne in mind, however, that, with non-aerodynamically shaped entrances, the higher

Table 8.1 Recommended capture velocities.

Source conditions	Typical situations	Capture velocity (m s^{-1})
Released into still air with no velocity	Degreasing tanks, paint dipping, still-air drying	0.25–0.5
Released at a low velocity or into a slow moving airstream	Container filling, spray booths, screening and sieving, plating, pickling, low-speed conveyor, transfer points, debagging	0.5–1.0
Released at a moderate velocity or into turbulent air	Paint spraying, normal conveyor transfer points, crushing, barrel filling	1.0–2.5
Released at a high velocity or into a very turbulent airstream	Grinding, fettling, tumbling, abrasive blasting	2.5–10.0

the air velocity, the greater the degree of turbulence created by the inlet. Turbulence often results in pollutants escaping the extract and entering the worker's breathing zone.

The shape of the extraction inlet will be dictated by the shape of the workplace and the area over which the pollutants are released. If the suction inlet area is too large, air distribution across the face may be uneven, allowing pollutants to escape capture over certain parts of the emission area. If the larger face dimension exceeds 1.5 m, it is advisable to provide twin duct offtakes or split the area with two hoods. It is advisable for flow splitters to be fitted to any hood in which the velocity distribution is expected to be uneven. Table 8.2 shows the shapes and uses of different suction inlets.

8.2.1 Low-volume, high-velocity extract systems

This technique is useful for extraction on portable hand-held power tools, such as grinders, circular saws and sanders. The principle is to place the suction inlet as close as possible to the point of release of the particles. The capture velocity should be greater than the velocity of the particle as it leaves the tool. The closer the inlet to the point of release, the less volume flow required and the smaller the ductwork. For hand-held tools, the ducting must be light and flexible, and is made of plastic ribbed with reinforcing material, and no larger in diameter than the hose of a domestic vacuum cleaner. The collected pollutants are usually particles of metal or wood, which are collected in an industrial type of vacuum cleaner. The whole unit is therefore portable and self-contained.

Table 8.2 Suction inlet shapes and uses.

Shape	Description and pressure loss calculations	Uses and features
	Canopy hood Pressure loss = 0.25 × duct p_v + filter loss (if fitted)	Suitable for pollutants having a natural upward current, i.e. hot processes, cooking. Unsuitable if workers need to lean over the process. Overhead access is difficult
	Side hood (open faced) Pressure loss = 0.25 × duct p_v	Suitable for bench work, but has an uneven velocity profile, i.e. the air velocity is higher at the top. Access to workplace available on three sides
	Side hood (slotted) Pressure loss = 1.8 × slot p_v + 0.25 duct p_v	Suitable for bench work. The slots provide a more even face velocity profile. Access to workplace available on three sides

Continued on p. 274

....

Table 8.2 *Continued*

Shape	Description and pressure loss calculations	Uses and features
	Enclosure (can be open faced as illustrated, but can have a sliding front as with fume cupboards) Pressure loss = 0.25 × duct p_v + filter loss (if fitted)	Provides greater containment as the pollutants are released inside and should not escape if the face velocity is sufficient. Access is limited to front only. Some turbulence can be expected due to entry of air at the edges of the enclosure, which can be minimised by aerofoil-shaped sides
	Booth with top extract and bottom supply through a perforated or gridded work surface Extract pressure loss = 0.25 × duct p_v	Provides good capture of internally produced pollutants and ensures low entry velocities through opening, thus minimising turbulence. Careful design is required to balance air flow rates to ensure a 10–25% excess of extract over supply. This ensures a small inflow at the mouth
	Slot, defined as having an aspect ratio of more than 5 : 1 Pressure loss = 1.8 × slot p_v + 0.25 × duct p_v	Has good access all round; suitable for surfaces of tanks or where pollutant release is spread over an area rather than from a point. Capture distance is limited

Continued

Table 8.2 *Continued*

Shape	Description and pressure loss calculations	Uses and features
	Double slot with extraction from two sides Pressure loss $= 1.8 \times$ slot p_v $+ 0.25 \times$ duct p_v	Has good access all round; suitable for surfaces of tanks or where the pollutant is spread over a wide area. A double slot will always provide better capture than a single one
	Extract hood with supply slot Extract pressure loss $= 1 \times$ face p_v $+ 0.25 \times$ duct p_v	Suitable for control over very wide surfaces as the supply of air can sweep the pollutants into the extract. Careful design is required to balance airflow rates to ensure that more air is captured than supplied. Also the 10° expansion of a jet of air must be borne in mind when sizing the extract hood
	Portable hood on flexible duct Pressure loss $= 0.25 \times$ duct p_v	Suitable for sources of pollution that are moving, such as welding on a large workpiece
	Curved slot Pressure loss $= 1.8 \times$ slot p_v $+ 0.25 \times$ duct p_v	Suitable for extracting closely around containers

Continued on p. 276

Table 8.2 *Continued*

Shape	Description and pressure loss calculations	Uses and features
	Extract annulus Pressure loss = 1.8 × annular p_v + 0.25 × duct p_v	Suitable for extracting around discharge pipes and outlets
	Evacuated containers Pressure loss = 0.65 × duct p_v	Suitable for sources of emission which are released at very high velocities. An evacuated container is placed in the path of the particles as they are emitted. Capture velocities of about 10 m s^{-1} are required

p_v is the velocity pressure at the stated position.

The performance of many of the above suction inlets can be improved by the addition of a flange fitted around the periphery of the inlet. This has the effect of limiting the zone of influence to the immediate area in front of the inlet. The effect this has on the capture velocity and distance is shown on p. 277.

8.2.2 Suction inlet performance

With straight-sided hoods and slots, centre-line velocities in the area in front of the inlet can be predicted. They are dependent upon the aspect ratio of the inlet, the mean face velocity and the distance from the hood. The relationship developed by Fletcher (1977) is given in the expression:

$$\frac{V}{V_0} = \frac{1}{0.93 + 8.58\alpha^2}$$

where $\alpha = XA^{-1/2}(W/L)^{-\beta}$, $\beta = 0.2(XA^{-1/2})^{-1/3}$, V is the centre-line velocity at distance X from the hood mouth, V_0 is the mean velocity at the face of the hood, L is the length of the hood, W is the width of the hood and $A = LW$.

The volume flow rate through the hood can be calculated by assigning V_0 to the required capture velocity and X to the designed capture distance. The volume flow Q is then obtained from:

$$Q = V_0 A$$

This formula also applies to the relationship between the volume flow rate, cross-sectional area and air velocity in ducts. The solution of the

Fletcher equations can be simplified by using the nomogram provided in Fig. 8.3.

The addition of flanges to the hoods will increase the centre-line velocities by up to 25% for hoods with a low aspect ratio, but by up to 55% with a slot of aspect ratio 16 : 1. The optimum flange widths are in the region of $A^{-1/2}$.

If capture distances are too great, the required face velocities to provide a suitable capture velocity can become excessive. For example, to provide a capture velocity of 1 m s^{-1} at a distance of 1 m from the mouth of a 200×1000 mm slot would require a face velocity of 66 m s^{-1}, which is unrealistic.

The prediction of velocities away from the centre line is difficult. In general, however, they will be less than the centre-line velocity on either side.

Unfortunately, the theoretical prediction of centre-line velocities assumes that the surrounding areas are free from disturbing air currents, which is often far from the case, particularly if there is a regular movement of people and vehicles in the vicinity of the source of pollution. In addition, the edges of the hood, the workpiece and the worker all contribute to local air turbulence, which can result in pollutants being drawn out of the capturing airstream and into the workplace and the breathing zone of the worker. In an ideal workplace, the entries to hoods should be of aerofoil shape to minimise turbulence.

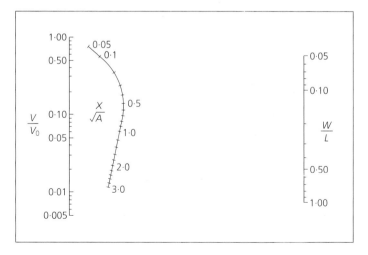

Fig. 8.3 Nomogram for the solution of the Fletcher equations. Crown copyright is reproduced with the permission of the Controller of The Stationery Office.

In practice, one of the few situations in which aerofoil shapes are used is in modern fume cupboards, where they have been shown to be successful in minimising the escape of pollutants. It is possible to add aerofoils to the entrances to older fume cupboards, and they have been shown to improve capture.

8.2.3 Ducts and fittings

Air is conveyed from the extract inlet to the point of discharge in ducts, which take a route to suit the needs of the building in which they are housed. In so doing, fittings, such as bends and changes of section, are required to assist in negotiating obstructions and to accommodate items of equipment, such as filters and air cleaners. The remaining parts of the system employ straight ducts. The shapes and sizes of the ducts depend upon the configuration of the workplace and the building, and the desired velocity of the air inside the ductwork. There are several factors that should be considered when deciding upon the cross-section of the ducts, and usually a compromise is made between them. For a given volume flow rate, the larger the duct, the lower the air velocity inside, and the less energy absorbed in overcoming friction. Such a duct is, however, high in capital cost. A circular cross-section is more economical in material than a rectangular one, but, in some buildings, the space available into which the duct can be placed is more suited to the rectangular shape.

If dust or larger particles are to be conveyed, it is important to ensure that they do not settle out and deposit inside the ducts to cause an obstruction or, in the case of flammable dusts, become a potential explosion hazard. The correct transport velocity is therefore required to minimise deposition.

The *transport velocity* is the minimum air velocity within the duct necessary to maintain the particles airborne. Table 8.3 gives some recommended transport velocities.

If only gases and vapours are to be carried, transport velocities are not important, and the air velocity becomes a matter of economics or acoustics. Optimum velocities are usually between 5 and 6 m s^{-1}, but, if noise levels are not to be obtrusive, 5 m s^{-1} should be the maximum.

In extract ventilation design, the volume flow rate (Q) is determined first by virtue of the requirements of the suction inlet. Then, having decided upon the duct velocity (V), the cross-sectional area (A) is determined from the expression:

$Q = VA$

Table 8.3 Recommended transport velocities.

Pollutant	Transport velocity (m s^{-1})
Fumes, such as zinc and aluminium	7–10
Fine dust, such as lint, cotton fly, flour, fine powders	10–12.5
Dusts and powders with low moisture contents, such as cotton dust, jute lint, fine wood shavings, fine rubber dust, plastic dust	12.5–17.5
Normal industrial dust, such as sawdust, grinding dust, food powders, rock dusts, asbestos fibres, silica flour, pottery clay dust, brick and cement dust	17.5–20
Heavy and moist dust, such as lead chippings, moist cement, quicklime dust, paint spray particles	Over 22.5

Ducting is usually made of galvanised sheet steel, but a variety of other materials can be used, including brick, concrete, polyvinyl chloride (PVC), fibreglass, canvas, plastic and stainless steel. Where the air contains corrosive materials, galvanised metal is unsuitable, and a corrosion-resistant material must be used.

8.2.4 Pressure losses

Air requires a pressure difference for it to flow, and it will always flow from the higher to the lower pressure. The source of motive power is either natural or by means of a fan. Pressure is a type of energy which appears in two forms, static (p_s) and velocity (p_v), and the sum of these is known as the total pressure (p_t). Static pressure is exerted in all directions by a fluid that is stationary, but, if it is moving, it is measured at right angles to the direction of flow to eliminate the effects of velocity. Static pressure can be either positive or negative in relation to atmospheric pressure: on the suction side of a fan, it is usually negative and, on the delivery side, it is normally positive. This is illustrated using the U-tube gauges shown in Fig. 8.4.

Velocity pressure is the kinetic energy of a fluid in motion, and is calculated from the following expression:

$$P_v = \frac{\rho v^2}{2}$$

where ρ is the air density and v is the air velocity.

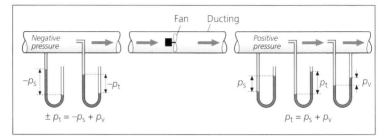

Fig. 8.4 Examples of typical liquid-filled manometer readings on either side of a fan showing the effect of positive and negative pressure.

If the standard air density at 1.2 kg m^{-3} is used, the above expression becomes:

$$p_v = 0.6v^2$$

If v is in metres per second, p_v will be in pascals. These expressions are widely used in airflow measurement and in the calculation of pressure losses in ductwork systems.

8.2.5 Reynolds number

In a pipe through which fluid flows, the relationship between the energy absorbed and the rate of flow depends upon the character of the flow. At low velocities, a non-turbulent flow exists, which is termed 'laminar' or 'streamlined' flow, where the energy absorbed is proportional to the velocity of the fluid. At higher velocities, a turbulent flow exists, in which the energy absorbed is proportional to the square of the fluid velocity. The character of the flow is determined by the following variables:

- μ, the dynamic viscosity of the fluid;
- ρ, the density of the fluid;
- v, the velocity of the fluid;
- D, the diameter of the pipe.

These variables combine together to form a dimensionless number, known as the Reynolds number (Re), which may be calculated from the equation:

$$Re = \frac{vD\rho}{\mu}$$

In general, with $Re < 2000$, laminar flow exists and, with $Re > 4000$, turbulent flow exists. Between these limits, flow conditions are variable. In most engineering applications, $Re > 4000$, and it is assumed that the energy absorbed is proportional to the square of the velocity. The exception to this general statement is in air filtration, where air velocities can be very low within the filter medium, and Re approaches 2000.

The energy losses due to friction are expressed as a pressure loss, which can be calculated or obtained from charts and nomograms. With regard to straight lengths of ducting, the pressure loss can be obtained in pascals per metre, using the nomogram given in Fig. 8.5. As the duct sides are parallel, there is no change in air velocity from one end to the other. The pressure losses obtained from the nomogram are therefore both total and static. The losses in most fittings are calculated by multiplying the velocity pressure at a point in the fitting by a factor determined empirically for the geometrical shape of that fitting. The

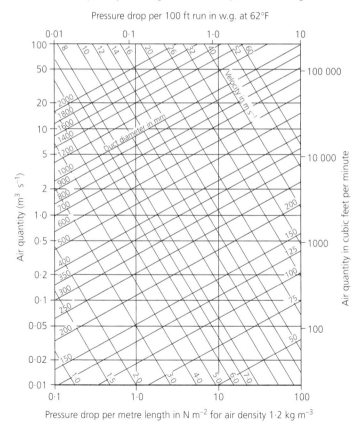

Fig. 8.5 Nomogram for calculating airflow in round ducts (plotted on logarithmic scales). (Taken from CIBS Guide Section C4, published by the Chartered Institute of Building Services (CIBS).)

resulting pressure loss is in total pressure. It is important to work in total pressure for ventilation calculations, because fittings and changes of section have changes in static pressure within them, sometimes resulting in a gain of static, but a loss of total, pressure. Working in total pressure throughout avoids any confusion.

8.2.6 Fan required

In order to establish the duty of a fan to draw air through the system, it is necessary to sum the individual pressure losses from each of the components, starting from the suction inlet and working towards the fan (see Fig. 8.6). If there are components on the delivery side of the fan, it is also necessary to add the pressure losses on that side. Similarly, if a filter or dust collector is installed, the pressure loss of that component must be included. This will be obtainable from the manufacturer, and should be quoted both for a clean unit and for the time when the filter needs changing or cleaning, the latter higher pressure being included in the calculation. Having summed all the pressure losses involved throughout the system (this should include the discharge velocity pressure), the fan can be chosen from manufacturers' catalogues to handle the chosen volume flow rate at the total pressure calculated.

It is not unusual with extract systems to add several branches, all feeding to a single duct and fan. When this occurs, the pressure needed to specify the fan is normally taken as that required to bring the air from the inlet furthest from the fan through the system to the discharge point. Sufficient pressure will be available to overcome the resistance of the intermediate branches, i.e. those nearer the fan. Indeed, there may be an excess of pressure, making it necessary to restrict the intermediate branches in order to prevent an excess of airflow from passing through them to the detriment of the furthest branch. This results in the multibranched system being out of balance, a common fault with many industrial systems which have been in use for some time. Balancing can be achieved by installing adjustable dampers in the intermediate branches, or by making those branches higher in resistance by design. The damper method has the disadvantage of being thrown out of balance by injudicious tampering unless the damper handles are locked in the balance position. In addition, if dust is to be carried in the duct, the dampers can act as a depository, such that unwanted accumulations of dust can build up, making the damper unworkable, and causing an unnecessary obstruction in the duct. Inherent balancing by design is therefore preferred. When designing a system, it is useful to draw a sketch of the layout, labelling each junction at which the air changes

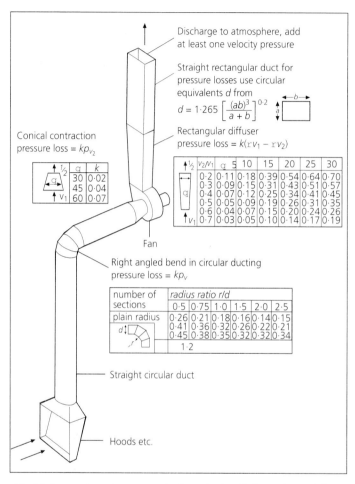

Fig. 8.6 Pressure losses in components of an extract ventilation system. p_v is the velocity pressure, the subscript referring to the position as indicated in the diagram accompanying each fitting. For fan, see p. 287; for pressure losses, see Table 8.2; for hoods, etc., see pp. 273–6.

speed or direction, or where two air streams meet, by assigning the change point with a number or letter of the alphabet. In this way, each section can be identified as, for example, 3–4 or E–F. A table should be drawn up with headings as shown in Table 8.4.

The table should be filled in section by section, starting from the inlet furthest from the fan, using the design information selected as appropriate to the requirements of each section. It is not necessary to

Table 8.4 Headings for table to be used in designing an extract system.

Section	Length (m)	Volume flow ($m^3 s^{-1}$)	Duct dimension (mm)	Duct area (m^2)	Air velocity ($m s^{-1}$)	Velocity pressure (Pa)	Loss factor (k)	Pressure loss per metre ($Pa\ m^{-1}$)	Section pressure loss (Pa)	Cumulative pressure loss (Pa)

complete every column for each section, as they do not all apply, and it may be necessary to leave some sections until after the following section has been designed. The last column on the right of the table is the sum of the pressure losses accumulated from the beginning, and this provides a statement of the pressure inside the duct at that point, in relation to the atmosphere. Thus, if a connection was to be made to the atmosphere at that point, the pressure difference available to overcome the resistance of the connecting branch is known.

8.3 Dilution ventilation

There are many situations in industry where it is impracticable to extract at source by means of a hood or enclosure. Typical situations include:
- where the source of emission is very large, e.g. the manufacture of boats in glass-reinforced plastic (GRP);
- where the source is moving, e.g. in a production line where products are hanging from a moving conveyor;
- where the presence of a hood or enclosure would impair the transfer of products.

Control can be achieved by passing large quantities of air over the source to dilute it to a safe level or to divert it into an unoccupied space.

It is necessary to decide on the volume flow rate of air to dilute the emission to a chosen concentration, and for this the following equation should be used:

$$Q = \frac{R}{C}$$

where Q is the required diluting volume flow rate in cubic metres per second, R is the rate of emission of the pollutant in milligrams per second and C is the chosen concentration in milligrams per cubic metre. This equation assumes that the diluting air stream and the pollutants are evenly mixed.

The chosen concentration can be the published occupational exposure limit or a certain fraction of it. For example, if the pollutant has a maximum exposure limit (MEL), it is suggested that the chosen concentration should be as low as reasonably practicable, for example 25% of the published value. The rate of emission is more difficult to determine, and may be related to the rate of usage during a working period and how much of the pollutant is released into the workroom atmosphere.

For example, in the manufacture of items in GRP, the resin emits styrene; the suppliers of this resin are able to predict how much styrene is released for a given surface area during the curing process. A typical value of normal pigmented polyester resin is an emission rate of 50 g of styrene per hour per square metre of exposed surface. Thus, if 100 m^2 of GRP is emitting, the rate of emission will be 5000 g h^{-1} or approximately 1400 mg s^{-1}. Therefore, to dilute that to 25% of the published MEL for styrene (430 mg m^{-3}), i.e. 108 mg m^{-3}, a volume flow rate of 1400/108 = 13 m^3 s^{-1} is required.

The method of introducing diluting air into the workroom needs some care. Supply grilles designed to create high velocities may provide good mixing, but would be unpopular with the workforce as cold draughts may occur. Low-velocity displacement ventilation, with the diluting air being heated to, for example, 16°C and introduced at floor level, will gently displace the pollutant with little discomfort to the workforce.

8.3.1 Summary of the aims of both dilution and extraction ventilation

1 Do not draw or blow the contaminated air towards the face of the worker.

2 Place the extract as close to the source of pollution as possible.

3 Enclose as much of the source as is consistent with the work process.

4 Direct dilution ventilation so that the source of emission is entrained away from the occupied areas.

5 Discharge polluted air in such a way that it does not re-enter the building or adjacent buildings. High discharge stacks improve dispersion and minimise weather effects.

6 Make allowances for outside wind effects to prevent blowback of extracted air.

7 Make allowances for buoyancy effects of the release gases or vapours, i.e. hotter or less dense substances tend to rise when in a concentrated form, whilst colder, heavier substances tend to fall. There is also a tendency for a concentrated pollutant released into still or slow moving air to form a layer on the floor or in the roof, according to its density relative to air, the removal of which is difficult, and which can lead to dangerous accumulations if the material is toxic or flammable. This phenomenon only occurs when air is stagnant. Under normal operating circumstances, where there is movement of people and products, there is sufficient turbulence to mix the heavy vapour with room air, such that the density of the mixture is little different from that of air, and no sedimentation will occur.

8 If it is important to contain the polluted air in the room in which it is released, this can be achieved by extracting 10–15% more air than supplied.

9 Do not discharge toxic or harmful substances into the atmosphere without rendering them harmless.

10 Certain gases and vapours are flammable, and their handling may come under special regulations or codes requiring flameproof equipment. Due regard must be taken of this.

8.3.2 Legal requirements

Specific mention of ventilation of the workplace is made in the following Acts and Regulations, although many others call for ventilation.

- Health and Safety at Work, etc. Act 1974.
- Factories Act 1961, Section 4.
- Offices, Shops and Railway Premises Act 1956, Section 7.
- Coal and Other Mines (Ventilation) Regulations 1956 (SI 1956 No. 1764).
- Coal and Other Mines (Locomotive) Regulations 1956 (SI 1956 No. 1771).
- Highly Flammable Liquids and Liquefied Petroleum Gases Regulations 1972 (SI 1972 No. 917).
- Control of Substances Hazardous to Health Regulations 1994 (SI 1994 No. 3246).

8.4 Choice of fan

Having decided upon the volume flow rate to pass through the ventilation system, and the pressure or suction required to overcome friction losses through the system, it is necessary to select a fan capable of providing that duty. Fan manufacturers publish catalogues from which the correct fan can be chosen. The performance figures are often presented by means of graphs, known as characteristic curves, which show the relationship between pressure and volume flow. It is necessary to select the fan so that the duty point lies on the curve at the fan's most efficient operating condition. This will be indicated on the curve or by the manufacturer.

Most fans used in industrial ventilation are of two types: *axial flow* and *centrifugal*. Axial flow fans normally consist of a multibladed propeller-type rotor inside a cylindrical casing, often of the same diameter as the ducting. The electric motor is usually inside the casing and in the air stream being moved. These fans tend to be noisy, and are limited in the amount of pressure they develop, such that they are not suited to high-resistance systems, e.g. those containing fabric or centrifugal filters. Some have a bifurcated arrangement, so that the motors remain outside the air stream and are suitable for systems carrying hot air or flammable vapours.

Centrifugal fans are capable of developing much higher pressures, and are best suited to high-resistance systems. They can be described as having a paddle-wheel type of impeller, rotating inside a volute-shaped casing, such that air leaves the fan at right angles to the direction in which it enters. They are normally quieter than axial flow fans. Motors are normally outside the airstream, and may be directly coupled to the shaft of the impeller or connected by means of a drive, such as a V-belt or gearbox.

Many fan motors used in industry are powered by a 380–440 V three-phase electrical supply. The direction of rotation is dictated by the way in which the terminals are connected. Should they be connected wrongly, the fan will run in reverse. This could occur on installation or after routine maintenance. With axial flow fans, reversal will result in air flowing in the opposite direction, and is usually noticed and rectified. However, the flow in centrifugal fans is not reversed when the motor turns in the wrong direction, but results in a greatly reduced airflow. As the air continues to flow in the correct direction, the error is not noticed, and may continue for long periods of time, with the consequent reduction in control efficiency. Most good fan makers indicate the correct direction of rotation on the casing, but, if this is not marked, it is possible to determine the correct direction by examining the fan casing. It enlarges in the direction of rotation.

The COSHH Regulations 1994 in the UK require a thorough examination and test of ventilation systems that control substances hazardous to health to be made at regular intervals, varying between 1 and 14 months, depending upon the substance or operation that is being ventilated (Regulation 9).

8.5 Air cleaning and discharges to the atmosphere

8.5.1 Air cleaning

Environmental pressures are already placed upon employers to limit the amount and concentration of toxic substances discharged to the atmosphere, and certain registered works are required by law to do so. These pressures are reinforced by a more wide-ranging law (Environmental Protection Act) which came into force in the early 1990s. Therefore, attention should now be turned to limiting the emissions from ventilation systems that contain substances hazardous to health.

The removal of particles from discharged air involves various alternative principles, the choice of which is dictated by the size, nature and concentration of the particles. Large, dry particles in a high concentration from, for example, a woodworking shop are best dealt with by a centrifugal method, such as a cyclone. Small, dry particles from, for example, a lead smelter would best be removed by a fabric filter, such as a bag house. Dusts that can be easily charged electrically can be removed by electrostatic means. Sticky or wet dusts will require methods involving wet scrubbing, which, although cleaning the discharged air, may lead to a secondary problem of wet sludge disposal.

The removal of gases and vapours from discharged air is generally more difficult, as the pollutant is in molecular form, and does not respond to the physical forces that can capture airborne particles. Chemical adsorption and absorption are the principles employed. Wet absorption involves passing the gas-laden air through extended wetted surfaces and sprays of water or chemical solutions. Adsorption normally uses activated charcoal beds through which the gas-laden air passes, the pollutant being adsorbed onto the minute pores in the charcoal. Thermal oxidation techniques are also being developed. To achieve a high degree of cleaning, all techniques are bulky and costly to purchase and operate.

Air cleaning techniques absorb energy from the extracted air. This must be taken into account when choosing the correct fan for the job. Adding air cleaning later will invariably involve upgrading the performance of the fan to cater for the extra resistance to airflow that the device provides.

8.5.2 Discharges to the atmosphere

Any ventilation system that discharges air horizontally to the atmosphere will, at some time or another, encounter external wind pressures. Sometimes the direction and velocity of the outside wind will result in a reversal of the airflow in the ventilation system, and pollutants will be scattered internally rather than be extracted. Such systems require weather covers to prevent blowback, but these devices can result in polluted air remaining close to the buildings and being re-entrained into them. It is far better to discharge vertically as high as permissible with a high efflux velocity. Conical weather covers should be removed as they tend to bring pollutants down to ground level to be re-entrained into adjacent buildings. Suitable alternatives are available to prevent rain and snow from entering the discharge stack.

8.6) Energy and cost implications of ventilation systems

The energy needed to provide ventilation can be divided into that required to overcome air friction in the hardware and that required to heat the replacement air, where air is discharged to the atmosphere. In most cases, and at most times of the year, the latter is far more costly.

The costs of providing motive power to overcome the friction of moving air through a ventilation system can be calculated from the fan power formula knowing the cost per electrical unit the user is being charged by the electricity supplier.

8.6.1 Power and efficiency definitions

The *air power (total)* is the theoretical power required for a volume of air to move against a resistance, and is calculated from:

$$P_a = Qp_t$$

where P_a is the air power (total), Q is the volume flow rate and p_t is the total pressure required to move that flow rate. If Q is in metres per second and p_t is in Pascals, the resulting power will be in Watts.

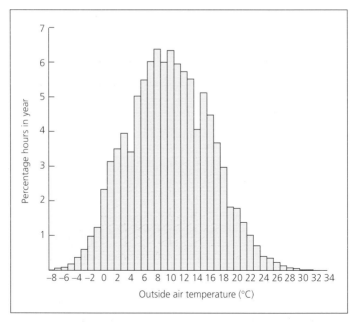

Fig. 8.7 Annual frequency of hourly values of air dry bulb temperatures, Heathrow Airport, London, 1949–1976.

The *fan efficiency (total)* is the ratio of the air power (total) to the input power at the shaft of the fan impeller.

The *fan power (total)* is the power required at the shaft of the fan impeller to move the air against the resistance. It is calculated from:

$$P_t = \frac{Qp_t}{\eta}$$

where P_t is the fan power (total) and η is the fan efficiency (total).

Where extracted air is discarded to the atmosphere, the energy required to provide heated replacement air will depend upon the outside air temperature and the designed inside air temperature. In Britain, meteorological records are available for many sites, from which estimates of the number of hours in a year at a particular air temperature have been made. Figure 8.7 gives such values for a typical south of England site.

In order to establish the amount of energy required to heat 1 m³ s⁻¹ of outside air to inside designed conditions, the chart in Fig. 8.8 can be used in conjunction with the cost of the fuel being used for heating the workplace.

To use the chart in Fig. 8.8, the vertical lines represent outside air temperatures and the inclined lines represent those inside. From the

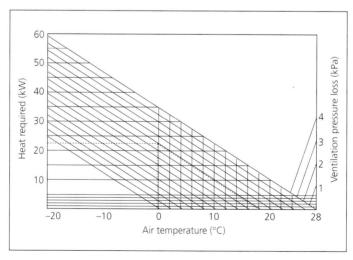

Fig. 8.8 Chart for estimating energy requirements for heating 1 m³ s⁻¹ of air from outside to inside air temperature; also shows energy equivalent of ventilation pressure loss. (After Gill, 1980.)

position at which any two intersect, the power required can be read horizontally on the left-hand column. An example (represented by the broken lines) is shown: outside air, 0°C; inside air, 18°C; power required to heat 1 $m^3 s^{-1}$ of air, 22.5 kW; thus, for every hour that the air is drawn in, the energy required would be 22.5 kWh. The running costs can then be estimated, based upon the type of fuel used.

To use the pressure loss ordinate, the theoretical power required to overcome the frictional resistance of a system can be found by reading horizontally from the position at which the ventilation pressure loss line intersects with the top, inclined, outside temperature line. Example: a ventilation system whose pressure loss is 2.5 kPa for a flow rate of 1 $m^3 s^{-1}$ will give a theoretical power requirement of 2.5 kW. Thus, for every hour that it is operated, it will require a theoretical power of 2.5 kWh. The true power will take into account the efficiency of the fan and, if the fan is electrically driven, the cost can be obtained.

9 Personal Protection of the Worker

9.1) Introduction

If control at source or during transmission is not possible, or if extra safeguards are required, the worker must be protected. This can be performed in one of three ways, depending on the nature of the contaminant.

1 By washing the worker in a stream of uncontaminated air, thus displacing any airborne pollutants.

2 By segregation or separation, using a shield or air-conditioned enclosure.

3 By providing personal protective clothing.

9.1.1 Displacement

This depends upon the creation of a diffuse, clean airflow over the worker and towards the work, carrying away the work products, preferably towards some form of extraction system. The provision of work station supply ventilation has corresponding economies in the volume of air required in comparison with a system ventilating the whole building. Care must be taken to ensure that local turbulence is minimised, so that effectiveness of control is maintained. This technique is most suited to well-defined work stations.

Thermal comfort of the worker must be considered, so that the combination of air temperature and velocity is such that cold draughts are not experienced at the work station. To this end, supply diffusers must be chosen carefully, and the supply air temperature must be accurately controlled to suit the air velocity directed at the worker. This is particularly important when air is discharged from above and behind the worker, as the back, neck and back of the head are the parts of the body most sensitive to draughts. It is important to remember that even air at a temperature above that of a normal room can feel cold if it is flowing at a sufficiently high velocity. Figure 9.1 shows the relationship between air velocity and temperature and the part of the body affected.

Figure 9.1 shows the number of people complaining of discomfort as a percentage of the total number tested. As an example, it can be seen that a draught of 0.2 m s^{-1} at a temperature of 1°C below ambient room temperature, blowing on the occupants' necks, will give a feeling of uncomfortable coolness to 20% of the room occupants, whereas the same draught blowing on the ankle region will cause discomfort to only 5%.

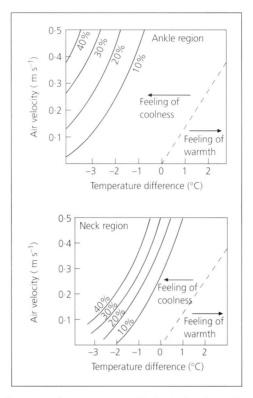

Fig. 9.1 Percentage of room occupants objecting to draughts on the ankle and neck region.

9.1.2 Enclosing or shielding the worker

Isolating the worker from an uncongenial or toxic environment is a technique which is often adopted when the working process is too large or too expensive to control at source or in the transmission stage. Isolation cubicles can be used to protect from noise, ionising radiation, heat and cold, as well as from airborne toxins. In most cases, the enclosure will require ventilation and, possibly, air-conditioning, and the amounts of air required will need to be calculated. As a general rule, each person enclosed will require 10 l of fresh air per second, but this amount can be varied, depending upon the size of the enclosure and whether or not smoking is permitted. For example, a small enclosure containing one person who smokes would require a fresh air rate of 25 l s^{-1}, whereas a spacious enclosure in which no smoking takes place could be ventilated with as little as 5 l s^{-1} per person.

9.1.3 Personal protection

The organs of the human body that are vulnerable to attack from external sources are the eyes, the ears, the skin and the respiratory system. In the case of the first three, a barrier or attenuation device should be worn over the organ being protected. With regard to airborne pollutants, respiratory protection involves the wearing of a device that either cleans the polluted air to a safe level or provides a stream of uncontaminated air from a separate source.

At this juncture, it must be pointed out that Regulation 7 of the Control of Substances Hazardous to Health (COSHH) Regulations 1994 specifically states that control should be secured by measures other than by the provision of personal protective equipment (PPE), but, where other means are not preventive or do not provide adequate control, then, in addition to those measures, suitable PPE shall be provided adequately to control exposure. The Regulations require that the PPE provided must be suitable for the purpose and conform to a standard approved by the Health and Safety Executive (HSE).

Examples of situations in which the use of PPE may be necessary include the following:

• where it is not technically feasible to achieve adequate control by other measures alone, control should be achieved by other methods as far as reasonably practicable and then, in addition, PPE should be used;

• where PPE is required to safeguard health until such time as adequate control is achieved by other means;

• where urgent action is required, such as in a plant failure, and the only practical solution is to use PPE;

• during routine maintenance operations.

In most cases, PPE appears to offer a cheap alternative solution to the provision of engineering control methods. On closer scrutiny, however, the management problems that are created by its introduction make this alternative less attractive. In order to make the decision to use personal protective devices routinely, it is necessary to hold discussions involving trade unions or workers' representatives and, once the decision to go ahead has been made, arrangements must be put in place for the education and training of the users. A complete back-up system of purchasing, storage, cleaning, repair, inspection, testing and replacement must also be established. Moreover, the reaction of the worker to being asked to wear the devices may involve financial inducements and changes in contract conditions before adoption, and management supervision may need to be strengthened.

European legislation

Late in 1989, the Council of European Communities published two important Directives regarding PPE. The first (89/656/EEC) sets out the minimum health and safety requirements for the use by workers of PPE in the workplace, and required member states to implement it by December 31, 1992. Details of this Directive can be seen in the Official Journal (OJ) of the European Communities No. L 393/19. The purpose of the second (89/686/EEC) is to harmonise the European standards of PPE through the European Committee for Standardisation (CEN). This Directive can be found in OJ No. L 399/19, and was required to be implemented by December 31, 1991.

9.2 Eye and face protection

Protection must be provided to guard against:
- the impact of small particles projected at a low velocity;
- the impact of heavy particles at a high velocity;
- the splashing of a hot or corrosive liquid;
- the contact of the eyes with an irritating gas or vapour;
- a beam of electromagnetic radiation of various wavelengths, including laser beams.

Each harmful agent may require a particular form of eye protection, which may be unsuitable for another agent. In some cases, the protection may need to be extended to the whole face. Whatever hazard or hazards exist, the protective device must be carefully chosen to suit.

9.2.1 Legal requirements
- Health and Safety at Work, etc. Act 1974.
- SI 1974 No. 1681, Protection of Eyes Regulation made under Section 65 of the Factories Act 1961, requiring employers to provide eye protection and shields to persons employed in specified processes, and embracing many industrial situations.

9.2.2 Standards
Various standards for eye protection have been produced to assist in obtaining the correct specification to suit the harmful agent.

British Standard (BS) and BS EN
- *BS EN 169*. Specification for filter for personal eye-protection equipment used in welding and similar operations.

- *BS EN 170*. Specification for ultraviolet filters used in personal eye-protection equipment.
- *BS EN 171*. Specification for infrared filters used in personal eye-protection equipment.
- *BS 679*. Specification for filters, cover lenses and backing lenses for use during welding and similar operations.
- *BS 2092*. Specification for industrial eye protectors.
- *BS 4110*. Specification for eye protectors for vehicle users.

American National Standards Institution (New York)
- ANSI 287.1, Standard Practice for Occupational and Educational Eye and Face Protection 1968.

9.2.3 General points
Eye protection takes the form of spectacles, goggles or face shields, all of which are available from a wide range of manufacturers and suppliers, in a wide range of sizes. Suitability for the hazard and comfort must be the overriding factors in choosing the particular device, as the users must have complete confidence in the protection it provides and must not be forced to remove it to relieve discomfort during the operation for which protection is required. A preoccupation with discomfort may also distract from the task in hand and lead to errors and accidents. A good range of suitable forms of protection should therefore be made available for the user to choose the one to suit the shape of his/her face. This may mean having products from more than one manufacturer available.

Some of the problems involved in the use of eye protectors are given below. Several can be overcome by suitable selection, but certain problems are inherent in the use of such devices.

1 They may not guard against the hazard.
2 They may not fit properly.
3 They may be uncomfortable due to uneven pressure on the face.
4 They will restrict the field of view.
5 Spectacles worn for correction of vision may interfere with the wearing of eye protectors and vice versa. Whilst safety spectacles with corrective lenses are available, their suitability is limited to minor eye hazards.
6 Optical services and follow-up may be necessary to deal with problems of refraction of light.
7 Eye protectors may interfere with the wearing of respiratory and/or hearing protection. Where more than one organ is to be protected, an integrated, combined protective device may therefore be more suitable.

8 Due to discomfort, the wearer may be tempted to remove the protector from time to time, with a consequent loss of protection for that period.

9 Fitting, cleaning, inspection and replacement procedures are necessary.

10 Training may be required for users and for maintenance staff.

9.2.4 Types available

Safety spectacles are only suitable for low-energy hazards, but are available in a wide range of sizes to suit the face. Types: clear, clip-on, prescription, tinted (anti-flash).

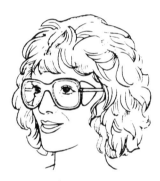

Goggles are suitable for a wide range of hazards, but are limited in fittings from any one manufacturer. Types: chemical, dust, gas, gas welding, general purpose, molten metal.

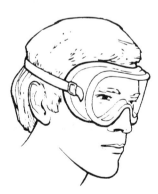

Shields are suitable to protect the eyes or the whole face; they can be attached to a helmet or a headband, but may be hand-held. Types: eye, face, furnace viewing, welding.

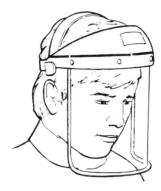

Skin and body protection

Skin protection includes guarding hands, feet and body against:

- damage from dermatitic or corrosive agents;
- absorption into the body via the skin;
- radiant heat;
- cold;
- ionising and non-ionising radiation;
- physical damage.

The material used for the gloves, apron or garment must be suited to the purpose and must be chosen carefully.

9.3.1 Legal requirements

- Health and Safety at Work, etc. Act 1974.
- SI 1950 No. 65, The Pottery (Health and Welfare) Special Regulations.
- SI 1948 No. 1547, The Clay Works (Welfare) Special Regulations.
- SI 1980 No. 1248, The Control of Lead at Work Regulations.
- SI 1985 No. 1333, Ionising Radiation Regulations.
- SI 1994 No. 1657, The Control of Substances Hazardous to Health Regulations.

9.3.2 Standards and codes, BS and BS EN

Hand protection

- *BS EN 374*. Part 1. Protection gloves against chemicals and micro-organisms: terminology and performance requirements.
- *BS EN 388*. Protection gloves against mechanical risks.
- *BS EN 407*. Protection gloves for thermal risks.
- *BS EN 420*. General requirements for gloves.

- *BS EN 421*. Protective gloves for ionising radiation including contamination and direct exposure to radiation.
- *BS EN 455*. Medical single-use gloves.
- *BS EN 511*. Protection gloves for cold.
- *BS EN 60903*. Insulating protective gloves for working with electricity.
- *BS 2606*. Specification for X-ray protective gloves for medical diagnostic purposes up to 150 kV peak.

Foot protection

- *BS EN 344*. Requirements and test methods for safety, protective and occupational footwear for professional use.
- *BS EN 345*. Specification for safety footwear for professional use.
- *BS EN 346*. Specification for protective footwear for professional use.
- *BS EN 347*. Specification for occupational footwear for professional use.
- *BS 2723*. Specification for fireman's leather boots.

Body protection

- *BS EN 340*. Protection clothing: general requirements.
- *BS EN 470*. Part 1. Protective clothing for use in welding and allied processes: general requirements.
- *BS EN 702*. Protection clothing — protection against heat and flame; test method — determination of the contact heat transmission through protective clothing or its materials.
- *BS 3783*. Specification for X-ray lead–rubber protective aprons for personal use.
- *BS 7182*. Specification for air-impermeable chemical protective clothing.
- *BS 7184*. Recommendation for selection, use and maintenance of chemical protective clothing.

9.3.3 Types available

Hand protection

Materials	Protection	Gloves
Asbestos	Abrasion	Armoured
Cotton	Chemical	Chain-mail
Leather	Electrical	Disposable
Moleskin	Fire/flame/heat resistant	Electrician's

Continued

Hand protection *Continued*

Materials	Protection	Gloves
Neoprene	General purpose engineering	Gauntlets, hand pads
Nitrile		
Nylon	Hygiene	Mitts
Polythene	Low temperature	Reversible
PVA	Radiation	Surgical, X-ray
PVC-impregnated cotton		
PVC		
Rubber		
Terrycloth		
Terylene		

PVA, polyvinyl acrylate; PVC, polyvinyl chloride.

Foot and leg protection

Anti-static footwear	Knee pads
Boots and shoes	Leggings
Chemical footwear	Moulded footwear
Clogs	Non-slip footwear
Cold-storage footwear	Over boots and over shoes
Conductive footwear	Rubber ankle boots
Foundry boots	Soles and heels
Gaiters/spats	Thigh boots
Knee boots	

Body protection

Materials	Protection	Garments
Asbestos	Buoyant	Aprons
Chain-mail	Chemical	Armlets and sleeves
Cotton (denim, etc.)	Exposure	Capes
Glass fibre	Fire/flame/heat resistant	Coats and jackets
Leather	High-visibility fluorescent	Disposable gloves
Melton	Ionising radiation	Hoods and sou'westers
Moleskin	Proofed	
Neoprene	Quilted	Overalls
Nylon, terylene	Ventilated	Suits — hot entry
Paper and disposable		Trousers
Plastic coated		
Polyurethane		
PVC		
Wool		

9.3.4 General points

1 Protective clothing materials may be attacked and degraded by contact with chemicals (permeation leading to degradation leading to penetration). Protective clothing designed to withstand chemicals comes in a variety of forms and materials, each with its own characteristics with regard to resistance to chemical permeation. Permeation rates with different manufacturers' garments may vary even with the same material. Therefore, it is important to know the breakthrough times before selection.

2 Whilst the material may be suitable, seams and joints in garments may allow the passage of particles, liquids and/or vapours. This can be aggravated by the bellows action of body movement within a clothing assembly. In addition, continual flexing of the material allows liquids to pass through more readily.

3 Protective clothing, particularly a whole-body garment, sets up a microclimate, inside which the loss of body heat may be limited, causing discomfort and leading to possible stress. Some such garments can be ventilated.

4 Some garments restrict the movement of limbs, which slows the worker and increases fatigue.

5 Provision must be made for changing, cleaning and storage of protective clothing.

6 Impervious gloves must be sufficiently long to tuck under a sleeve to prevent materials from spilling inside.

7 Low temperatures may make certain plastic materials too stiff to be usable.

8 Caution must be exercised in the use of latex gloves, especially in those with a history of allergy.

9.4 Respiratory protection

The choice of equipment in this field is vast, ranging from the simple disposable dust mask to the full, self-contained breathing apparatus, and there is much confusion as to which device to use for a particular hazard. As the wrong choice may seriously affect the health of the wearer, and could lead to asphyxiation, advice from an expert is required. In addition, user training is essential, whatever device is chosen, and servicing and cleaning facilities must be provided.

9.4.1 Legal requirements
• Health and Safety at Work, etc. Act 1974.

- Factories Act 1961, Section 30.
- SI 1956 No. 1768, Coal and Other Mines (Fire and Rescue) Regulations 1966.
- SI 1961 No. 1345, The Breathing Apparatus, etc. (Report on Examination) Order.
- SI 1987 No. 2115, The Control of Asbestos at Work Regulations.
- SI 1980 No. 1248, The Control of Lead at Work Regulations.
- SI 1950 No. 65, as amended by SI 1963 No. 879 and SI 1973 No. 36, The Pottery (Health and Welfare) Special Regulations.
- SI 1960 No. 1932, The Shipbuilding and Ship-Repairing Regulations.
- SI 1994 No. 3246, Control of Substances Hazardous to Health Regulations.

9.4.2 Standards and codes, BS and BS EN

- *BS EN 132*. Respiratory protective devices — definitions.
- *BS EN 133*. Respiratory protective devices — classification.
- *BS EN 134*. Respiratory protective devices — nomenclature of components.
- *BS EN 135*. Respiratory protective devices — list of equivalent terms.
- *BS EN 136*. Part 10. Parts for full face masks for respiratory protective devices: specification for full face masks for special use.
- *BS EN 137*. Specification for respiratory protective devices — self-contained open-circuit compressed air breathing apparatus.
- *BS EN 139*. Respiratory protective devices — compressed air-line breathing apparatus for use with full face mask, half mask or mouthpiece assembly — requirements, testing, marking.
- *BS EN 141*. Specification for gas filters and combined filters used in respiratory protective equipment.
- *BS EN 143*. Specification for particle filters used in respiratory protective devices.
- *BS EN 146*. Respiratory protective devices: specification for powered particle filtering devices incorporating helmets or hoods.
- *BS EN 147*. Respiratory devices: specification for power-assisted particle filtering devices incorporating full face masks, half masks or quarter masks.
- *BS EN 149*. Specification for filtering half masks to protect against particles.
- *BS EN 371*. Specification for AX gas filters and combined filters against low boiling organic compounds used in respiratory protective equipment.
- *BS EN 372*. Specification for SX gas filters and combined filters against specific named compounds used in respiratory protective equipment.

- *BS EN 400*. Respiratory protective devices for self-rescue — self-contained closed-circuit breathing apparatus — compressed oxygen escape apparatus — requirements, testing, marking.
- *BS EN 401*. Respiratory protective devices for self-rescue — self-contained closed-circuit breathing apparatus — chemical oxygen (KO_2) escape apparatus — requirements, testing, marking.
- *BS EN 402*. Specification for respiratory protective devices for escape — self-contained open-circuit compressed air breathing apparatus with full face mask or mouthpiece assembly.
- *BS EN 403*. Specification for filtering respiratory protective devices with hood for self-rescue from fire.
- *BS EN 404*. Respiratory devices for self-rescue — filter self-rescuer.
- *BS EN 405*. Respiratory protective devices — valved filtering half masks to protect against gases or gases and particles.
- *BS 4275*. Recommendations for the selection, use and maintenance of respiratory protective equipment (RPE) (inc. nominal protection factor (npf)).
- *BS 4400*. Method for sodium chloride particulate test for respiratory filters.
- *BS 4667*. Part 4. Specification for breathing apparatus — open-circuit escape breathing apparatus. Part 5. Specification for breathing apparatus — closed-circuit escape.
- *BS 7170*. Specification for respiratory protective devices: self-contained closed-circuit compressed oxygen breathing apparatus.
- *BS 7309*. Specification for mouthpiece assemblies for respiratory protective devices.
- *BS 7355*. Specification for full face masks for respiratory protective devices.
- *BS 7356*. Specification for half masks and quarter masks for respiratory protective devices.

9.4.3 Types available

The efficiency of respiratory protection in the removal of contaminants is expressed as the npf, which is defined as the ratio of the concentration of the contaminant present in the ambient atmosphere to the calculated concentration within the facepiece when the respiratory protection is being worn, i.e.:

$$npf = \frac{\text{concentration of contaminant in the atmosphere}}{\text{concentration of contaminant in the facepiece}}$$

The npf is used to determine the degree of protection required, knowing the concentration of pollutant in the workplace and the required concentration inhaled by the worker. However, actual protection factors, commonly referred to as effective or workplace protection factors (epf or wpf), are often much lower than the quoted npf.

Respirators

These operate by drawing the inhaled air through a medium that will remove most of the contaminant. For dust and fibres, the medium is a filter which is replaced when dirty, but, for gases and vapours, the medium is a chemical adsorbent specifically designed for the gas or vapour to be removed. The medium is carried in a canister or a cartridge for ease of handling and renewal. Extreme caution must be observed to ensure that the correct medium is used for the pollutant in question; where dust and fibres are concerned, it is important to consider the size range of the particles to be removed in order to select the appropriate filter medium. Filters are also available for combinations of dust, gases and vapours. It is important to note that respirators do not provide any protection from an atmosphere deficient in oxygen.

Disposable respirators are manufactured from the filtering material; some are suitable for respirable-sized dust. The facepiece is at a negative pressure as the lung provides the motive power; npf ≈ 5.

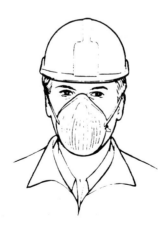

Half-mask respirators are manufactured from rubber or plastic, and are designed to cover the nose and mouth; they have a replaceable filter cartridge. With the appropriate cartridge fitted, they are suitable for dust, gas or vapour. The facepiece is at a negative pressure as the lung provides the motive power; npf ≈ 10.

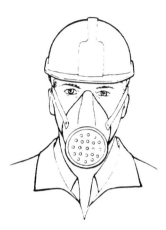

Full-facepiece respirators are manufactured from rubber or plastic, and are designed to cover the mouth, nose and eyes. The filter medium is contained in a canister directly coupled or connected via a flexible tube. With the appropriate canister fitted, they are suitable for dust, gas or vapour. The facepiece is at a negative pressure as the lung provides the motive power; npf ≈ 50.

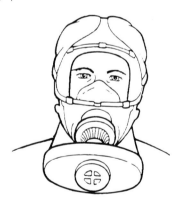

Powered respirators with a half mask or full facepiece are made of rubber or plastic, maintained at a positive pressure, as the air is drawn through the filter by means of a battery-powered fan. The fan, filter and battery are normally carried on the belt, with a flexible tube to supply the cleaned air to the facepiece; npf ≈ 500.

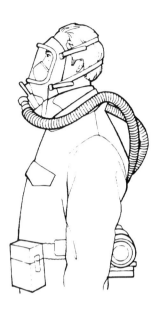

Powered visor respirators have a fan and filters carried in a helmet, with the cleaned air blown down over the wearer's face inside a hinged visor. The visor can be fitted with side shields, which can be sized to suit the wearer's face. The battery pack is normally carried on the belt. A range of filters and absorbents is available, and a welder's type is also produced; npf ≈ 1–20. It is worth noting that, for both powered respirators and powered visor respirators, because the air is drawn into

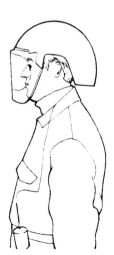

the filter(s) either in the small of the back or nape of the neck, the air is often cleaner than that found in the breathing zone. Therefore, although the npf may be low, the epf or wpf may be much higher.

There are many variations in the types of the above devices, and manufacturers' catalogues and advice should be sought before a choice is made.

Breathing apparatus

This provides a supply of uncontaminated air from a source which is either drawn from fresh air or compressed air, or is supplied from a high-pressure cylinder carried by the wearer.

In a *fresh air hose apparatus*, a supply of fresh air is fed to a facepiece, hood or blouse via a large-diameter flexible tube. The motive power is provided either by a manually or electrically powered blower, giving a positive pressure in the facepiece. It is important to establish a suitable fresh air base for the blower and, if manually operated, two operators should be present; npf ≈ 50.

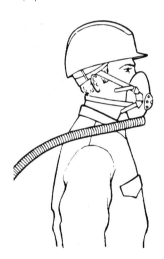

A *compressed air-line apparatus* supplies air via a reducing valve to a facepiece, hood or blouse. If the normal factory compressed air supply is used, it is necessary to filter out contaminants, such as oxides of nitrogen, carbon monoxide and oil mists, from the air before introducing it to the wearer. Specially designed air compressors for breathing apparatus are preferred, as these use special lubricating oils to minimise air contamination; npf ≈ 1000.

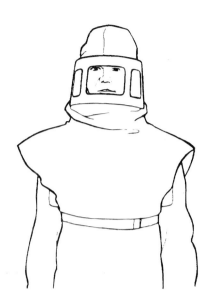

Self-contained breathing apparatus uses cylinders of air or oxygen, feeding a mouthpiece or facepiece, via a pressure-reducing valve. Open-circuit sets contain sufficient air or oxygen for a duration of use of between 10 and 30 min. Closed-circuit sets, which recirculate and purify exhaled breath, can last up to 3 h; npf ≈ 2000.

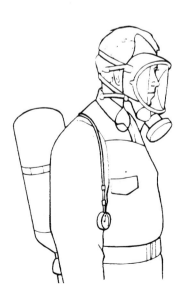

9.4.4 General points

With negative pressure facepieces, the success of the device depends largely upon the adequacy of the seal between the wearer's face and the edge of the facepiece. The sizes and shapes of human faces vary so widely that it is important to have a range of sizes available to suit every wearer. Unfortunately, this type of respirator is unsuitable for men who wear beards, even with as little as 2 days of growth. BS 5108 suggests that the following negative pressure test will reveal leaks both around the facepiece and elsewhere in the device:

> To ensure proper protection, the facepiece fit should be checked by the wearer each time he puts it on. This may be done in this way: Negative pressure test. Close the inlet of the equipment. Inhale gently so that the facepiece collapses slightly, and hold the breath for 10 seconds. If the facepiece remains in its slightly collapsed condition and no inward leakage of air is detected, the tightness of the facepiece is probably satisfactory. If the wearer detects leakage, he should re-adjust the facepiece, and repeat the test. If leakage is still noted, it can be concluded that this particular facepiece will not protect the wearer. The wearer should not continue to tighten the headband straps until they are uncomfortably tight, simply to achieve a gas-tight face fit.

Respiratory protection is generally uncomfortable to wear, particularly those forms which use the lungs to provide the motive power and have negative pressure facepieces. As the resistance of the filter has to be overcome by the wearer's lungs, the higher the resistance, the less comfortable the apparatus, and the greater the temptation to remove it for some temporary respite. This problem can be exacerbated when the work rate of the individual is high. It has been shown that the removal of the respirator, even for a short period of time, can seriously reduce the degree of protection given — the higher the npf, the more pronounced this reduction.

In order to maintain an effective protection factor, all devices, with the exception of disposable ones, require cleaning and inspection after use. The manufacturer should advise on the life of the canister or cartridge, taking into account the environment in which it is being used, and this must be replaced at the interval recommended. If the mass of contaminant the cartridge/canister is capable of adsorbing is quoted, then, by combination of the average airborne concentration, duration of exposure and breathing rate, the appropriate replacement date can be calculated. However, care needs to be taken if the interval between wearing periods is long, as the concentration of the contaminant within the adsorbent will homogenise rather than progressing across the cartridge/canister as a 'concentration front' (see Fig. 9.2). Central maintenance procedures are preferable to allowing the wearers to

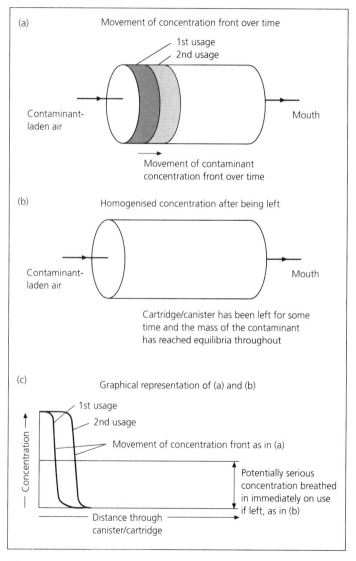

Fig. 9.2 Movement of concentration front over time.

service their own, as nominated responsible persons can build up an expertise on care and maintenance, apply routine tests and keep records on the respirators.

Wearer training and practice are essential, even with the simplest respiratory devices, but, with breathing apparatus, training courses must be extensive and thorough. No person should be allowed to wear a set, unless he/she is seen to be fully conversant with the apparatus, and knows the procedures to adopt in cases of emergency. The mines' rescue services and the fire brigades have the greatest expertise and experience in the use of self-contained non-aquatic breathing apparatus in the UK.

9.5 Hearing protection

Regulation 7 of the Noise at Work Regulations 1990 (see p. 172) requires that the exposure of employees to noise should be reduced as far as reasonably practicable by means other than the use of personal ear protectors. However, Regulation 8 requires that suitable and efficient personal ear protectors should be made available to all employees who are likely to be exposed to daily levels of noise between the 'first' (85 dB(A)) and 'second' (90 dB(A)) action levels. If employees are likely to be exposed to levels above the 'second' or 'peak' (140 dB) action levels, the employer shall provide suitable and efficient hearing protectors which, when worn properly, should reduce the levels to below those action levels.

Because noise is produced over a range of frequencies, the choice of hearing protection must be based upon the measured spectrum of the noise to be attenuated. Hearing protectors are either ear-muffs, which cover the ears, or ear-plugs, which are inserted into the ear canals. Within these two groups, however, there are several subdivisions. The ear-muffs can have several degrees of attenuation, whilst the ear-plugs can be of a variety of materials, both disposable and reusable. Figure 9.3 shows attenuation data for four types of hearing protection, and illustrates the importance of frequency.

It is recommended that hearing protection should be used if the workplace noise levels cannot be reduced to below 85 dB(A). The degree of protection provided should be such that the level at the worker's ears is below 85 dB(A).

9.5.1 Legal requirements

- Health and Safety at Work, etc. Act 1974.
- SI 1989 No. 1790, Noise at Work Regulations.

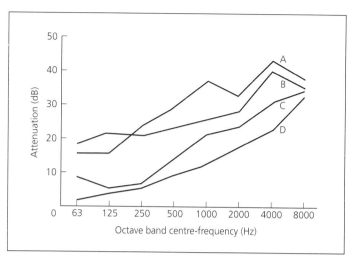

Fig. 9.3 Comparison of the attenuation data for four hearing protectors: A, high-attenuation ear-muff; B, disposable expanding polyurethane foam ear-plugs; C, low-attenuation ear-muff; D, disposable ear-plugs.

9.5.2 Standards

- BS 5108, Method of Measurement of Attenuation of Hearing Protectors at Threshold 1983.
- BS 634, Industrial Hearing Protection. Part 1: Specification for Ear-muffs 1984. Part 2: Specification for Ear-plugs 1988.

9.5.3 Types available

Ear-muffs

These consist of a cup-shaped cover over each ear, held in place by a spring-loaded headband. To ensure a good seal around the ear, the cups are edged with a cushion filled with liquid or foam. The degree of attenuation is affected by the material of the cup and its lining, and the success of the device depends upon the quality of the seal around the ear. The duration for which ear-muffs perform to specification can be very limited (i.e. months).

Ear-plugs

These can be of a variety of materials:

Disposable plugs	Reusable plugs
Glass down	Permanent moulded plastic
Plastic-coated glass down	Paste-filled rubber
Wax-impregnated cotton wool	Paste-filled plastic
Polyurethane foam	

All reusable plugs require washing after use and a sterile place for storage. Disposable plugs are available commercially in wall-mounted dispensers or in cartons containing several days' supply for one person. If noise exposure is extreme, it is possible to use ear-plugs in combination with ear-muffs.

9.5.4 Theoretical protection

To calculate the degree of protection given by hearing protectors, it is necessary to measure the sound spectrum of the noise emitted at the workplace, using octave band analysis. If the result is required in dB(A), the A-weighting values at each mid-octave frequency should be subtracted from the measured sound to provide a 'corrected level'; each mid-octave level can then be added together, according to Fig. 9.4.

The assumed protection of the hearing protector, also expressed in mid-octave values, should then be subtracted from the corrected level, and the result added as before to produce the estimated dB(A) at the wearer's ear. This can best be illustrated with an example (Table 9.1). As with respiratory protection, hearing protection can be uncomfortable,

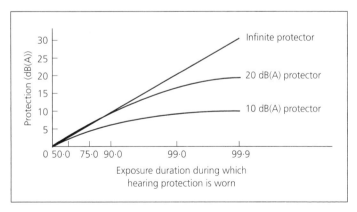

Fig. 9.4 The effects of removing hearing protectors for short periods of time. Comparison of the protection afforded by hearing protectors which reduce the instantaneous sound level by 10 dB and 20 dB. (After Else, 1974.)

Table 9.1 Example of calculation to find the degree of attenuation provided by a particular ear-muff against a typical industrial noise.

		Octave band mid-frequency (Hz)							
		63	125	250	500	1k	2k	4k	8k
Measured sound pressure level (SPL) of typical noise	dB	92	96	102	101	98	97	94	93
A-weighting correction (see p. 167)	dB	−26	−16	−9	−3	0	+1	+1	−1
Corrected level (measured SPL minus correction)	dB	66	80	93	98	98	98	95	92

Approximate summation of levels (see Fig. 5.9)

66, 80 → 80
93, 98 → 99
98, 98 → 101
95, 92 → 97
80, 99 → 99
101, 97 → 102
99, 102 → 104 dB(A)

Estimated level of noise unprotected: 104 dB(A)

		63	125	250	500	1k	2k	4k	8k
Ear-muff attenuation, mean of measurements	dB	—	13	20	33	35	38	47	41
Standard deviation (SD)	dB	—	6	6	6	6	7	8	8
Assumed protection of ear-muff (mean minus SD)	dB	—	7	14	27	29	31	39	33
Corrected level (from above)	dB	66	80	93	98	98	98	95	92
Levels at the ear (corrected level minus protection)	dB	66	73	79	71	69	67	56	59

Approximate summation of levels (see Fig. 5.9)

66, 73 → 74
79, 71 → 80
69, 67 → 71
56, 59 → 61
74, 80 → 81
71, 61 → 71
81, 71 → 81 dB(A)

Estimated level of noise at ear with protection: 81 dB(A)

particularly if worn for long periods, as the wearer may feel enclosed and isolated and, with ear-muffs, perspiration can build up around the seals. Although ear-muffs provide the greatest amount of attenuation, they are easy to remove and replace. Therefore, wearers are tempted to remove them to ease discomfort. It has been shown that the removal of hearing protection, even for short periods, will reduce the overall protection substantially, the effect being increasingly more pronounced as the noise levels increase. This effect is illustrated in Fig. 9.4, from which it can be seen that protection giving 20 dB(A) attenuation when worn 100% of the time will only give an effective 10 dB(A) protection when worn 90% of the time. If noise levels are much in excess of 90 dB(A), protection must therefore be worn continuously to maintain levels of below 85 dB(A) at the ear, averaged over the whole shift.

It can be seen from this that better overall protection may be provided by using a lower degree of attenuation from, for example, glass down ear-plugs, which may be more comfortable and more acceptable and so not be removed during the shift, than by using a higher degree of attenuation with less comfort, e.g. ear-muffs.

Servicing and replacement facilities must be provided for ear-muffs, because they will deteriorate with time, in particular at the seals, which become distorted and harden with age. A range of hearing protection should also be made available, so that wearers can choose the type that is most comfortable for them.

As with all forms of personal protective devices, adequate training must be given, so that the wearers can understand the reasons for providing these devices. In-house training programmes should be implemented, and can be aided by films and/or tape/slide presentations. Hearing protection manufacturers can assist with audio-visual aids and explanatory leaflets. Routine audiometric measurements on workers can provide an opportunity to make contact with them and to encourage them to wear hearing protection.

10 Special Issues in Occupational Health

10.1 Introduction

In addition to the occupational health issues presented in the previous chapters, the occupational health practitioner is faced with other problems which cannot always be neatly classified under section headings. This chapter constitutes a series of short accounts of aspects of occupational health of current interest. Psychosocial aspects are now of sufficient importance to warrant a chapter of their own (Chapter 11).

10.2 Working hours

The health issues related to working hours involve two aspects:
1 shift work;
2 long working hours.
Both of these working practices can be construed as involving 'unsociable' hours. That is, employees are, for one reason or another, required to work outside the limits considered by most people to be 'normal'. In practice, this equates to a 7–8-h stint between the hours of 09.00 and 17.00 for 5 days of the week.

10.2.1 Shift work

Shift work is practised by about 20% of the workforce in most countries. The need for shift work is threefold.
1 *Societal*. Services and emergencies.
2 *Technical*. Continuous process industries.
3 *Economic*. Optimal plant utilisation.
  There are various types of shift work:
- two or three shifts in a 24-h period;
- rotating or fixed shifts;
- rapid or slow rotation shifts;
- forward or backward rotation shifts;
- 8-, 10- or 12-h shifts.

  There is no doubt that rotating shift work — particularly those systems involving night work — leads to various disruptions to normal life. These include:
- *biological*: circadian dysrhythmia, cardiovascular disorders, gastrointestinal disorders;
- *psychosocial*: fatigue/sleep loss, lowered performance, increased accidents;
- *individual*: perhaps greater variation than group effects; dependent on domestic/social circumstances and coping strategies.

10.2.2 Long hours of work

Although many of the effects of rotating shift work are now well known, the effects of long working hours have received much less attention in the scientific literature. Long hours include the manager working a 50–70-h week, or the shop-floor employee working a 12-h shift for more than four shifts a week.

Fatigue has been recognised as an effect of 12-h shifts, but other putative effects, such as ill health, increased accident rates and poor performance, are less well documented and the issue is, as yet, unresolved. A particular problem here is that although the 12-h shift usually means 3–4 days off each week, it also allows for a second job to be undertaken — often in clandestine circumstances. This makes it difficult to assess the harm caused by just 3 days of 12 h.

For the manager working long hours per week, there are virtually no studies which can answer the health effect issue. Either the studies have not been executed, or the populations studied so far are rather special groups with factors that prevent any generalisation to the issue as a whole.

Nevertheless, the European Commission has promulgated a Directive on Working Time (93/104/EC), which attempts to restrict working hours in terms of both weekly total and hours to be worked in any day. There are negotiable exceptions to the Directive, but, despite the recent protestations of at least one member state (!), there is every reason to believe that health and safety issues are an important reason to restrict working hours.

10.3 Workplace injury incidents

In Great Britain, about 600 people are killed as a result of workplace incidents every year; in addition, about 1.4 million suffer injuries. In terms of fatalities, approximately 60% are employees, 15% are self-employed and 35% are members of the public. Table 10.1 provides an overview of the percentages of the types of incident that cause fatalities and major injuries.

It is evident that the rank order of incidents causing fatalities is different from that causing major injury (Table 10.2). It is also worth noting that incidents classified as 'other kind of accident' would have been ranked sixth for fatalities ($\approx 6\%$) and ninth in major injuries ($\approx 4\%$), and that the fifth and sixth most prevalent major injuries are 'injured while handling, lifting or carrying' ($\approx 7\%$) and 'struck against something fixed or stationary' ($\approx 4\%$). A cautionary note is that only about 30% of

....

Table 10.1 Approximate percentages of fatal incidents and injuries.

Type of incident	Fatalities (%)	Rank order	Injuries* (%)	Rank order
Falls from heights	22.5	1	22	2
Struck by moving vehicle	14	2	4	=7
Struck by moving/falling object	13	3	13	3
Trapped by something collapsing/overturning	7.5	4	1	10
Contact with moving machinery	6.5	5	10	4
Contact with electricity/electrical discharge	5.5	6	1.5	9
Drowning or asphyxiation	3.5	7	—	—
Exposure/contact with harmful substances	2.5	8	4	=7
Explosion	2	9	—	—
Fire	1.5	10	0.5	11
Slip, trip or fall on some level	1.0	11	29	1

*Major injuries are defined under Reporting of Injuries, Diseases and Dangerous Occurrences Regulations (RIDDOR), and include fractures, amputations, losses of consciousness and any injury resulting in immediate admittance to hospital (>24 h).

Table 10.2 The proportion of fatalities and major injuries by nature of injury.

Nature of injury	Fatalities (%)	Rank order	Major injuries (%)	Rank order
Fracture	18	1	72	1
Injuries of more than one nature	15	2	1.5	7
Contusion (bruise)	13	3	2	5
Poisonings and gassings	7	4	1	=9
Concussion and internal injuries	6	5	1.2	8
Other injuries caused by contact with electricity	5	6	—	—
Burns	4.5	7	4.5	3
Lacerations and open wounds	2	8	3.5	4
Amputation	—	—	9	2
Superficial injuries	—	—	1.5	6
Sprains and strains	—	—	1	=9

all reportable incidents to employees are reported, with the figure falling to about 5% for the self-employed.

The figures in both tables are approximate (certainly for fatalities as the numbers are, fortunately, small), and major incidents (such as Piper Alpha, 1988) could alter the proportions and rank order. However, these figures are presented to provide a feel for the types of incident and their outcome.

10.3.1 Safety management

Over the last few years, there has been a shift away from the prevention of repetitions of accidents (reactive prevention) (which is easier, but unreliable) towards proactive prevention, where the probabilities of a range of unwanted outcomes are considered and an integrated control plan is implemented.

Workplace incidents are very rarely caused by a single unsafe act or condition, but, more commonly, by a combination of factors. An 'unsafe act' can include human actions which are unintentional, i.e. 'unintentional errors', and intentional risky behaviour, i.e. 'violations'. However, it could be said that it is unsafe acts by an individual or group, often remote in time and place from the workplace, that create conditions where unsafe acts by the workforce can lead to accidents. These remote errors by managers have been referred to as 'latent' or 'decision' failures, and those by the workforce at risk as 'active' failures.

10.3.2 Proactive safety management

Programmes to prevent workplace incidents must address the following four elements of the accident causation process.

1 *Multicausality.* It must be recognised that most accidents have multiple causes, and that, to identify and prevent their occurrence, it is necessary to investigate all aspects of an organisation, and attempt to alter its perception of occupational health and safety.

2 *Active and latent failures.* An active failure is one in which the error has an immediate adverse effect (equivalent to an unsafe act), whereas a latent failure may exist within an organisation for some time and may only manifest itself when combined with appropriate active failures (unsafe acts/conditions).

3 *Skill-, rule- and knowledge-based errors, and violations.* Skill-based errors are 'lapses' in highly practised and routine tasks. If an individual assesses a situation and makes the wrong decision, this is a rule-based error, and knowledge-based errors are those in which there is no rule to cope with a situation. Violations are when an individual deliberately undertakes a task contrary to the rule.

4 *Hazard identification, risk assessment and preventive action.* The avoidance of latent failures necessitates the identification of hazards, the assessment of risk and the selection, implementation and measurement of the preventive actions taken. Clearly, it is implicit that individuals must recognise and accept responsibility and have the appropriate knowledge and skills to recognise, evaluate and control.

The Management of Health and Safety at Work Regulations 1992 and the Health and Safety Executive's publication, Successful Health and Safety Management (HS(G) 65, 1991), state four key functions for the management of health and safety.

1 *Policy and planning.* Determine goals, quantifiable objectives/priorities and a programme of work capable of achieving the objectives. The relative success of this programme must then be measured and, if appropriate, revised.

2 *Organisation and communication.* Clearly defined responsibility and lines of two-way communication must be determined.

3 *Hazard management.* Hazards must be identified and their risks assessed. Appropriate control measures must be determined, implemented and reviewed over time.

4 *Monitoring and review.* It is essential that steps 1, 2 and 3 are not only in place, but are in use and are seen to work in the conflicting world of commerce.

10.3.3 Safety culture

It is possible that an organisation may have all of the relevant parts of a safety programme in place, but that the culture associated with safety may be inappropriate or even poor. Organisations with a positive safety culture have a number of crucial elements, as reported by the Confederation of British Industry (CBI) in their report 'Developing a Safety Culture':

- importance of leadership and the commitment of the Chief Executive;
- the executive safety role of line management;
- involvement of all employees;
- openness of communication;
- demonstration of care and concern for all those affected by the business.

Researchers at the US Nuclear Regulating Commission (NUREG) state that the key predictive indicators of safety performance are as follows, in rank order.

1 Effective communication, leading to commonly understood goals and means to achieve these goals at all levels in the organisation.

2 Good organisational learning, where organisations are tuned to identify and respond to incremental change.

3 Organisational focus; simply the attention devoted by the organisation to workplace health and safety.

4 External factors, including the financial health of the parent organisation, or simply the economic climate within which the company is working and the impact of regulating bodies.

It should be evident from the foregoing that the basic philosophy and elements of workplace incidents (safety) are not dissimilar to those of occupational health. Although, perhaps, considering the immediacy of workplace incidents, the success (or failure) of intervention of safety management is much more obvious than it is for good occupational health practice.

Repetitive strain injury (RSI)

10.4.1 Synonyms
- Repetitive motion injuries.
- Cumulative trauma disorder (CTD).
- Occupational overuse syndrome (OOS).
- Work-related repetitive movement injury (WRRMI).
- Work-related upper limb disorders (WRULDs).

10.4.2 Definition
The definition of the condition is controversial and confusing. Repetitive strain injury was first used to refer to pain and discomfort in the upper limbs from work tasks that involved repetitive movements and/or constrained postures. Usage of the term was then widened to include similar effects involving the lower limbs. Arguments against the use of the term 'repetitive strain injury' include the lack of evidence of 'injury', the inappropriateness of the word 'strain' and the fact that static loads without repetitive movements can also produce similar clinical effects. Other synonyms proposed later confined the use of the term to the upper limbs, and included effects arising only from work activity (see above). The term 'non-specific forearm pain' has been proposed for cases of vague forearm pain with no evidence of clearly identified disease.

The wrists and elbows are the common sites of involvement. The term RSI encompasses a variety of clinical entities, all of which can present with pain and discomfort, are associated with repetitive movements and are attributed to or made worse by work factors/activities:
- tenosynovitis;
- de Quervain's disease;
- peritendinitis crepitans;
- carpal tunnel syndrome (wrists);
- epicondylitis (elbow joints).

10.4.3 Clinical features

• Persistent pain and discomfort of the muscles, tendons or soft tissues of the limbs.

• Swelling, tenderness and other features indicating inflammation may be present, especially in the acute stages.

• Crepitus may be present on examination.

• Tingling sensation and numbness, especially with accompanying peripheral nerve involvement.

The symptoms can be acute, recurrent or chronic.

10.4.4 Relevant exposures

• Dynamic load — repeated, frequent movements of the limbs over a prolonged period (as over an 8-h working day with limited rest periods).

• Movements throughout the full range of motions at the joints, e.g. from pronation to supination and back.

• Awkward postures and/or postures at the extremes of the range of movement, e.g. hyperflexion or hyperextension, or ulnar/medial deviation at the wrist.

• Static load — e.g. using the limbs to support weight, or holding the limbs against force or pressure, for sustained periods of time.

10.4.5 Other contributory factors

The extent to which some of these factors contribute to the occurrence of RSI remains debatable.

• *Non-occupational factors*. Where repetitive movements and other relevant exposures also occur from non-occupational activity, such as hobbies or household chores, these exposures can contribute to the clinical effects. However, with hobbies, in particular, there is a degree of control over discontinuation of these non-occupational activities if necessary. Similar control may not be available in carrying out work tasks.

• *Previous injury* affecting the same sites may predispose to pain and discomfort. This depends on the nature and severity of the previous injury.

• *Individual susceptibility*. Some cases have been described in part-time rather than full-time workers, and sometimes in those with relatively minor manual tasks but not in others with considerable physical effort in the performance of work duties. This suggests that work activity is not the only determining factor in the development of RSI.

• *Psychological overlay* — especially with monotonous work, where a bonus is paid depending on work output or if work performance is affected by peer pressure from supervisors or team members. The presentation and persistence of symptoms can also be affected by concurrent psychosocial stress.

• *Financial compensation*. Schemes for providing monetary benefits for work-related illnesses have been thought to contribute to the reporting of cases. This includes state-administered schemes as well as civil court claims. The extent may also be related to the perceived difficulty or ease of obtaining benefits.

10.4.6 Extent of the problem

In developing countries, such as those in the Far East, RSI seems to be relatively rare, whereas in Australia there was an apparent epidemic followed by a decline. Many reasons have been suggested for the decline, including effective measures of prevention and intervention and a change in the compensation scheme. In the UK, there is a steady reporting of cases, with tenosynovitis being the second most common prescribed occupational disease after occupational dermatitis.

Some occupations and industries with a high prevalence of RSI are:

• poultry processing;
• electronics assembly;
• mechanical components assembly line;
• data processing;
• telephonists;
• checkout operators at supermarkets and stores.

RSI is more common in women and in blue-collar workers.

10.4.7 Treatment

Clinical treatment provides varying degrees of relief from persistent symptoms. Treatment regimes vary depending on the severity, site and clinical findings. Procedures that have been tried include:

• surgery;
• rest with immobilisation of the affected area;
• physiotherapy;
• analgesics and non-steroidal anti-inflammatory drugs (NSAIDs);
• local injection with hydrocortisone;
• ultrasound;
• infrared treatment;
• acupuncture.

Where there are contributory factors in the system of work, these treatment procedures are less likely to be effective unless accompanied by improvements in job design, or in the ergonomics of work stations.

10.4.8 Prevention

- Attention to ergonomics at the workplace.
- Proper design of machinery, tools and equipment.
- Adequate information, instruction and training of operators.
- Sufficient rest periods during the working day. Views on this vary from prescriptive rest breaks of 5 min every 1–2 h to a general recommendation of not having a system of mandatory rest periods, but allowing flexibility in the system of work to enable employees to take rest breaks as needed. Arguments against the latter include the difficulty of managerial control when individuals are away from their work area, and work procedures that do not allow much flexibility, thereby making it difficult for employees to take a break even when needed, e.g. working on tracking computer data in real time.
- Job rotation with a variety of job tasks requiring a range of different physical activities and effort. Systems of rotation could include different jobs during a shift or different jobs on a week-to-week basis.
- Prompt response and clinical support for those who develop symptoms.
- Pre-placement assessment of those with previous musculoskeletal problems.

10.5 Occupational health for health-care workers

10.5.1 Introduction

Health-care workers form the largest occupational group in many countries. In the UK, the health service is the largest employer of labour, and the National Health Service is probably the largest employer in Europe. The job categories in health care are varied. They include:

1 staff dealing directly with patient care, e.g.
  - doctors, nurses, midwives;
  - scientific officers;
  - laboratory and physiological measurement technicians;
  - pharmacists;
  - physiotherapists;
  - ambulance crew;
2 ancillary and support staff, e.g.
  - administrative and clerical personnel;
  - porters, painters, drivers;
  - laundry, catering and maintenance staff.

There are also trainee grades for some of the above groups. From an occupational health perspective, it is essential to consider health and safety aspects for all staff, including trainees and students, locum grades and patients, visitors and volunteer workers.

The areas of work are also varied, and include sites within hospitals, clinics, public areas and even homes of patients (e.g. for visits by domiciliary health-care staff, general practitioners and ambulance staff). It may also be possible for some health-care facilities to be provided in supermarkets and shopping centres! The traditional work areas include:

- operating theatres
- X-ray departments;
- outpatient departments;
- wards (e.g. medical and surgical, intensive care, coronary care);
- laboratories, mortuaries and post-mortem rooms;
- dental surgeries;
- general practice premises;
- offices;
- kitchens.

The range of hazards is considerable.

10.5.2 Physical hazards

- Ionising radiation is present in radiology departments, and also in clinics and dental surgeries where X-rays are taken. In countries in which mobile vans provide mass miniature radiography, there is a potential for staff to be exposed to ionising radiation. Radioisotopes used for treatment or investigation represent an unsealed source of radiation.
- Nuclear magnetic resonance has become increasingly used in diagnosis. This can affect those who use cardiac pacemakers. The long-term effects of exposure to magnetic fields are, as yet, unknown.

10.5.3 Chemical hazards

- Sensitisers and allergens, such as acrylates (used in orthopaedics and dentistry) and glutaraldehyde (used to sterilise endoscopes). Latex gloves have also been identified as a cause of respiratory and skin problems in health-care staff.
- Toxic chemicals are used in laboratories, although the amounts employed tend to be in much smaller quantities than in industrial processes. Examples include xylene in histopathology laboratories and formaldehyde in the same laboratories and in post-mortem rooms and mortuaries.
- Narcotic gases include the anaesthetic agents. Nitrous oxide, halothane, enflurane and cyclohexane are four such agents that have

been allocated an occupational exposure limit (OEL) in the UK. In the main, this is due to the possible effects in recovery room personnel, anaesthetists and anaesthetic assistants who are exposed to exhaled anaesthetic gases from patients on a daily basis. Scavenging devices and improved local and general ventilation in operating theatres and recovery rooms have helped to reduce the exposures to below the OELs. Nitrous oxide is present together with oxygen in Entonox, which is a gas used for analgesia. There are concerns that the availability of Entonox in ambulances may facilitate its abuse as a recreational drug.

• Cytotoxic drugs are used for treating patients with cancer. Some of these are alkylating agents; others act as anti-metabolites or inhibit deoxyribonucleic acid (DNA) enzymes. Because of their action on cellular DNA, contact with these drugs by health-care staff should be kept to a minimum. Staff at risk of exposure include pharmacists, nurses and doctors, who have to prepare and administer the drugs, and cleaners, who dispose of waste from patients who have been given these drugs, and who are also responsible for the removal of soiled and contaminated bedding and linen.

10.5.4 Mechanical and ergonomic hazards

• Low back pain in nurses is a well recognised cause of long-term sickness absence in this group of health-care staff. Part of this may be related to the inappropriate lifting of patients in awkward situations. Contributory factors include the heavy and/or struggling patient, crowded and narrow work areas, lack of lifting aids and poor techniques for lifting and carrying loads. Training in manual handling is important, and attention to assessment of the task, with the provision of assistance when needed, could reduce the incidence of back pain.

10.5.5 Biological hazards (see also Chapter 6)

Blood-borne infections, such as hepatitis B, hepatitis C and human immunodeficiency virus (HIV), can be acquired by health-care staff from contact with infected blood and body fluids. This may occur from needlestick injuries, which are common in medical and nursing staff. Laboratory staff who have to process blood samples sent from abroad, or research staff working on specific infectious agents, have been known to develop certain exotic infections, such as malaria, toxoplasmosis, scrub typhus and Rocky Mountain spotted fever. Pathologists and post-mortem technicians are at risk of tuberculosis (TB).

Occupational health services for health-care staff have systems for screening new categories of staff for their immune status before they begin work. The aim of screening is twofold. Firstly, to protect the staff against occupational infections, and, secondly, to ensure that patients are not put at risk. Immune status for hepatitis B, TB and rubella is usually determined. If staff are not immune, vaccination can confer protection. Where indicated, determination of carrier status and advice on safe systems of work, or redeployment when necessary, will reduce the risk to patients.

10.5.6 Psychosocial hazards (see also Chapter 11)

Stress among health-care workers is well recognised. Some of the contributing factors are:

- long hours of work, e.g. for junior medical staff;
- unsociable hours, e.g. shift system for nurses and interrupted meal or rest breaks (to respond quickly to emergencies) for paramedics and ambulance crew;
- dealing with very sick or dying patients and their families, e.g. care assistants and hospice staff;
- having to make decisions on matters of life and death;
- organisational change;
- conflict between ensuring the best care for patients vs. the costs of treatment;
- coping with busy schedules, having to study and prepare for professional examinations, allocating sufficient time for their families and meeting repayment costs of medical school loans, e.g. doctors in training.

As the causes of stress are often multifactorial, efforts to reduce stress may be of limited success, or may only appear to succeed temporarily. The efforts by the occupational health service include trying to eliminate or reduce identified causes, and providing counselling and support for the individual to cope with stress. The former is fraught with difficulties, especially if the management system is thought to be the main contributor to stress in the staff. If difficulties with spouses or family, or financial problems, are identified, these factors are outside the influence of the occupational health service and, sometimes, out of the control of the individual.

Violence and assaults on health-care staff are becoming of increasing concern to occupational health departments in the health service. Certain groups of staff are more at risk from verbal and physical threats. These groups include:

- receptionists;

- accident and emergency staff;
- ambulance crews;
- general practitioners on house calls;
- community nurses;
- prison services' medical and nursing staff.

The source of these threats may be patients, their relatives or members of the public. The reasons are varied and include:

- frustration from waiting for medical attention when they perceive that they are an emergency and should be attended to immediately;
- anger at what they feel is inappropriate or unsuccessful treatment;
- attempts to obtain drugs or medicines from the health-care staff;
- staff on shift duties going to and from work unaccompanied at different times of the day and night.

Attempts to reduce the likelihood of violence and assault to staff have focused on:

- better training of health-care staff in dealing with the public, with emphasis on communication skills;
- breakaway techniques for coping with physical threats;
- improved security in hospitals and at staff quarters;
- counselling and support for victims of violence and assaults.

10.6 Audit and quality improvement in occupational health

10.6.1 Introduction

Audit and quality improvement principles have been successfully introduced in occupational health to improve the delivery of occupational health services. A number of factors have contributed to this development, including economic, professional, social and legal considerations.

Economic

The rising cost of health care has focused attention on ensuring that the maximum value is gained from the use of health-care resources. Pressure on occupational health services to demonstrate that they are providing cost-efficient and effective services is a part of this general trend. In addition, occupational health services often face pressures from their employers to demonstrate that they do make a contribution to the economic success of the host organisation. Audit and quality improvement are sometimes used as a means of enhancing the efficiency and effectiveness of services, primarily for economic reasons.

Professional

The wide variations which exist between occupational health departments in the methods by which they undertake common practices have caused occupational health professionals to question the basis of their practice, and to seek evidence on which to base their practice. Audit and quality improvement have been used to identify, investigate and address variations in common practices, such as pre-employment assessment or the management of cases of sickness absence, for the purpose of improving professional performance.

Social

The consumers of health care (as individuals or organisations) are now much better informed about choices in health care than they were previously, and expect to be involved in decision making. Health-care professionals are encouraged to become more open and accountable to their clients. Audit and quality improvement processes have been used to widen the involvement of customers in the planning and delivery of occupational health care. This approach has been successful in increasing the uptake of services.

Legal

The increasing trend towards litigation in health care has led to the need to record and document practice more rigorously than in the past. Clear criteria for the delivery of services, professional standards and records of audit can help to protect the practitioner as well as the user of occupational health services.

10.6.2 Professional audit

Medical and clinical audit is the systematic, critical analysis of the quality of care, including the use of resources and the resulting outcome and quality of life for the patient. It can involve audit of the structure, process or outcome of care, and commonly is undertaken by setting standards and measuring performance against those standards.

Audit spiral

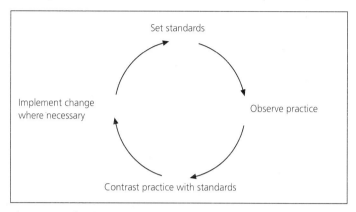

The process of audit is iterative, and opportunities to improve further the quality of care should be sought as a continuous process. Standards which are set by the professionals involved are used to improve services; therefore, it is essential that the standards which are adopted are based upon the best evidence available. Peer-reviewed research papers, guidance documents and evidence of effectiveness should be used to support standard setting. Once standards are set, these must be reviewed regularly and must not be allowed to become obstructions to improvements in the future.

10.6.3 Quality principles

The recipients of health care, i.e. patients, clients or organisations, expect the professionals delivering health care to be trained and competent. How, when and at what cost they deliver health care are open to negotiation, and those using or paying for the service expect to play a role in negotiating the type of service with which they are to be provided. The principles of quality management can be used to underpin the planning and delivery of services. These principles are described below.

Customer identification

Quality management systems require services to be customer orientated. Customers of an occupational health service will include those who are paying for the service, those who are using the service and those who may be affected by the service. Interactive management presentations, staff surveys and user groups can be employed to help to identify and involve customers of the service.

Needs assessment

A structured needs assessment should be conducted to identify the actual as opposed to the perceived needs of the organisation. A dialogue between service providers, purchasers and users needs to be established, so that clear expectations and priorities can be identified. Occupational health professionals may need to educate the customers as part of the process of needs assessment, but must also be prepared to listen and respond to the needs of their clients.

Critical success factors

The occupational health service needs to agree with its customers the factors which are critical to its own success, i.e. those factors which the service must achieve in order to meet the customer's expectations. Experience suggests that there should be no more than eight critical success factors which can be used as goals for the service to achieve.

Key processes

Having established what the service is intended to achieve, the key processes which will be used to attain these goals should be identified and reviewed to improve their efficiency and effectiveness. Some practices may have to be curtailed and new ones introduced.

Performance indicators

In order to manage the delivery of services, it is necessary to have some means of measuring the quantity and quality of services delivered. Performance indicators need to be realistic, clearly defined and capable of being measured objectively. The information provided by the performance indicators can be used to monitor progress and lead to the correction of faults. It is essential that performance indicators are reviewed regularly by providers, purchasers and users of the service.

Occupational cancer

Volumes have been written on this subject, but space allows only the briefest survey here. A short historical account is followed by an annotated list of some of the characteristics of occupational cancer, and by some lists indicating the probable and possible human carcinogens of occupational origin.

10.7.1 Historical perspective

The first recognised association between cancer and occupation was made in 1775 by Percival Pott, a surgeon at St Bartholomew's Hospital, London. He noted an increased incidence of scrotal cancer in chimney sweeps, and, rejecting the venereal aetiology popular in his day, thought that the tumour was more likely to be due to soot. Further observations later linked other components of fossil fuel with skin cancer — notably of the scrotum — but it took many long and arduous laboratory experiments before the link was confirmed experimentally in the first quarter of the twentieth century. The compounds implicated were all polynuclear aromatic hydrocarbons, examples of which include the following:

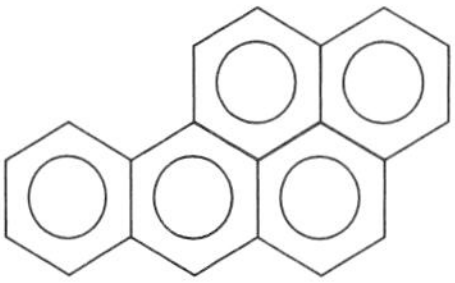

Benzo(α)pyrine

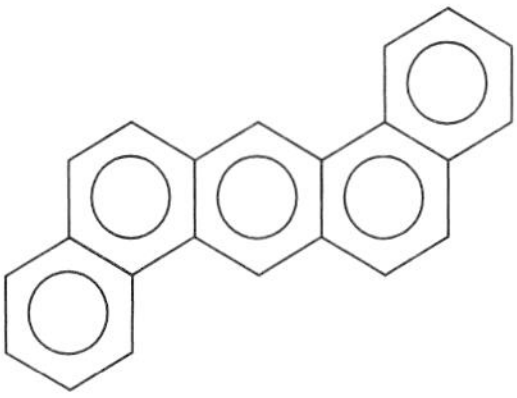

Dibenz(α,β)anthracene

In 1895, Rehn described bladder tumours in workers in the aniline dye industries. Subsequently, a range of aromatic amines have been noted to be bladder carcinogens. Examples include the following:

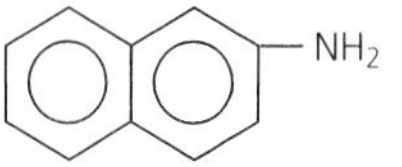

2-Naphthylamine

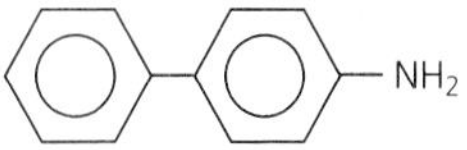

4-Aminobiphenyl

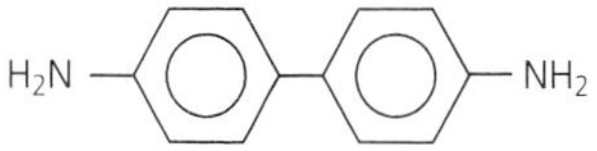

Benzidine

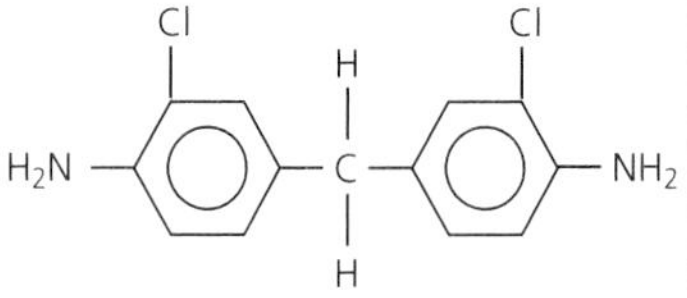

Methylene-bis-O-chloraniline

Despite the length of time that has elapsed since the discovery of these carcinogens, workers are still contracting tumours from these or similar agents, and will continue to do so. This is partly due to the legacy of a long latent period (sometimes exceeding 40 years), partly because effective substitutes of such materials have not always been available and, in some cases, such as benzene and vinyl chloride monomer, society has chosen to continue to use these agents — albeit more safely.

10.7.2 Theories of chemical carcinogenesis

Chemicals form the bulk of the occupationally related carcinogens, and it is important to distinguish between the different classes. In brief, two broad groups are postulated. *Genotoxic* carcinogens pose a clear qualitative hazard to health as they are capable of altering cellular genetic material, and thus should theoretically cause cancer after a single exposure. On the other hand, *epigenetic* carcinogens seem to be without direct effect on genetic material and to require high or prolonged exposure for effect. The genotoxic carcinogens probably have no safe threshold; the epigenetic carcinogens may have.

A tentative classification, which seems reasonable in animal models, can be expressed as shown in Table 10.3.

Table 10.3 Classification of chemical carcinogens.

Type	Mode of action	Example
Genotoxic		
Direct action	Interacts with DNA	Bis(chloromethyl)ether
Secondary action	Requires conversion to direct type	2-Naphthylamine
Inorganic	Affects DNA replication	Nickel salts
Epigenetic		
'Solid state'	Mesenchymal cell effects	Asbestos
Hormone	Endocrine effect ± promoter	Diethylstilboestrol
Immunosuppressor	Stimulates certain tumour growth	Azathioprine
Co-carcinogen	Enhances genotoxic types when given at same time	Ethanol
Promoter	Enhances genotoxic types when given subsequently	Bile acids

10.7.3 Characteristics of occupational carcinogens

Tumours of occupational origin are usually indistinguishable, histopathologically and symptomatically, from non-occupational tumours. Nevertheless, there are some characteristics of note.

1 They tend to occur earlier than 'spontaneous' tumours of the same site.

2 Exposure to the putative agent is repeated, but not necessarily continuous.

3 The latent period is 10–40 years.

4 The tumours are often multiple in a given organ.

5 Despite widely differing estimates of the proportion of all cancers caused by occupation, the true figure probably lies in the range of 3–8%. However, if one adds in the interaction of occupational exposures with other risk factors, e.g. asbestos and cigarette smoking, the range doubles to 5–15%. For some shop floor groups in some industries, and for some tumour sites, such as lung and bladder, the risks can rise to 20–40%. Multiple chemical exposures, which are the norm in modern industry, make it, however, exceedingly difficult to isolate particular individual chemicals as the guilty parties. The role of synergism is probably important, although still largely unquantified.

10.7.4 Known or suspected occupational carcinogens

The length of the list and its individual members vary according to which organisation has compiled it. Perhaps the most widely accepted list is that of the International Agency for Research on Cancer (IARC). They regularly review the evidence for carcinogenicity of compounds and processes, where published data exist suggesting a cancer effect. Their evaluations depend on animal data, short-term mutagenicity tests and human evidence, with the greatest weight given to sound epidemiological evidence.

The compound or chemical is then graded for evidence of carcinogenicity into one of four categories:

- sufficient;
- limited;
- inadequate;
- lacking.

The overall evaluation has five groupings.

- *Group 1*. The agent (mixture) is carcinogenic to humans. The exposure circumstance entails exposures that are carcinogenic to humans.
- *Group 2A*. The agent (mixture) is 'probably' carcinogenic to humans. The exposure circumstance entails exposures that are 'probably' carcinogenic to humans.
- *Group 2B*. The agent (mixture) is 'possibly' carcinogenic to humans. The exposure circumstance entails exposures that are 'possibly' carcinogenic to humans.
- *Group 3*. The agent (mixture, exposure circumstance) is not classifiable as to its carcinogenicity to humans.
- *Group 4*. The agent (mixture, exposure circumstance) is probably not carcinogenic to humans.

Table 10.4 IARC list of Group 1 carcinogens (1997) (Vols 1–68).

Chemical	Industrial process	Medicinal	Other
4-Aminobiphenyl	Aluminium production	Azothioprine	Aflatoxins
Arsenic and arsenic compounds	Auramine (manufacture)	N,N-Bis(2-chloroethyl)-2-naphthylamine	Alcohol
Asbestos	Boot and shoe manufacture	Chlorambucil	Betel nut (with tobacco)
Benzene	Coal gasification	Cyclosporin	Solar radiation
Benzidine	Coke production	Cyclophosphamide	Tobacco
BCME	Haematite mining (U/G) (with radon exposure)	Melphalan	
CMME		Methyl CCNU	
Chromium compounds (hexavalent)	Iron and steel founding	MOPP	
Coal tar pitches	Isopropyl alcohol manufacture (strong acid process)	Myleran	
Coal tar	Magenta (manufacture)	Oestrogens (some steroidal and non-steroidal)	
Dioxin (TCDD)	Painting	Oral contraceptive (combinations)	
Ethylene oxide	Rubber industry	Phenacetin (in analgesic mixtures)	
Erionite	Wood (furniture and cabinet making)	Tamoxifen*	
Inorganic acid mists (strong) containing sulphuric acid		Thiotepa	
Mineral oils (untreated and mildly treated)		Treosulfan	
Mustard gas			
2-Naphthylamine			
Nickel compounds			
Radon (and its decay products)			
Silica (crystalline)			
Shale oils			
Soots			
Talc (containing asbestos)			
Vinyl chloride			

BCME, bis(chloromethyl)ether; CMME, chloromethyl methyl ether; CCNU, lomustine; MOPP, mustine, vincristine, procarbazine, prednisolone; U/G, underground.
*But *prevents* breast cancer.

Table 10.5 Occupations recognised as presenting a carcinogenic risk.

Industry	Occupation	Site of tumour	Likely carcinogen
Agriculture, forestry, fishing	Farmers, seamen	Skin	Ultraviolet light
	Vineyard workers	Lung, skin	Arsenical insecticides
	Mining arseniferous ores	Lung, skin	Arsenic
	Iron ore	Lung	? Radon
	Tin	Lung, bone marrow	? Radon
	Asbestos	Lung, pleura and peritoneum	Asbestos
	Uranium	Lung	Radon
Petroleum	Wax pressmen	Scrotum	Polynuclear aromatics
Painting	Painter	Lung, ? bladder	?
Metal	Aluminium production	Bladder, ? lung	Polynuclear aromatics
	Copper smelting	Lung, ? sinonasal	Arsenic
	Chromate production	Lung, ? sinonasal	Chromium compounds
	Chromium plating	Lung	Chromium compounds
	Ferrochromium production	Lung	Chromium compounds
	Iron/steel production/founding	Lung	Benzo(a)pyrene
	Nickel refining	Nasal sinuses, lung	Nickel compounds
	Pickling operations	Larynx, lung	Acid mists
Transport	Shipyards	Lung, pleura and peritoneum	Asbestos
Chemicals	BCME and CMME production	Lung	BCME, CMME
	Vinyl chloride production	Liver	VCM
	Isopropyl alcohol (manufacture by strong acid method)	Paranasal sinuses	? Acid mists
	Chromate pigment production	Lung	Chromium compounds
	Dye manufacture and users ⎫		
	Auramine manufacture ⎭	Bladder	Aromatic amines

Continued on p. 342

Table 10.5 *Continued*

Industry	Occupation	Site of tumour	Likely carcinogen
	Poison gas manufacturers	Lung	Mustard gas
	Inorganic acid mists (strong) containing sulphuric acid	Larynx, lung	Sulphuric acid
Rubber	Rubber manufacture	Lymphatic and haemopoietic systems, bladder	Benzene, aromatic amines
	Calendering, tyre curing and tyre building	Lymphatic and haemopoietic systems	Benzene
	Cable makers, latex producers	Bladder	Aromatic amines
Construction, maintenance	Insulators, demolition engineers	Lung, pleura and peritoneum	Asbestos
Leather	Boot and shoe makers	Nose, bone marrow	Leather dust, benzene
Wood pulp and paper	Furniture makers	Nasal sinuses	Wood dust
Electric/electronics	Engineers	Bone marrow, brain	? Fluxes, ?? EMF
Health-care industry	Pharmaceutical manufacturers Pharmacists Nurses	Bone marrow	Cytotoxic drugs
	Radiologists/radiographers	Bone marrow	Ionising radiation
	'Patient carers'	Hepatoma Kaposi's sarcoma Non-Hodgkin's lymphoma	Hepatitis B and C HIV
	Sterilisation unit	Lymphatic and haemopoietic systems	Ethylene oxide

VCM, vinyl chloride monomer; EMF, electromagnetic field.

In addition to (or in conjunction with) the list in Table 10.4, there are studies that suggest links between certain tumours and certain industries or materials. Table 10.5 lists the occupations recognised as presenting a carcinogenic risk.

Some infectious agents of occupational relevance are now on the list as well:

- hepatitis B and C;
- *Schistosoma haematobium*;
- human papillomavirus (HPV) 16 and 18;
- HIV-1;
- human T-cell lymphotrophic virus 1 (HTLV-1).

The lists are, however, heavily dependent on the quality of the epidemiological studies.

Undoubtedly, future research will reveal new carcinogens (see Table 10.6), but it is to be hoped that some of the present group will become historical relics. Pre-market testing of new chemicals may help to limit the carcinogenic load for future generations of workers, whilst substitution or stringent environmental control should lessen the impact of known carcinogens. The problem is not an easy one to solve but, whereas tumours related to lifestyle are difficult to control, and many tumours are of unknown aetiology, all occupationally related cancers are, by definition, theoretically preventable.

Table 10.6 In the past 5 years (to 1997), the following chemicals/processes are amongst those which have been classified as Group 2A in the IARC evaluations.

Chemical	Process/occupation	Other
Acrylamide	Hairdresser/barber	UVA, B and C
Formaldehyde	Occupational exposure to art glass	
Tetrachloroethylene	manufacture	
Trichloroethylene		
Styrene-7,8-oxide		
Vinyl fluoride		

11 Psychosocial Aspects of the Workplace

In recent years, there has been increasing emphasis on the psychological well-being of people in the workplace. Improved conditions at work, and in society as a whole, have raised expectations about what now constitutes a healthy workplace. Rightly, this now includes freedom from psychological as well as physical harm. Moreover, there is plenty of evidence to suggest that psychological conditions at work are getting worse, as other conditions improve.

11.1 Occupational stress

Psychological stress usually occurs when there is an imbalance between the demands made upon an individual and their perceived ability to meet these demands. In the workplace, stress may result from situations of high demand, where the individual feels unable to cope, but also from situations in which the work is monotonous and repetitive, providing little or no challenge or interest. For some individuals, understimulation may be as stressful as overstimulation. A particularly important factor is control. People's mental health, both in general and in the workplace, is influenced strongly by their perception of control over factors affecting their situation.

11.2 The effects of stress

Although it is difficult to ascribe specific health effects to the presence of psychosocial hazards, it is increasingly accepted that psychological stressors are likely to contribute to a range of problems. These may be psychological (how people feel), behavioural (what people do as a result of how they feel) or physical (disease in which stress is a contributory factor).

An individual suffering from stress may exhibit a number of the following symptoms or behaviour patterns:

- irritable, aggressive or obsessive behaviour;
- lack of concentration;
- nervousness or panic attacks;
- depressive symptoms, such as excessive tiredness and apathy;
- feelings of alienation;
- lack of confidence;
- indecision;
- lack of attention to safety procedures;
- sexual and general relationship difficulties;
- increased alcohol consumption;

- increased smoking;
- eating disorders;
- sleeping difficulties;
- poor time-keeping;
- frequent short-term absences.

In addition, the effects of stress may manifest themselves as a range of non-specific somatic physical symptoms. The most commonly reported are:

- headache;
- backache and other musculoskeletal problems;
- sweating;
- nausea;
- dizziness;
- palpitations.

These symptoms are frequently reported when individuals suspect the presence of a physical or chemical hazard. The hazard may not in fact be present, or exposure may be insufficient to result in harm. The symptoms may not therefore be directly related to the hazard in question. When they are related, however, they may be intensified by a range of psychosocial influences, such as the attitudes of management, the media or health professionals. In this sense, psychosocial factors can heighten a worker's response to potential hazards in the working environment and, as a result, the exact nature of the relationship between hazard and health can be difficult to disentangle.

In addition, some specific health problems have been linked to stress, notably:

- mental health problems (anxiety, depression);
- cardiovascular problems;
- depression of the immune system (vulnerability to infection).

11.3 Special problems

11.3.1 Post-traumatic stress disorder (PTSD)

In some occupations, e.g. the emergency services, employees are likely to be exposed to traumatic events. Some individuals may, as a result, suffer from PTSD, a syndrome characterised by the following:

- intrusive recollections of the incident (flashbacks);
- avoidance of stimuli associated with the incident;
- symptoms of anxiety and depression (e.g. excessive nervousness, social withdrawal).

This is a recognised psychiatric condition which may become chronic and disabling, and which requires specialist help.

11.3.2 Chronic fatigue syndrome/myalgic encephalomyelitis (CFS/ME)

Recent estimates suggest that this condition may occur in 1–3% of the population. As the name suggests, it is characterised by ongoing excessive fatigue, which is made worse by any physical or mental effort. The existence, definition and cause of the condition are all controversial. Possible causes include:

- viral infection;
- muscular disorder;
- immune dysfunction;
- psychological distress.

Current evidence suggests that it has multiple causes, but that psychological factors play a major role. As such, it may occur in psychologically vulnerable individuals in the workplace who are under stress. CFS is difficult to treat and needs sensitive management, usually involving specialist psychiatric help.

11.3.3 Multiple chemical sensitivity (MCS)

Like CFS, this condition is controversial. Individuals report intolerance to a range of chemicals at exposure levels far below those which would affect most people. They report a wide range of symptoms, affecting many different organs of the body, and for which there is usually no accepted medical explanation. The problem is usually triggered by perceived exposure to one specific chemical, often in the workplace, and then becomes generalised to other substances. As with CFS, psychological factors are thought to play a major role; treatment is difficult and specialist help is required.

11.4 Personality characteristics

Certain behaviour patterns may influence an individual's susceptibility to the effects of stress.

11.4.1 Type A and Type B

The Type A behaviour pattern is characterised by:

- a high need for achievement;
- competitiveness;

- aggression;
- restlessness;
- impatience.

This is in marked contrast to the Type B personality who tends to be calm and relaxed, and to place a higher value on enjoying activities than on demonstrating achievement. When exposed to high levels of stress, the high-achieving Type A is more prone to develop stress-related illness, particularly heart disease.

11.4.2 External–internal locus of control

Individuals with a highly developed internal locus of control have a strong belief in the influence of their own decisions on their personal circumstances. By contrast, those with a strongly external locus of control believe more readily that their situation is determined largely by chance, and have a tendency towards feelings of powerlessness in their lives. Such individuals appear to be very vulnerable when faced with highly stressful situations.

11.5 Coping strategies adopted

These may be:
- adaptive (confront the problem, seek solutions);
- maladaptive (avoid the problem, e.g. alcohol, substance abuse, sickness absence).

Maladaptive strategies offer only short-term solutions, and may in themselves result in further health problems. Stress management training tends to emphasise adaptive strategies.

11.6 Causes of stress

A number of factors have been identified as potential sources of stress in the workplace.

Job content:
- work overload;
- time pressure/deadlines;
- work difficulty;
- work underload.

Work organisation:
- shift working;
- long, unsociable, unpredictable hours;

- change, restructuring.

Organisational culture:
- communications (management/workers);
- participation in decision making;
- feedback;
- resource provision;
- support.

Work role:
- role clarity;
- role conflict.

Interpersonal relationships:
- communication;
- harassment (racial, sexual);
- bullying;
- verbal/physical abuse.

Career structure:
- underpromotion;
- overpromotion;
- threat of redundancy;
- pay structure.

Physical environment:
- noise;
- temperature;
- lighting;
- space;
- ergonomics;
- exposure to hazards.

Home–work interface:
- childcare responsibilities;
- transport problems;
- relocation problems.

Some of these problems may be potentially soluble (e.g. role clarity, support); others may be intrinsic to certain work situations (e.g. potential for violence or verbal abuse).

11.7 Managing occupational stress

The way stress is managed in the workplace depends on the identified cause. The assessment of sources and levels of stress in an organisation can be carried out by questionnaire.

11.7.1 Primary intervention

Where sources of stress are identified which are potentially avoidable, they should be reduced by organisational change that targets the specific causes.

In addition, organisational measures can reduce intrinsic problems, such as the threat of violence, e.g. the introduction of safe systems of work such as call-back procedures.

11.7.2 Secondary intervention

Where jobs are inherently stressful, e.g. those involving emergency or social services, inspection or other contact with the public, it is often appropriate to train workers in specific stress management techniques. These might include training in assertiveness skills and aggression management to reduce exposure to stress and increase feelings of control, and training in relaxation skills to minimise the effects of stress. In many occupations, personal stress management training may be regarded as a useful addition to, although not a substitute for, primary intervention.

11.7.3 Tertiary intervention

This consists of counselling services for individuals suffering severe effects of stress. It is also appropriate for specific problems, such as PTSD, alcohol abuse and non-occupational difficulties which may be affecting an individual's work performance.

Ideally, good management of psychosocial problems in the workplace will contain all three elements.

12 Legal Aspects of Occupational Health

12.1 Introduction

This chapter outlines some of the ways in which the law may affect the employment of people with health problems, and the services available to them to help them to return to work. There are three major legal sources — the common law, statute and European Directives and Recommendations.

12.2 Common law

The English legal system is based on the common law. This system developed from the decisions of the judges, whose rulings over the centuries have created precedents for other courts to follow, and these decisions were based on the 'custom and practice of the Realm'. The common law can be contrasted with statute law (passed by Parliament) and equity (the body of rules administered by the Court of Chancery).

The system of binding precedent means that any decision of the House of Lords (the highest court in the UK) will bind all the lower courts, unless the lower courts are able to distinguish the facts of the current case, and argue that the old decision cannot apply due to the difference in the facts of the two cases.

The common law covers both the criminal and civil law. The law of negligence has grown out of the common law and forms part of the civil law of torts (civil wrongs).

For centuries, the common law courts have held employers liable for negligence if the employers have not taken reasonable care of the health and safety of their workers.

12.2.1 Common law duties of employers

At common law, the employer has an obligation to take reasonable care of all his/her employees, and to guard against reasonably foreseeable risks of injury. These duties are judged in the light of the 'state of the art' of knowledge of the employer — either that which he/she knew or ought to know.

12.2.2 Standard of care of occupational health specialist

The standard of care expected of a professional person, e.g. an occupational health specialist, is set out in a case which established the so-called 'Bolam' test[1], where McNair J held that the test of the ordinary man's standard of care is judged by the action of the man in the street, i.e. the man on the top of the Clapham omnibus.

However, in the case of a specialist, the standard of care is higher:

- … Where you get the situation which involves the use of some special skill or competence, then the test whether there has been negligence or not is not the test of the man on the top of the Clapham omnibus, because he has not got this special skill.
- The test is the standard of the ordinary skilled man exercising and professing to have that special skill.
- A man need not possess the highest expert skill at the risk of being found negligent.
- It is well-established law that it is sufficient if he exercises the ordinary skill of an ordinary competent man exercising that particular art.
- … There may be one or more perfectly proper standards; and if a medical man conforms with one of those proper standards then he is not negligent.
- A doctor is not guilty of negligence if he has acted in accordance with a practice accepted as proper by a responsible body of medical men skilled in that particular art.
- Put the other way round, a doctor is not negligent, if he is acting in accordance with a practice, merely because there is a body of opinion that takes a contrary view.
- At the same time, that does not mean that a medical man can obstinately and pig-headedly carry on with some old technique if it has been proved to be contrary to what is really substantially the whole of informed medical opinion.
- Otherwise you might get men today saying:

---

[1] *Bolam* v. *Friern Hospital Management Committee* [1957] 1 WLR 582. In *Eckersley and others* v. *Binnie & Partners*, reported in Health and Safety Information Bulletin 149, Bingham LJ held that:

'A professional man should command the corpus of knowledge which forms part of the professional equipment of the ordinary member of his profession. … He should be alert to the hazards and risks inherent in any professional task he undertakes to the extent that other ordinarily competent members of his profession would be alert. He must bring to any professional task he undertakes no less expertise, skill and care than other ordinarily competent members of his profession would bring, but need bring no more. The standard is that of the reasonable average. The law does not require of a professional man that he be a paragon combining the qualities of a polymath and prophet.'

'I don't believe in anaesthetics. I don't believe in antiseptics. I am going to continue to do my surgery in the way in which it was done in the eighteenth century.'

That clearly would be wrong …

12.2.3 Duty to inform and warn of risks to health and safety

Employers, through their medical advisers, in certain cases are under a duty to inform and warn their workers, including prospective employees, of the potential dangers and inherent risks of the job, so that they can make an informed choice as to whether or not to accept the job. This warning does not, of course, cancel out the employer's duty to take all such care as is reasonable to guard against reasonably foreseeable risks of injury. What this does is to inform the employee and to give him/her the choice which, if left uninformed, he/she would not have.

In some cases, it may act as a defence to an employer in a claim for negligence under the principle of 'volenti non fit injuria', i.e. that the individual knew about the risk, understood the exact nature of that risk and accepted that risk. In employment situations, it has rarely proved to be a successful defence because, in order to be able to accept a risk, there must be no duress. If the threat is to be dismissed or to accept a particular risk at the workplace, then the courts would not be slow to disallow the defence of 'volenti'.

In one of the several cases brought against Bernard Matthews for work-related upper limb disorders (WRULDs), Mrs Mountenay and others[2] successfully argued that she had never been given sufficient warning of the inherent or potential dangers of various upper limb disorders that could obtain from eviscerating chickens on piecework, having to work at a particularly fast pace with no regular rest breaks, etc. At the end of this chapter, there are some guidelines for employers and occupational health practitioners as to the kind of warnings that should be provided where the work involves repetitive movements.

In another leading case, *Stokes and others* v. *Guest, Keen & Nettlefold*[3], the company was found liable for the scrotal cancer which eventually killed several of its workers. The company had employed a doctor who also lectured in industrial medicine, but he had failed to warn the men of the dangers of cancer associated with working with the oils

---

[2] *Mountenay (Hazzard) and others* v. *Bernard Matthews plc* (Unreported) 4.5.93 Norwich County Court (HSIB 215, November 1993).
[3] *Stokes and ors* v. *Guest, Keen & Nettlefold* [1968] 1 WLR 1776.

which covered their overalls, as he had not wanted 'to alarm the men'. He could and should have circulated a leaflet to the workers warning them of the dangers of scrotal warts. He should also have instituted periodic medical examinations. The employer was held to be vicariously liable for this act of negligence on the doctor's part.

The duties are summarised as follows.

1 A duty on an employer to take positive steps to ensure the safety of his/her employees in the light of the knowledge which he/she has or ought to have.

2 A right of the employer to follow current recognised practice unless in the light of common sense or new knowledge this is clearly unsound.

3 Where there is developing knowledge, a duty to keep reasonably abreast with it and not be too slow in applying it.

4 Where the employer has greater than average knowledge of the risk, a duty to take greater than average precautions.

5 A duty on the employer to weigh up the risk (in terms of the likelihood of the injury and the possible consequences) against the effectiveness of the precautions to be taken to meet the risk and the cost and inconvenience.

12.2.4 Balancing the risk

In deciding what is 'reasonably practicable' to do in terms of eliminating risk and in determining what is reasonably foreseeable in terms of injury, the courts have determined a test which balances the quantum of risk against the time, trouble and expense that the employer must go to to avert that risk. The greater the risk to health or safety, the greater the time, trouble and expense the law requires of the employer.

In a leading case involving the National Coal Board[4], the Court of Appeal held that the employer could only discharge his duty of care where the time, trouble and expense that he had gone to to avert the risk was grossly disproportionate to the risk involved. The Court held that the term 'reasonably practicable' meant:

> … a narrower term than 'physically possible' … (it) implies that a computation must be made by the owner in which the quantum of risk is placed on one scale and the sacrifice involved in the measures necessary for averting the risk (whether in money, time or trouble) is placed on the other, and that, if it be shown that there is *a gross disproportion* between them, the risk being insignificant

---

[4] *Edwards* v. *National Coal Board* [1949] 1 All ER 743, Court of Appeal.

in relation to the sacrifice, the defendants discharge the onus on them.

12.2.5 Constructive knowledge

Ignorance is no defence in law. However, if one member of the employer's staff knows about a risk or health or safety problem, then whether this is shared with the employer or not, the employer is deemed to know about it. This is called 'constructive knowledge'.

The courts will look at the state of knowledge at the time of the alleged act of negligence in judging whether the employer ought to have acted.

12.2.6 The state of the art

Employers are not expected to be prophets, nor are they expected to remain ignorant of the growing knowledge of health and safety matters. Nor are they permitted to ignore advice and information given to them by their occupational health experts merely because no other employer in their industry appears to know about the issues, or be concerned enough to take any action.

In the noise-induced deafness cases, the courts have investigated just what employers knew about noisy environments back in the 1950s despite the fact that the Ministry of Labour pamphlet on 'Noise and the Worker' was not published until 1963.

In *Baxter* v. *Harland & Wolff plc*[5], the employer was held liable for noise-induced deafness prior to 1963 — as far back as 1953. Here the employer failed to *'seek out knowledge of facts which are not in themselves obvious'.*

Harland & Wolff had not sought or heeded medical, scientific and legal advice between 1953 and 1963 — despite there being evidence of several incidents in the naval shipyards in Devon before the Second World War of noise-induced deafness problems, and medical reports and papers on this in the early 1950s. There was produced in evidence an advertisement in *The Lancet* on April 28, 1951 of an ear-plug — Sonex V-51R.

> With hindsight it seems strange that so little was available during the decade of the 1950s by way of ear protection — whether this was due to lack of confidence in the product or lack of market opportunity due to disinterest amongst employers in noisy industries is impossible to say ...

---

[5] *Baxter* v. *Harland & Wolff plc* [1990] IRLR 516.

The employer was held to be negligent because of its:

> lack of interest and apathy ... . The defendants knowing that noise was causing deafness among their workmen should have applied their minds to removing or reducing the risk ... sought advice ... and pooled ideas with others in the industry as to how to tackle a real problem which was injuring though not disabling a large number of their employees ... .
>
> In a matter affecting the whole trade every possible idea might be pooled, every suggestion tested and every conceivable course tried in order that, in the interests of all concerned, the maximum degree of safety might be achieved ... .

12.2.7 Greater duty of care — 'eggshell skull' principle

The employer owes a higher duty of care to any particularly vulnerable employee with a known, pre-existing medical condition. In other words, you take your victim as you find him. Those with an eggshell skull physique are more vulnerable to serious injury than others of robust physical health. Those with a fragile personality may suffer far greater psychological damage than those with a robust personality.

This is defined as the 'eggshell skull' principle, and a classic example of this can be seen in the case of *Paris* v. *Stepney Borough Council*[6].

Here the Council employed a labourer with only one eye. The Council failed to ensure that he was wearing eye goggles and, as a result, he suffered an injury to his other eye at work and was blinded. The House of Lords held that his employers owed him a much higher duty of care as he was an individual with extra susceptibility to serious injury.

It will therefore be vital for employers to take informed advice from qualified occupational health professionals regarding the fitness or otherwise for work, any disabilities which might affect the work or the health and safety of the individual or others and whether any special arrangements or precautions or restrictions ought to be made. Failure to pursue adequate pre-employment medical checks — by properly qualified and trained occupational health staff — may lead to a successful claim for negligence against the employer.

12.2.8 Duty owed for mental breakdown

In several recent cases, the courts have extended the principle of the employer's common law duty to psychiatric injury, and, in a case which

---

[6] *Paris* v. *Stepney Borough Council* [1951] 1 All ER 42.

went to the House of Lords (non-employment), the negligent party was held liable for the onset of chronic fatigue syndrome which the plaintiff alleged returned because of the car accident (*Page* v. *Smith*, Times Law Report, 4 May 1991)!

Although not the first case to establish an employer's duty of care to look after the mental well-being of employees, it was the first successful claim for damages: *Walker* v. *Northumberland County Council* [1995] IRLR 35.

In this case, John Walker was a senior social worker in charge of four teams of social workers, dealing with, *inter alia*, child abuse cases. He lost his job after suffering two mental breakdowns. The Council was held liable for the second of his nervous breakdowns, and ordered to pay damages for his lost career and his permanent psychological impairment.

In finding the Council negligent for the second nervous breakdown, the High Court held that they had failed to foresee that he was unable to cope with the workload and the work following his first mental breakdown. His workload became heavier and heavier with no help or guidance from the Council. Mr Walker literally collapsed with a second breakdown — this time unable to continue working for good.

The High Court held that the Council ought to have anticipated this, and should either have provided him with a deputy who was as experienced as him, or should have permanently reduced his workload. By continuing to employ him after the first breakdown, and by requiring him to work under even more pressure, the Council had failed in their duty to take care of his mental health. The Court helpfully discussed what 'standard' of care was appropriate in such a case. It held that:

> The defendant County Council was in breach of the duty of care owed to the plaintiff as his employer in respect of a second mental breakdown which he suffered as a result of stress and anxiety occasioned by his job as Area Social Services Officer responsible for an area with a very heavy workload, including an increasing incidence of child abuse cases.
>
> An employer owes a duty to his employees not to cause them psychiatric damage by the volume or character of the work which they are required to perform. Although the law on the extent of the duty on an employer to provide an employee with a safe system of work and to take reasonable steps to protect him from risks which are reasonably foreseeable has developed almost exclusively in cases involving physical injury to the employee, there is no logical reason why risk of injury to an employee's mental health should be excluded from the scope of the employer's duty.

What is reasonable depends upon the nature of the relationship, the magnitude of the risk of injury which was reasonably foreseeable, the seriousness of the consequences for the person to whom the duty is owed of the risk eventuating and the cost and practicability of preventing the risk.

Having regard to the reasonably foreseeable size of the risk of repetition of Mr Walker's illness if his duties were not alleviated by effective additional assistance and to the reasonably foreseeable gravity of the mental breakdown which might result if nothing was done, I have come to the conclusion that the standard of care to be expected of a reasonable local authority required that, in March 1987, such additional assistance should be provided if not on a permanent basis, at least until restructuring of the Social Services had been effected and the workload on Mr Walker thereby permanently reduced.

When Mr Walker returned from his first illness, the Council had to decide whether it was prepared to go on employing him in spite of the fact that he had made it sufficiently clear that he must have effective additional help if he was to continue at Blyth Valley. It chose to employ him, but provided no effective help.

In so doing, it was in my judgement acting unreasonably and therefore in breach of its duty of care …

12.2.9 Post-traumatic stress disorders (PTSDs)

In cases in which workers are in highly stressful occupations, such as the rescue services, medical services and social work, the employer must be particularly mindful of the mental strain and trauma of the job and take steps accordingly.

Similarly, workers who are at risk of violent attacks are entitled to be treated sympathetically when they have been traumatised by such an event.

Many banks and building societies, transport companies and hospitals are well aware of the effects of such events upon their workers, and train their staff in how to deal with violent customers and patients, and offer counselling, support and paid sick leave after such attacks.

In one highly publicised case, the Court of Appeal showed considerable sympathy to workers suffering nervous shock as a result of a traumatic event at work.

In *Frost and others* v. *Chief Constable of South Yorkshire*[7], several

[7] *Frost and others* v. *Chief Constable of South Yorkshire* [1997] IRLR 173.

police officers, who were present at the Hillsborough football stadium at the time of the tragic deaths of many fans, sued their employer for the psychological damage that they suffered on that day. The Court of Appeal held that:

> An employer owes a duty of care to avoid exposing an employee to unnecessary risk of physical or psychiatric injury. There is no justification for treating physical and psychiatric illness as different kinds of injury for the purposes of that duty.
>
> The duty exists by reason of the employer/employee relationship.
>
> … In the Hillsborough case there was a breach of the duty of care in respect of those plaintiffs who were at the football ground in the course of duty, within the area of risk of physical and psychiatric injury dealing with the dead and dying and who were thus exposed by the employer's negligence to the exceptionally horrific events which occurred.

12.2.10 Liability for pre-existing chronic fatigue syndrome (CFS)

The principle at common law that you take your victim as you find him was well illustrated in the case (not involving an employer) of *Page* v. *Smith*[8]. Here, a negligent motorist was held liable for the victim's nervous shock and for his CFS which he had had in a mild form, but which he argued had been triggered off in a more serious form following the accident.

As a result, he recovered damages for mental distress as an exacerbation of his current condition (CFS). The House of Lords held that:

> … The judge had said that it was well established that the defendant must in law take the plaintiff as he found him. Once it is established that ME existed and that a relapse or recrudescence could be triggered by the trauma of an accident, and that nervous shock was suffered by the plaintiff who was actually involved in the accident, it became a foreseeable consequence …
>
> If liability had been established for nervous shock the defendant would have been liable for all the consequent mental injury sustained by the victim even though it was unforeseen and of a kind that would only be suffered by someone who was particularly vulnerable.

---

[8] *Page* v. *Smith*, House of Lords *The Times* May 1, 1994.

> That was the point at which the tortfeasor had to take his victim
> as he found him and the principle of the eggshell skull was to be
> applied …

12.2.11 Stress and other mental disorders
The courts have now recognised that an employer owes a duty of care
not only for the physical well-being of the employee, but also for the
mental well-being. Conditions such as CFS[9] have been the subject of
recent publications in the medical press (see Chapter 11). It will become
more important than ever that occupational health specialists understand
these conditions and advise their employers accordingly.

12.2.12 Employees' duties
At common law, employees have implied duties, including the duty to
work with reasonable care and competence and to serve their employer
loyally and faithfully.

Statute

12.3.1 Health and Safety at Work, etc. Act 1974
The Health and Safety at Work, etc. Act (HASWA) 1974 imposes
statutory duties on all employers in the UK to take reasonable care of
their employees' health and safety. HASWA 1974 supplements and, in
some cases, supersedes former statutory enactments such as (part of) the
Factories Act 1961, the Offices, Shops and Railway Premises Act 1963,
the Mines and Quarries Act 1954, etc.

Detailed regulations made under HASWA 1974, imposing criminal
liability, can be heard in the Magistrates Courts. The Magistrates Courts
have the power to impose a fine of up to £5000, or up to £20 000 for
breaches of Sections 2–6 and breaches of Improvement or Prohibition
Notices — increased from £5000 to £20 000 under the Offshore Safety
Act 1992 — or to commit to prison for up to a 6-month term. For more
serious breaches of HASWA 1974, the Crown Court has the power to
impose an unlimited fine or a term of imprisonment.

HASWA 1974 currently imposes only criminal liability. Both the
company and individual managers and employees can be prosecuted for
breaches of their statutory duties. There is provision in HASWA 1974

---

9 'Chronic fatigue syndrome', Report of the Joint Working Group of the Royal
Colleges of Physicians, Psychiatrists and General Practitioners, October 1996/CR54.

(Section 47) to extend the jurisdiction of the Act to permit employees injured at work to sue in the civil courts, under HASWA 1974, for their injuries, but this has not happened to date.

Employees who are injured at work as a result of a breach of any other statutory duties can sue in the civil courts, as the other statutory enactments impose both civil and criminal liability.

The Act covers everyone at work, including independent contractors and their employees, the self-employed and visitors, but excludes domestic servants in private households.

12.3.2 Employer's statutory duties

HASWA 1974 imposes general duties on employers in Section 2 to take reasonable care so far as reasonably practicable of the health, safety and welfare at work of their employees, and to ensure so far as reasonably practicable that:

1 there is a safe system of work;

2 there is a safe place of work;

3 staff are given information, instruction and training on matters of health and safety and are adequately supervised;

4 there is a safe system for the handling, storage and transport of substances and materials; and

5 there is a safe working environment.

Although there is no specific mention of a duty to conduct pre-employment medical examinations, part of a safe system of work could be interpreted as ensuring that the staff recruited are able to perform their duties. Thus, adequate medical data on new members of staff will be essential. However, due care must be taken of the employer's duties under the Disability Discrimination Act 1995.

12.3.3 Employees' statutory duties

Employees have duties under Sections 7 and 8 to take reasonable care to ensure the health and safety of themselves and others, to cooperate on any matter on health and safety and to do nothing which could endanger their health and safety or those of others.

Part of this duty includes the duty to inform the employer truthfully when requested for information on matters concerning medical history. Failing to disclose, when requested, material information about previous or current medical conditions may result in a finding of fair dismissal should the employer take the decision to dismiss the employee for this reason (see below in section on 'Unfair dismissal', p. 366).

12.3.4 The institutions

The Health and Safety Commission (HSC) was set up under HASWA 1974 as a tripartite body (Government, Confederation of British Industry (CBI) and Trades Union Congress (TUC)), and is responsible for policy. The Health and Safety Executive (HSE) is responsible for enforcing the Act. There are several divisions, the largest of which is the Factory Inspectorate (HMFI). The Employment Medical Advisory Service (EMAS) is the field force of the medical division of HSE.

Enforcement of the Act in relation to offices is carried out by Environmental Health Officers who are employed by the local authorities. Their powers are the same as the Factory Inspectors.

12.3.5 Employment protection legislation

(i) Right not to be discriminated against or dismissed

Employees have statutory protection from being unfairly dismissed and unlawfully discriminated against because they have raised matters of health and safety concerns to their employer[10].

(ii) Unfair dismissal

Employees have been given protection from unfair dismissal provided that they satisfy certain qualifying conditions, such as 2 years' continuous service, under the normal retirement age, etc., save for dismissals for inadmissible reasons such as pregnancy, where there is no service requirement.

Claims for unfair dismissal are heard by industrial tribunals. The tribunals are chaired by a person who is legally qualified (solicitor or barrister of at least 15 years' standing), and include two lay members (one appointed by the Employers' Organisations and one appointed by the TUC). The lay members direct the chair as to good industrial practice and the chair directs the lay members as to points of law. Appeals on points of law or a perverse decision lie with the Employment Appeal Tribunal (EAT), then on to the Court of Appeal and, finally, the House of Lords.

---

[10] Section 44 of the Employment Rights Act 1996 provides protection from any detriment applied to an employee who raises health and safety complaints, and Section 100 renders it an inadmissible reason for dismissal to dismiss on such grounds.

The Employment Rights Act 1996[11] sets out five potentially fair reasons for dismissal — one being 'capability', which covers ill health. Lying about health at the pre-employment stage has been held to constitute another fair reason for dismissal, namely 'some other substantial reason of a kind such as to justify the dismissal of an employee holding the position which that employee held'.

Employers must advance factual evidence of the ill health disabling the individual from performing the job for which they were employed to do, in order to justify the dismissal. Tribunals also have to be satisfied that the employer acted reasonably in treating that reason as a sufficient reason for dismissal. The tribunals have given guidance as to what constitutes reasonable conduct on the part of the employer in this regard. Whether or not any decision to dismiss is deemed fair or unfair, recent protection against discrimination on grounds relating to disability may also be relevant (see Section 12.7). For example, employers should specify the allegations if misconduct is alleged, carry out a thorough investigation and hold a disciplinary hearing, to allow the employee to state his or her case.

(iii) Evidence of ill health

Most employers initially rely upon medical statements (MED 3) from the employee's general practitioner (GP). The tribunals, however, require full medical evidence in the form of medical reports from either the GP, specialist consultant or the occupational health practitioner.

The mere fact that the individual is not disabled from all the duties does not affect a decision to dismiss for ill health, as long as the individual is unfit to perform some of the duties. This was stated in the case of *Shook* v. *London Borough of Ealing*[12]. Miss Shook was employed as a trainee residential care assistant, who strained her back and was off work for some 9 months. She was declared unfit to carry out her duties of residential social worker because of the bending and lifting which was involved in her job, and this was confirmed by both her GP and the Council's Medical Officer. She was eventually dismissed, having been offered alternative posts which she had rejected.

She argued that her employers did not have any fair reason to dismiss

[11] Section 98 provides for five potentially fair reasons for dismissal. 'Capability' is provided for in Section 98(2)(a) and 'some other substantial reason' is provided for in Section 98(1)(b). Acting reasonably, which is the other half of the equation, is a requirement with which the tribunal must be satisfied, as a neutral burden, under Section 98(4).

[12] *Shook* v. *London Borough of Ealing* [1986] IRLR 46.

her because she was not disabled from all her contractual duties, as her contract actually provided for a very wide flexibility and mobility clause and she worked in numerous posts within the Social Services Department of the Council.

The Court of Appeal ruled that the dismissal was fair and rejected this argument:

> ... The Tribunal were entitled to reject the submission that an employee is not incapacitated from performing ... the work that they are employed to do unless he is incapacitated from performing every task which the employers are entitled by law to call upon him to discharge ...
>
> ... However widely that contract was construed, her disabilities related to her performance of her duties thereunder, even though her performance of all of them may not have been affected ...

(iv) Medical evidence and medical reports

In assessing the fitness or unfitness for work, and the prognosis as to the return date to work of an employee off sick, the tribunals have made it clear that employers should not rely upon medical certificates alone. A full medical report should be sought by the employer or the occupational health physician or nurse (if there is one). Employers are required to inform the doctor of the purpose of the medical report sought. It is not regarded as fair to request a medical report without first making its purpose clear. In most cases, employers will state that the report is required in order to plan for the work in the department and administer the sick pay scheme(s). Doctors should always ensure that they are clear as to why the employer is seeking such a report, and write to ask if it is not clear before carrying out the examination!

Those employers without any occupational health personnel should advise the doctor as to the reasons for their enquiry, the basic job functions of the individual and the length of the absence to date. The employer is required to obtain the prior, written informed consent to do this from the employee. If the medical report is being sought from the employee's GP or own specialist, the employer is required under the Access to Medical Reports Act 1988 to inform the employee of his/her rights under that Act (which include the right to see the report before it is sent to the employer, and the right to refuse to allow the report to be sent to the employer).

Employees are now entitled to see their medical records (made from November 1, 1991) — this includes occupational health records as well as the GP records and hospital records (Access to Health Records Act 1990).

The questions asked by the employer of the occupational health physician or nurse, once the full report has been received from the specialist or GP, should be limited to the following list.

1 When is the likely date of return to work?

2 Will there be any residual disability upon return to work?

3 Will it be permanent or temporary?

4 Will the employee be able to render regular and efficient service?

5 If the answer to question 2 is 'Yes', what duties would you recommend that your patient does not do and for how long?

6 Will your patient require continued treatment or medication upon his/her return to work?

(v) Conflicting medical advice

In some cases, employers receive conflicting medical opinions — the employee's own specialist or GP stating that the individual is unfit to return to work and the occupational health practitioner confirming that the individual is fit to return to work.

In such a dilemma, the tribunals have made it clear that employers are entitled to rely upon the view of their occupational health practitioner unless:

1 the occupational health practitioner has not personally examined the individual, but has merely written a report on the basis of the medical notes;

2 the occupational health practitioner's report is woolly and indeterminate!;

3 the continued employment of the individual would pose a serious threat of health or safety to the individual or others; and

4 the individual has been treated or is being treated by a specialist and no report has been received by that specialist.

The tribunals have accepted that an unreasonable refusal by an individual to return to work following the advice of the occupational health practitioner constitutes misconduct on the part of the employee. Here, the reason for dismissal is refusing to obey a lawful and reasonable instruction.

(vi) Disclosure of medical notes

As discussed above, employees are entitled under the Access to Medical Reports Act 1988 to see any medical report prepared by a medical practitioner who is responsible or has had responsibility for their clinical care. There is considerable debate and confusion, because of the ambiguity of the wording of the Act, whether occupational health practitioners' reports come within the ambit of the Act. It is clear that, once an occupational health practitioner or a member of his/her staff has 'treated' an employee, the Act will apply to all subsequent medical reports[13].

In a case of dismissal for refusing to return to work, the medical notes made by the occupational health practitioner may be ordered by the court to be disclosed to the individual. This may include the notes made by the occupational health practitioner to the consultant and to the management of the company.

In *Ford Motor Co Ltd* v. *Nawaz*[14], Mr Nawaz had been off sick for some 18 months with a bad back. He was eventually sent to an independent consultant who had stated that there was no evidence of any neurological symptoms. Dr Dhanapala, one of Ford's occupational health practitioners, wrote a report to management based on this consultant's report. When Mr Nawaz refused to return, continuing to send in medical statements, he was dismissed for unauthorised absence.

He sought the outside consultant's medical report (which would now not be covered by the Access to Medical Reports Act 1988) and Dr Dhanapala's notes. The EAT confirmed an Order for Discovery of these documents and stated:

> The Industrial Tribunal had not erred … in ordering discovery of certain medical reports … notwithstanding the appellants' policy of never disclosing medical reports to lay people.
>
> The test for discovery is whether the documents are necessary for the fair disposal of the claim, not whether it is a matter of company policy that such documents be disclosed or the ultimate value of the document to the claimant. What has to be determined is whether it is right and fair in the light of the issues which arise in a case for the applicant to have sight of the documents which are sought.

(vii) Consultation with the employee

The tribunals have ruled that, in the normal case, the employer should contact the employee, either by telephone or personally, ideally by visiting them at home by appointment, to consult the employee about the incapacity, to discuss any possible return date, to discuss the continuation or otherwise of company benefits and state benefits, to

---

[13] Advice from the British Medical Association (BMA), 1988 and June 26, 1989.

[14] *Ford Motor Co Ltd* v. *Nawaz* [1987] IRLR 163.

discuss the employment of a temporary or permanent replacement and to discuss the future employment or termination of employment.

Consultation in this case takes the place of warnings, which employees are entitled to receive in poor performance or misconduct cases. This was stated in a number of leading cases — *East Lindsey District Council* v. *Daubney*, *Spencer* v. *Paragon Wallpapers Ltd* and *Williamson* v. *Alcan Foils*[15].

There may, however, be exceptional cases in which the tribunal views the lack of consultation as still rendering a subsequent dismissal fair. These are rare. In one such case, *Eclipse Blinds Ltd* v. *Wright*[16], the Managing Director received a very pessimistic medical opinion concerning the state of health, and possibility of return to work, of the company's receptionist, who had been off sick for some time with a bad back. The Managing Director felt it was not in her best interests to speak to her personally because she did not realise the seriousness of her illness. He decided instead to write to her to inform her that a permanent replacement had been employed and that her services were to be terminated.

The Court of Appeal concluded that:

… The Industrial Tribunal must determine, as a matter of fact and judgement, what consultation was necessary or desirable in the known circumstances of a particular case.

… The test applied by Lord MacDonald refers to consultation being expected in 'the normal case' …

… The test espoused by PHILLIPS J was that consultation is necessary unless there are 'wholly exceptional circumstances'.

The one is the converse of the other since, if a case is wholly exceptional, it is not normal …

(viii) Seeking suitable alternative employment

The tribunals expect an employer to consider all alternatives other than dismissal, and this includes looking for suitable alternative employment within the organisation or any associated employers. The duty also includes considering whether any modifications to the original job could be possible. This duty has become even more important as a result of the

---

[15] *East Lindsey District Council* v. *Daubney* [1977] IRLR 181; *Spencer* v. *Paragon Wallpapers Ltd* [1976] IRLR 373; *Lynock* v. *Cereal Packaging Ltd* [1988] IRLR 510.
[16] *Eclipse Blinds Ltd* v. *Wright* [1992] IRLR 133.

duty under Section 6 of the Disability Discrimination Act 1995 to make 'reasonable adjustments to the workplace' (see Section 12.7). Here the occupational health specialists may offer valuable advice to employers.

The leading cases cited above of *East Lindsey District Council* v. *Daubney* and *Spencer* v. *Paragon Wallpapers Ltd* confirm that failure to seek alternative employment will normally render any dismissal for ill health unfair. This proposition has received judicial approval in the Court of Appeal in the case of *P* v. *Nottinghamshire County Council*[17], where BALCOMBE LJ stated:

> In an appropriate case and where the size and administrative resources of the undertaking permit, it may be unfair to dismiss an employee without the employer first considering whether the employee can be offered some other job notwithstanding that it may be clear that he cannot be allowed to continue in his original job …

(ix) Absenteeism

Where an employee has taken excessive absences for persistent, short-term illnesses (normally unrelated), the courts and tribunals have ruled that the employer may have a fair reason for dismissal ('some other substantial reason of a kind such as to justify the dismissal of an employee holding the position which that employee held' — Section 98(1)(b) of the 1996 Act).

However, the tribunals have ruled in several cases[18] that the fairness of any such dismissal depends upon:

1 examining the absence record objectively, assessing and investigating the underlying reasons for the absences with the individual and measuring the amount and frequency of the absences against the company or department average; taking the absence record at face value will not be good enough;

2 warning the employee in a sympathetic, compassionate way and after attempting to understand the problems that the individual may be facing — these warnings should make clear that the continued absences are causing problems and that, if the individual cannot attend work more regularly, even though the absences are caused by genuine symptoms, the employment may be terminated; and

---

[17] *P* v. *Nottinghamshire County Council* [1992] IRLR 362.
[18] *International Sports Co Ltd* v. *Thomson* [1980] IRLR 340; *Walpole* v. *Rolls Royce Ltd* [1980] IRLR 343; *Lynock* v. *Cereal Packaging Ltd* [1980] IRLR 343.

3 giving the employee a disciplinary hearing and an opportunity to state their case, and a chance to appeal against any decision to dismiss.

Employers may ask their occupational physician to examine the individual to see whether there is any underlying medical problem which could explain all the absences. In many cases, no such confirmation can be given, because the doctor may not have ever seen the patient during any of these short absences and the symptoms have normally resolved before the employee is sent to the physician. Nevertheless, it is common for employers to confirm or otherwise whether there is an underlying medical problem in such cases.

(x) Interrelationship with the terms of the contract

Employers who offer long-term disability (LTD) or permanent health insurance (PHI) as part of their contractual benefits ought to be aware that a failure to consider offering such benefits in an appropriate case could well be challenged in the common law courts as a breach of implied obligation of good faith.

In a House of Lords case, *Scally* v. *Southern Health and Social Services Board*[19], the House of Lords ruled that there was a positive duty on employers to inform their staff of those valuable benefits to which the employee must make an application. This includes the option of making additional voluntary contributions (AVCs) to the pension, claiming sick pay, PHI or LTD, maternity rights, etc.

The issue of the option of an LTD or PHI scheme may also be viewed by the industrial tribunals as an important factor in any unfair dismissal case, because the tribunals could well decide that there was an alternative to dismissal which was not properly considered by the employer — thus rendering the dismissal unfair.

In three more recent cases[20], the courts have interpreted the inclusion of sickness payments, whether provided for under an insurance policy or the contract itself, in a liberal way, so as to give maximum protection to the employee.

In *Aspden* v. *Webbs Poultry & Meat Group (Holdings) Ltd*, SEDLEY J held that the fact that the employer had provided for a PHI scheme within the terms of the contract, and because the benefit of such a scheme depended upon the continuance of the employment relationship, there

---

[19] *Scally* v. *Southern Health and Social Services Board* [1991] IRLR 522.

[20] *Aspden* v. *Webbs Poultry & Meat Group (Holdings) Ltd* [1996] IRLR 521; *Adin* v. *Sedco Forex International Resources Ltd* [1997] IRLR 280; *Bainbridge* v. *Circuit Foil UK Ltd* [1997] IRLR 305.

was an implied term that the employer would not terminate the contract whilst the employee was incapacitated for work, save in cases of gross misconduct. Despite the fact that there was an express written term providing for notice to terminate the contract, SEDLEY J held that it was the mutual intention of both parties that this term would not operate so as to remove the employee's entitlement to benefit under the PHI scheme. Damages were therefore awarded against the employer for the ex-employee's loss of PHI benefits.

In *Adin* v. *Sedco Forex International Resources Ltd*, the Court of Session (Scottish equivalent of the Court of Appeal) held that an employer could not effectively block an employee's right to benefit under a sickness and disability plan by dismissing the employee on the grounds of ill health. In this case, a short-term disability plan covered existing employees, and long-term benefits became payable when short-term benefit ceased. The employers dismissed Mr Adin during the period of short-term benefit, and sought to rely upon the contractual right to dismiss for any reason.

However, the Court of Session held that the contractual provisions had to be read in the light of their purpose of providing income protection when an employee could not work due to illness or injury.

In *Bainbridge* v. *Circuit Foil UK Ltd*, the terms of the scheme gave the employer 'the right to terminate or amend it at any time without prior notice'. The scheme was funded under an insurance policy and the employer ceased paying the premium for that policy without notifying the employees.

When Mr Bainbridge claimed disability benefit under the scheme, he was told that it had been terminated. The Court of Appeal held that the words 'without prior notice' meant without notice in advance. However, termination of the insurance policy did not have the effect of terminating the employee's rights under the contract of employment. The result was that the employer was contractually bound to provide the benefits of the scheme until notice of termination or variation of the contract was given.

(xi) Check-list

Occupational health practitioners may wish to consider writing a check-list of questions to their patients, one of which could be:

• 'Does your employer offer LTD or PHI?'

If such a scheme exists, the doctor (whether GP or occupational health practitioner) ought to enquire of the employer whether the patient has been considered for such a scheme.

(xii) Early retirement on medical grounds

In some cases in which the employee is permanently incapacitated from any further full-time, permanent employment with the employer, the individual may be dismissed and given an early retirement pension. The common law courts have also indicated that the employer must act in good faith in deciding such cases — *Mihlenstedt* v. *Barclays Bank International*[21].

It will be important for medical practitioners to read the exact wording of any pension scheme in this regard, particularly if a medical examination is to be performed in order to assess eligibility. It would be wise for medical practitioners to require a copy of the sick pay scheme, PHI scheme and pension fund rules as they apply to early medical pensions.

(xiii) Medical decisions in LTD/PHI and early ill health pensions

Medical practitioners play an important part in determining whether or not the individual is awarded an early medical pension or permitted to enter the LTD/PHI scheme. It is therefore very important to read and understand the eligibility rules for such schemes. As far as the LTD/PHI schemes are concerned, one eminent occupational health practitioner stated that such a scheme could be likened, in his view, to a lay-by on a motorway, where the individual could rest until he could recover and return to work!

(xiv) Management decision to dismiss not medical

The tribunals have emphasised that the decision whether or not to dismiss an employee off sick and unable to work is a management decision and not a medical one. Doctors should therefore not be pressurised into making such decisions for management. However, the implications of the Disability Discrimination Act 1995 must now be taken into account before any decision to dismiss is taken in such cases (see Section 12.7).

(xv) Lying about medical condition(s)

Doctors should be wary about advising their patients to lie about medical conditions. such as mental illness, epilepsy, human immunodeficiency virus (HIV) or acquired immune deficiency syndrome (AIDS), alcoholism or

---

[21] *Mihlenstedt* v. *Barclays Bank International* [1989] IRLR 522.

drug addiction. Employees who are employed on the basis of false medical information given to the employer (or the occupational health team) can be fairly dismissed under the reason of 'some other substantial reason' (Section 98(1)(b) of the Employment Rights Act 1996).

The tribunals have upheld the dismissal of an insurance salesman who lied about his long history of mental illness — O'Brien v. *Prudential Assurance Co Ltd*[22] — and an employee who lied about his drug addiction despite the fact that he was being successfully treated — *Walton* v. *TAC Construction Materials Ltd*[23].

As far as the Disability Discrimination Act 1995 is concerned, Regulations have excluded controlled substances and alcohol addiction from the scope of the Act. Employees who have these addiction problems are not afforded any protection under this Act. It may therefore still be lawful to dismiss an employee who has lied about an addiction of this nature.

Finally, on this topic, there is material difference between falsifying information or lying at a pre-employment interview and failing to disclose information. The former is active, the latter is passive.

In one case, the courts have held that, as a general rule, there is no duty upon an employee to disclose voluntarily medical information that is not specifically requested. In *Walton* v. *TAC Construction Materials Ltd*, the EAT held that:

> … It could not be said that there is any duty on the employee in the ordinary case, though there may be exceptions, to volunteer information about himself otherwise than in response to a direct question.

12.4 Pre-employment medical examinations

12.4.1 Questionnaires

It is essential that suitable and relevant questions are addressed on the pre-employment medical questionnaires so that relevant and adequate information is gathered. In one unreported case, an occupational health physician applied for a post to work part of the time offshore, but failed to describe his hydrophobia on the pre-employment medical questionnaire, despite a question about mental illness. When he commenced employment and was required to undergo survival training

---

[22] O'Brien v. *Prudential Assurance Co Ltd* [1979] IRLR 140.
[23] *Walton* v. *TAC Construction Materials Ltd* [1981] IRLR 357.

in order to fly offshore, he refused point blank. He then disclosed his phobia and sought to argue that he had not been asked to disclose this condition. He also argued that he would fly with the aircraft, but refused to undergo the survival training. This was unacceptable to the employer who argued that his contract had either been frustrated or had been rescinded[24].

In another case, a prospective candidate from the Netherlands applied for an engineering post offshore and declared that she had used cannabis for social purposes, but had not taken the drug for over 2 years. However, at her interview, she declared that she had used the drug that weekend and would not be fit to fly offshore. The employer decided that the risk was too great despite the fact that, in the Netherlands, cannabis is not an illegal substance, and declined to recruit her.

12.4.2 Duty of care

In a recent unsuccessful claim for negligence against an eminent occupational physician[25], it was held that an occupational physician owes a duty of care to the subject of the medical examination as well as to the employer. The duty extends to taking reasonable care in carrying out a medical assessment in connection with a job offer, and in making a judgement as to the individual's suitability for employment by reference to the prospective employer's requirements.

In this case, the individual concerned had applied for the job of International Sales and Marketing Director. In view of the abnormal blood test results, the doctor concerned interpreted the results as indicating that the individual was likely to consume excessive amounts of alcohol in a work-related context. The doctor could not therefore recommend him to the company for a highly stressful and demanding job involving travel and business-related social occasions.

It was clear from the expert medical evidence presented in court that a substantial body of reasonable medical opinion would have arrived at the same conclusion when interpreting the results, and therefore the allegations of negligence in the interpretation of the results failed.

---

[24] Frustration of contract occurs where, through the fault of neither party and due to a supervening or intervening event, the contract becomes impossible to perform or radically different from that which was contemplated by the parties at the outset of the contract. Recession of a contract occurs where one party elects to rescind the contract where, for example, the other party has made a misrepresentation and is thus unable to perform (substantially) his part of the contract — see Treitel, *The Law of Contract*, 9th edn.

[25] *Baker* v. *Kaye* [1997] IRLR 219.

12.4.3 Duty to be honest

In a recent case brought before the European Court of Justice (ECJ) as a Court of Appeal from the Court of First Instance[26], the ECJ has ruled that prospective job candidates have the right to be informed of the exact nature of the tests to be carried out and to refuse to participate if they so wish.

In this case, a man had applied for a temporary post of typist with the European Commission. He had undergone a medical examination, but refused to be screened for HIV antibodies. After giving blood and undergoing the medical and disclosing his medical records, the medical officer ordered blood tests in order to determine the T4 and T8 lymphocyte counts. When these were below the normal ratio, the medical officer concluded that Mr X was suffering from a significant immune deficiency constituting a case of full-blown 'AIDS'. He was thus rejected on the grounds of his physical condition. His doctor was informed.

Mr X complained to the Court of First Instance that he had been subjected to an AIDS test without his consent, and sought an annulment that he was unfit for work and damages for the non-material damage that he had suffered.

The ECJ held that:

> The Court of First Instance had incorrectly held that, in view of the abnormalities found in the medical examination of the appellant as part of his application for a temporary post ... the Commission's medical officer was entitled to request that a T4/T8 lymphocyte count be carried out, notwithstanding that the appellant had expressly refused to undergo an HIV test. The manner in which the appellant had been medically examined and declared physically unfit constituted an infringement of his right to respect for his private life as guaranteed by Article 8 of the European Convention on Human Rights. The right to respect for private life, embodied in Article 8 and deriving from the common constitutional traditions of the member states, is one of the fundamental rights protected by the legal order of the Community. It includes in particular a person's right to keep his state of health secret.
>
> Although the pre-employment medical examination serves a legitimate interest of the Community Institutions and, if the person concerned, after being properly informed, withholds his consent to

---

[26] X v. European Commission [1995] IRLR 320.

a test which the medical officer considers necessary in order to evaluate his suitability for the post for which he has applied, the Institutions cannot be obliged to take the risk of recruiting him, nevertheless that interest does not justify the carrying out of a test against the will of the person concerned.

The right to respect for private life requires that a person's refusal to undergo a test be respected in its entirety.

In the present case, since the appellant expressly refused to undergo an AIDS screening test, that right precluded the administration from carrying out any test liable to point to or establish the existence of that illness in respect of which he had refused disclosure.

Yet it was apparent that the lymphocyte count in question had provided the medical officer with sufficient information to conclude that the candidate might be carrying the AIDS virus.

The Court of First Instance had wrongly considered that there was an obligation to respect a refusal by the person concerned only in relation to the specific test for AIDS and that any other test could be carried out which might merely point to the possible presence of the AIDS virus.

Therefore the decision of the Court of First Instance would be annulled to the extent to which it held that the medical officer was entitled to request a lymphocyte count, as would the decision of the Commission informing the appellant that he did not satisfy the conditions as to physical fitness for recruitment.

The appellant's claim for compensation for non-material damage suffered by him had correctly been dismissed by the Court of First Instance on the grounds that the correct administrative procedure under the Staff Regulations had not been followed in relation to it.

12.5 Duty of confidentiality and medical ethics

Finally, it is not possible in this chapter to discuss the ethical questions, such as the duty of confidentiality and medical ethics, in any detail[27].

---

[27] General Medical Council's former 'Blue Book' — *Professional Conduct and Discipline: Fitness to Practise*, April 1995 and '*Duties of a Doctor*' *Guidance from the General Medical Council*, 1995; '*Philosophy and Practice of Medical Ethics*', BMA, 1988; The UKCC for Nursing, Midwifery and Health Visiting 'Code of Professional Conduct', November 1984; and Faculty of Occupational Medicine '*Guidance on Ethics for Occupational Physicians*', 4th edn, published November 1993, reprinted with supplement in February 1997.

Suffice it to say that, although there is no legal protection from the invasion to privacy, medical staff are under very strict ethical codes of conduct, and can be struck off the medical register for serious breaches.

Employers are not entitled to require their staff to undergo medical examinations without obtaining, on each occasion, the informed written consent of the individual — this means ensuring the employee understands the nature of the examination and tests and the reasons for them. Medical staff are best placed to ensure completion of the written consent forms.

Employers must also, on each occasion, obtain the employee's written informed consent to the disclosure of the results or outcome to the company (a senior named individual).

Failure to obtain these written consents will mean that no such medical examination or disclosure should take place.

12.6) European law

12.6.1 General

As a member state[28], when Directives are adopted by the Council of Ministers[29], they bind the member states. This means that the member states and any emanation of the state, including nationalised industries and former public utilities, are bound by the Directives, and their employees may sue for breach of an article of the Directive directly in the UK tribunals against their employer. Private sector employers are not directly bound by any Directive. It is a requirement that the member state adopts the Directive into its national legislation within a laid down timescale.

12.6.2 Qualified majority voting (QMV)

Certain matters do not require a unanimous vote of all the member

---

[28] The United Kingdom of Great Britain and Northern Ireland acceded to the Treaty of Rome on January 1, 1973. There are now 15 full member states.
[29] The Council of Ministers is represented by the appropriate minister from each member state. Each member state has a block vote, with the number of votes depending on the size of its population. Four member states have ten votes each (UK, Italy, Germany and France). Except on matters of health and safety and product safety, the votes must be unanimous in order for a Directive to be adopted. However, in 1987, under the Single European Act, two articles of the Treaty of Rome were altered, Article 188A (worker health and safety) and Article 110A (product safety). Such matters may be adopted with qualified majority voting (QMV).

states in the Council of Ministers. Those matters which involve workers' health and safety (under Article 118a of the Treaty of Rome) and product safety (under Article 110a) require only QMV, 62 out of the possible 87 votes.

12.6.3 Recommendations

The Council of Ministers can make Recommendations which have a certain force, although they are not legally binding. European Union (EU) Resolutions and Recommendations have legal effect, in particular, where they are able to clarify the interpretation of national provisions adopted in order to implement them or supplement binding Community measures.

In *Grimaldi* v. *Fonds Des Maladies Professionnelles*[30], a labourer mainly working in mining and construction suffered from osteoarticular or angioneurotic impairment of the hand. He contended that this should be recognised as an occupational disease, because he argued that it was caused by using a pneumatic drill.

The Belgium Ministry of Social Security (Fund for Occupational Diseases) rejected his claim because, they argued, the origins of the disease were not occupational. The expert report requested by the Labour Court concluded that Mr Grimaldi was suffering from 'Dupuytren's contracture' which did not appear on Belgium's Schedule of Occupational Diseases.

Mr Grimaldi argued that he was suffering from an 'illness from overexertion of the peritendinous tissue' which does appear on the European Schedule of Occupational Diseases. However, despite the Recommendation of the Commission, that Schedule had not been incorporated into Belgian law.

The ECJ ruled that:

> In light of Article 189(5) of the Treaty of Rome which provides that Recommendations … shall have no binding force, the Commission's Recommendations on the adoption of a European Schedule of Occupational Diseases and on the conditions for granting compensation to persons suffering from occupational diseases do not in themselves confer rights on individuals upon which they may rely before the national courts. Recommendations are generally adopted by the Institutions of the Community when under the Treaty they do not have the power to adopt binding acts or when

[30] *Grimaldi* v. *Fonds Des Maladies Professionnelles* [1990] IRLR 400.

they think that it is not appropriate to issue more constraining rules.

Although the choice of form cannot change the nature of an act, in the present case there was no doubt that the acts in question were true Recommendations which, even in regard to those to whom they were addressed, did not aim at producing binding effects. Therefore they could not create a right on which individuals could rely before a national court. However, the Commission Recommendations could not be considered as lacking in legal effect. National courts were bound to take Recommendations into consideration in order to decide disputes submitted to them, particularly where they clarify the interpretation of national provisions adopted in order to implement them or where they are designed to supplement binding Community measures.

12.6.4 Working Time Directive

The Working Time Directive was adopted under the QMV system, and requires member states to legislate for maximum working hours of 48 in any 7-day period, with rest breaks and restrictions on the number of hours of work that can be performed at night. It was adopted on November 23, 1993 with the UK abstaining. All the provisions, save for 4 weeks of paid annual leave, should have been introduced as national legislation in the UK by November 23, 1996. The minimum 4 weeks of paid leave need not be implemented until late 1999.

The Directive provides that workers are entitled to:

- a minimum daily rest period of one consecutive hour in each 24-h period;
- a rest break where the working day exceeds 6 h;
- a minimum uninterrupted weekly rest period of 24 h;
- at least 4 weeks of paid annual leave;
- restrictions on night work, including an average limit of 8 h in 24 h;
- organisation of work patterns to take account of health and safety requirements and the adaptation of work to the worker;
- an average working limit of 48 h over each 7-day period, calculated over a reference period of 4 months.

The Directive is littered with 'derogations' which exempt certain types of worker. Firstly, there are some general exceptions which exclude workers involved in the air, at sea, on rail and road, in inland waterways and lake transport and in sea fishing and other work at sea, and the activities of doctors in training. The major provisions for which there are no derogations are the 4 weeks of paid annual leave and the 48-h working week. Secondly, there may, through national legislation or collective agreements, be workers who are exempt, such as those whose working time is not measured, e.g. senior management or other persons with autonomous decision-taking powers, family workers and workers officiating at religious ceremonies.

In addition, workers may agree to work longer hours than those laid down in the Directive. In other cases, workers must be given compensatory rest breaks if they work in excess of the 48-h week, e.g. those whose jobs involve travelling, such as sales people, those engaged in certain security or surveillance work, those whose work requires continuity of service or production, those whose jobs involve a foreseeable surge of activity, e.g. in tourism, agriculture, etc., and those who are employed in jobs where unforeseen circumstances occur or where there is an accident or imminent risk of an accident.

The UK Government rejected this Directive as having been placed on the wrong legal basis, i.e. it should not have been adopted on the basis of QMV, and unsuccessfully challenged the Council of Ministers in the ECJ early in 1997[31]. The ECJ held that the Working Time Directive had been adopted correctly as a health and safety measure on the basis of Article 118a of the EC Treaty to which the qualified majority procedure applied.

12.6.5 Other Directives on health and safety

In January 1992, the UK introduced the 'Six Pack'[32], implementing EU Directives on a range of health and safety matters. These Regulations made it mandatory for employers to carry out risk assessments where there are 'significant and substantial risks to health or safety' and to appoint 'competent' persons to assist the employer in this task. Employers are required to keep these risk assessments up to date and to keep records of them.

---

[31] *United Kingdom of Great Britain and Northern Ireland* v. *Council of the European Union*, Case C-84/94 [1997] IRLR 30.

[32] The Management of Health and Safety at Work Regulations 1992; Health and Safety (Display Screen Equipment) Regulations 1992; Personal Protective Equipment at Work Regulations 1992; Provision and Use of Work Equipment Regulations 1992; Manual Handling Operations Regulations 1992; Workplace (Health, Safety and Welfare) Regulations 1992.

12.7 Disability Discrimination Act 1995

12.7.1 General

Under legislation that came into force on December 3, 1996, discrimination on the grounds of disability or relating to disability has been made unlawful in the field of employment, provision of goods and services and education.

Briefly, in the employment field[33], if an individual has a disability as defined under the Act, it is unlawful for an employer to subject him/her to a detriment, i.e. refuse to employ, provide less favourable terms or conditions, dismiss, etc., unless the employer has made all such reasonable efforts to make reasonable adjustments to the workplace and this has not been reasonably practicable, and the reason for the treatment is material to all the circumstances of the case and substantial.

12.7.2 Meaning of disability

A person with a disability is defined[34] as a person who 'has or has had a physical or mental impairment which has a substantial and long-term adverse effect on his ability to carry out normal day-to-day activities'. Normal day-to-day activities are defined as ranging from mobility and manual dexterity to perception of the risk of danger and memory or ability to concentrate, learn or understand[35].

The Minister stated in the House of Commons that 'substantial' in this context meant 'more than minor'. The Act does not define physical impairment.

12.7.3 Mental impairment

'Mental impairment' is defined as[36] 'a mental illness which is a clinically well recognised mental illness'. This would therefore include all mental disorders within the International Classification of Diseases (ICD) or Diagnostic and Statistical Manual of Mental Disorders (DSM) classifications. It excludes[37] addictions to alcohol, nicotine or any other controlled substances. Whether the definition would cover illness such as

---

[33] Part 11 of the Disability Discrimination Act 1995.
[34] Section 1 and Schedule 1 of the Disability Discrimination Act 1995 and The Meaning of Disability Regulations 1996.
[35] Schedule 1, paragraph 4.
[36] Schedule 1, paragraph 1(1).
[37] The Meaning of Disability Regulations 1996, paragraph 3.

CFS is debatable, and the employer in such circumstances would need expert guidance.

12.7.4 Exclusions

Other conditions, such as[38] a tendency to set fires, a tendency to steal, a tendency to physical or sexual abuse of other persons, exhibitionism and voyeurism, are also excluded from the scope of the Act.

12.7.5 Severe disfigurements

Severe disfigurements are included within the definition of 'disability', save for tattoos and piercing of the body for non-medical purposes.

12.7.6 Perceived disability

Although the Minister was at pains to state that any 'asymptomatic conditions', such as HIV or carriers of the Huntington's chorea gene, would not be covered by the Act, there is great debate as to whether in fact this is the correct interpretation of the Statute. The clinical sign of a condition, which may render the individual symptomless for some time, may have been confused with the 'symptoms' of a disability. It is certainly possible for someone with HIV who is harassed at work to argue that they have suffered discrimination on the grounds of their perceived disability.

12.7.7 Meaning of 'long term'

'Long term'[39] means a condition that has lasted or is likely to last for 12 months or more. It includes periods of remission, where the condition ceases for a period of time to have a substantial adverse effect, or where the individual is being treated with medication or uses a prosthesis or other aid[40].

12.7.8 Unlawful discrimination

The Act makes it unlawful for employers to discriminate in any way in relation to a person's disability, i.e. at recruitment, in their terms and conditions of employment and by dismissing them. This would include not only direct discrimination, but also indirect discrimination, such as having policies which provide that only full-time workers will be employed, only workers who are willing to work long hours, only

[38] The Meaning of Disability Regulations 1996, paragraph 4.
[39] Schedule 1, paragraph 2.
[40] Schedule 1, paragraph 6.

workers who can drive, etc. These policies or rules, which appear neutral, have an adverse impact upon many more disabled people. If the employer cannot 'justify' them, he/she will be guilty of unlawful discrimination.

12.7.9 Duty to make reasonable adjustments

Once the employer knows (or could reasonably be expected to know) about a disability, and the disabled person is at a substantial disadvantage as compared with an able-bodied person, the employer must make reasonable adjustments to the workplace[41], such as modifying the job duties, altering the terms and conditions, modifying the equipment, etc.

12.7.10 Further defence of 'justification'

Even if it is not reasonably practicable to make those adjustments, the employer must still satisfy the industrial tribunal that the reason for the discrimination was 'both material to the circumstances of the case and substantial'[42], i.e. justifiable. So, for example, a person applying for a job as a court stenographer who has rheumatoid arthritis in his/her wrists and hands could justifiably be rejected for that job.

The concept of 'material' as a defence has been defined in a leading equal pay case[43] as meaning 'significant and relevant'.

12.7.11 Advice needed

Employers will be relying upon the advice of their experts to guide them during the pre-employment stages and when an employee who has been injured or has suffered a serious illness is due to return to work. Similarly, in ill-health dismissals, careful consideration of the employer's duties under this Act will have to be given if the employer is not to fall foul of this new anti-discrimination statute.

For further reading on this subject, readers are referred to an excellent publication written by Professor Brian Doyle[44].

---

[41] This key duty is in Section 6 of the Disability Discrimination Act 1995.
[42] Section 5(3).
[43] *Rainey* v. *Greater Glasgow Health Board* [1987] IRLR 86.
[44] Doyle B. *Disability Discrimination — The New Law*, 2nd edn. Jordans, 1997.

13 Sources of Information

13.1 Introduction

Information is an integral part of everyday life. We need information to function and make decisions in our personal, social and work roles.

The field of occupational health is diverse, and no one individual can be expected to have a comprehensive knowledge in all aspects of this subject. New legislation and the quest for information reinforce the need for an awareness of how and where to access occupational health information sources. This chapter aims to identify some of the publications and organisations which assist the occupational health practitioner to find the relevant information.

13.1.1 Libraries and information centres

There are various research and professional bodies, government departments, hospitals and some university departments which have libraries/information centres, either with collections or the means to access occupational health and related discipline material. Examples are: the Institute of Occupational Health, University of Birmingham; the Institute of Occupational Medicine, Edinburgh and the Health and Safety Executive Information Service.

13.1.2 Textbooks

Books are an important source of information. The book consulted will depend on the type and level of information required. For basic information on occupational health or industrial processes, a good source is the '*ILO Encyclopaedia of Occupational Health and Safety*'. Although textbooks are an important source of information, it should be borne in mind that they may be 1 or 2 years out of date as a result of the inherent delays in the process of writing, publishing and printing. Some textbooks are published in loose-leaf format, which enables them to be updated at regular intervals, thereby overcoming the 'out of dateness' syndrome. Examples are those published by Croner Publications: '*Croner's Health and Safety at Work*' and '*Croner's Health and Safety Case Law*'.

13.1.3 Regulations/legislation

The Health and Safety Commission (HSC) is the regulatory body in the UK for health and safety, and issues Approved Codes of Practice and Guidance Notes. The HSC issues consultative documents, which are proposals for future regulations, and invites comments from individuals and organisations on the content. A list of consultative documents is available from HSE Books. In the USA, the Occupational Safety and Health Administration (OSHA) ensures compliance with standards in the workplace and in the development of regulations. The National Institute for Occupational Safety and Health (NIOSH) produces a comparable set of consultative documents with those produced by the HSC.

13.1.4 Directories/yearbooks

There are a number of relevant directories and yearbooks produced by professional organisations or commercial publishers which are normally published annually. Examples include Croner Publications' '*The Health and Safety at Work Directory*', RoSPA's '*Health and Safety Manager's Yearbook*' and The British Library's '*Guide to Libraries and Information Units in Government Departments and Other Organizations*'.

13.1.5 Journals

There are numerous journals, which may also be referred to as periodicals or serials, published in the field of occupational health and allied disciplines. They range from the serious academic research journal to the 'newsy' journal. The former usually contains peer-reviewed research articles. Journals are published weekly, monthly, bi-monthly or quarterly. The less frequently published journals tend to concentrate on the findings of academic research. In the academic/research journals, literature reviews are found which are a summary of work normally carried out by an expert within his/her own field. A literature review is a concise form of information, but it must be borne in mind that the reviewer has to be relied upon to include everything and to report the findings accurately.

Examples of some occupational health journals include: '*Occupational Medicine*', a quarterly publication which covers national and international perspective articles on occupational disease, book reviews and details of occupational health seminars; '*Occupational Health Review*', a bi-monthly publication covering news items relating to occupational health/health and safety and abstracts of journal articles from other publications; '*Occupational and Environmental Medicine*' (formerly *British Journal of Industrial Medicine*), which is published monthly and covers articles relating to occupational and environmental medicine and toxicological studies of industrial chemicals; the '*American Journal of Industrial Medicine*', which is published six times per year and contains national and international articles relating to occupational medicine and environmental health; another American journal, the

'*Journal of Occupational and Environmental Medicine*', which is published monthly and is an international publication containing articles, selected reviews of the literature and a calendar of meetings; the '*Scandinavian Journal of Work, Environment and Health*', an international scientific journal published six times per annum with supplements on a particular theme; in addition to articles on occupational medicine, the topics covered include toxicology, epidemiology and sociology; book reviews and announcements of relevant conferences are also given; '*The Annals of Occupational Hygiene*', a bi-monthly international journal containing reviews and research papers on risks and hazards in the workplace; its coverage includes the effects of chemical, physical and biological agents, epidemiology, occupational toxicology and book reviews; the '*AIHA Journal*', which is published monthly by the American Industrial Hygiene Association; it contains national and international articles on all aspects of occupational hygiene; and '*Applied Occupational and Environmental Hygiene*', which is a monthly American journal; the articles are original research reports and case studies, covering occupational hygiene, occupational and environmental epidemiology and applied environmental chemistry.

13.1.6 Reports

These may emanate from an authoritative body, such as the Health and Safety Executive (HSE), NIOSH, the European Foundation for the Improvement of Living and Working Conditions (EFILWC) and other organisations. A report may be the published findings of research undertaken by an expert or group of experts commissioned by a government department on a particular topic.

13.1.7 Standards

Standards are published documents that have been produced by a group of experts, which contain specifications to be used as rules or guidelines to ensure that materials, services and processes are fit for their purpose. Most countries have a national standards institution.

British Standards Institution (BSI) — UK

This is the UK national body concerned with the certification and assessment of products, methods of testing, etc., and provides the recommended standards governing work equipment and machinery. (Although not legally binding, most employers conform to BSI specifications.) There are approximately 650 standards relating to health and safety. A catalogue containing a numerical and a subject index is produced annually, and is updated by a monthly supplement. The catalogue is available on a subscription basis to BSI members; BSI members can purchase British Standards at a discount rate or borrow British Standards from the BSI library. Non-members can purchase British Standards direct from BSI or their agents. British Standards are held in some city public reference libraries and also some university libraries.

American National Standards Institute (ANSI) — USA
This was founded in 1918, and is a private, non-profit, membership organisation supported by both the private and public sector organisations.

Comité Européen de Normalisation
This is the European committee for standardisation which acts to harmonise standards across Europe.

Deutsches Institut für Normung (DIN) — Germany
This is the German Institute for Standardisation; it is a registered association and not a government agency.

L'Association Française de Normalisation (AFNOR) — France
This is the state-approved organisation in France, which comes under the auspices of the French Ministry of Industry.

International Organization for Standardization (ISO)
This is a world-wide federation of national standards organisations from approximately 100 countries. One of its aims is to promote the development of standardisation to improve health, safety and environmental protection. The ISO produces a number of publications which include the ISO catalogue, standards handbooks, guides and newsletters. ISO on-line is an electronic information service provided by the ISO central secretariat, and is available on the World Wide Web.

13.1.8 Statistical information
There is no single source of statistical information in Great Britain on the full nature and extent of occupational ill health. A starting point is the *Guide to Official Statistics* published by the Office for National Statistics. This has a subject listing, and identifies the relevant statistical publication to consult. Examples of publications covering occupational health

statistics include: the '*Occupational Health. Decennial Supplement. OPCS Series DS No. 10*', which contains chapters on the occupational mortality of men and women, asbestos-related diseases and occupational and sickness absence; and '*Health and Safety Statistics*', published as a supplement to the HSC/E's annual report. Statistics prior to 1992/1993 were published as a supplement to the '*Employment Gazette*' produced by the Department of Employment. The HSE has units which deal with occupational ill health statistics and injuries arising from accidents in the workplace. Other countries also have centres for the collection of statistics. In France, this is performed by the Institut National de la Statistique et des Etudes Economiques (INSEE). In the USA, the Bureau of Labor Statistics (BLS) collects annual statistics on occupational injuries, and undertakes a census of fatal occupational injuries. Eurostat collects statistical data from the national statistical centres of the 15 member states of the European Union (EU). The statistics are grouped under nine subjects, including the environment and population and social conditions. Eurostat publishes an annual catalogue of all its publications, and some products are available electronically.

13.1.9 Theses/dissertations

These are unpublished documents of research undertaken as part fulfilment for first and higher degrees. The Association for Information Management (ASLIB) produces an index to theses accepted for higher degrees by the Universities of Great Britain and Ireland.

13.1.10 Audio-visual material

Visual presentation can help an individual to retain knowledge and can help to reinforce a health and safety message. Various organisations produce videos, slides and tape/slide presentations in the field of occupational health, such as RoSPA, the British Safety Council and the HSE.

13.1.11 Microfiche

The Barbour Index on microfiche provides access to health and safety documents for occupational health professionals. The information on Barbour contains full text of health and safety legislation, British Standards and HSE Guidance Notes. The Barbour Index is useful to those who have limited storage space and no easy access to library facilities.

13.2) Abstracting/indexing services

These aid in the location of references to publications, which are either in printed format or as databases. References to journal articles appear in the abstracting/indexing services any time from 2 months to 2 years after they were published.

13.2.1 Printed

An indexing service provides author, title and subject access to a particular journal title. For example the journal, '*Scandinavian Journal of Work, Environment and Health*', produces an annual cumulative index to articles that have appeared in that journal for a particular year. An abstracting service, however, cites references to more than one journal and includes an abstract of the article. One example is '*Selected Abstracts on Occupational Diseases*', produced by the UK Department of Social Security Library; it is published six times per annum.

13.2.2 Databases

A database is 'a collection of data or information, usually with a common subject theme', and may be available as a CD-ROM or on-line.

CD-ROM databases

With the increasing use of computers, printed indexing and abstracting sources are slowly declining. Most people have access to CD-ROM databases. (CD-ROM is an acronym for Computer Disk Read Only Memory.) These disks are similar to CD music disks, the obvious difference being that the former stores pages of text. There are bibliographic and full text databases; the former gives citations and abstracts to books, reports and journals in various subject areas; the latter provides publications in full on the database. There are numerous databases available on occupational health and related disciplines.

ACOEM/Physicians' Silver Platter

Occupational and environmental medicine. A bibliographic database that contains over 630 000 citations and abstracts from 1966 to the present from occupational and environmental medicine journals. It also includes the full text of the '*Journal of Occupational and Environmental Medicine*' from 1995 onwards, and a drug information handbook.

CHEMINFO

A full text database produced by the Canadian Center for Occupational Health providing details of the health effects of chemicals, personal protective equipment, trade names and regulatory requirements. Although the latter relates to Canadian legislation, the EU classification and labelling requirements have recently been introduced. The health hazard information is applicable in any country.

CINAHL

This is the database version of the printed '*Cumulative Index to Nursing and Allied Health Literature*', and contains references to nursing and allied health subjects. It is available from Silver Platter.

EuroOSH

A full text database produced by Chapman and Hall Electronic Publishing Division. It includes the occupational safety and health databases of the EU and member state legislation, with International Labour Organization (ILO) Conventions and Recommendations.

OSH-ROM

A bibliographic database produced by Silver Platter. There are four databases on OSH-ROM: CISDOC produced by the ILO; HSELINE produced by the HSE, UK; NIOSHTIC produced by NIOSH, USA; and MHIDAS developed by AEA Technology plc. There are approximately 350 000 records on these databases. The first three databases are extremely valuable when undertaking literature searches on topics pertinent to occupational health. The records date back to the 1970s, although there are earlier references which are considered to be of historical significance. The records contain citations and abstracts to journal articles, books and reports. The MHIDAS database is not as comprehensive, and provides limited details of chemical incidents that have occurred world-wide.

OSH-UK

A full text database produced by the HSE and published by The Stationery Office (formerly Her Majesty's Stationery Office, HMSO). It contains the full text of all HSE publications, including Approved Codes of Practice, Guidance Notes and leaflets and abstracts of British Standards relating to health and safety.

RTECS (Register of Toxic Effects of Chemical Substances)

Produced by the Canadian Center for Occupational Health, this is another full text database which provides information on chemicals and health hazards, and whether the substance has been investigated as a mutagen or carcinogen.

TOXLINE

This is produced by the USA National Library of Medicine and supplied by Silver Platter and CCINFO. It is an international bibliographic database which gives citations and abstracts to journal articles, books and reports. The records date from 1966 to the present day.

There are also textbooks now available on CD-ROM, e.g. the new edition of the '*ILO Encyclopaedia of Occupational Health*', '*SAX's Dangerous Properties of Industrial Materials*' and '*Hawley's Condensed Chemical Dictionary*'.

On-line databases

The term 'on-line' means that the database is searched via telecommunication lines to a remote host, e.g. Datastar in Switzerland, which hosts, amongst others, MEDLINE. The British Medical Association (BMA) library offers its members a MEDLINE service (for further details, contact the BMA). The advantage of using on-line databases is that they are usually updated monthly, compared with CD-ROM databases which are usually updated quarterly. The CD-ROM databases mentioned previously are also available as on-line databases.

- CISDOC. Provider: IRS Dialtech.
- HSELINE. Provider: IRS Dialtech, Knight Ridder Information Ltd.
- NIOSHTIC. Provider: Knight Ridder Information Ltd.

13.3 Internet

Another source of information is the Internet (INTERnational NETwork). In essence, the Internet is a large number of linked computer networks forming a global network — a communications network which is growing rapidly.

Information is available on a wide range of subjects via many different sources. You can use the Internet to:

- send e-mail all over the world;
- access library catalogues world-wide;
- access databases for references and abstracts — some are free of charge;
- join a mailing list for specialist subjects;
- consult specialist bulletin boards;
- find information on organisations/associations;
- consult journals, e.g. *British Medical Journal/The Lancet*.

Anyone can access or place information on the Internet. At present, there are no formal guidelines as to who places or what information is placed on the Internet. Therefore, the Internet should be used with caution; when using the Internet try to ensure that you use authoritative sites. Many professional organisations/associations have a 'home page' on the Internet giving details about that organisation and, in some cases, links to other sites. The Institute of Occupational Health (IOH) has its own home page on the Internet, which gives details of postgraduate courses and seminars organised by the IOH; the full text of the IOH's bulletin also appears.

The **W**orld **W**ide **W**eb is the hypertext system (contains links to documents) used for searching the Internet.

13.4 Organisations, associations and libraries

There are a number of organisations with an interest in occupational health. The HSE publishes a document entitled, '*Directory of Organisations Concerned with Health and Safety Information: UK and Worldwide*', which is available from HSE Books. These organisations provide information and advice on most aspects of occupational health.

13.4.1 Canadian Center for Occupational Health and Safety (CCOHS)

This is Canada's national centre for occupational health and safety information. It is a corporation governed by a council, and has representatives from government, labour and employees. Its aim is to provide health and safety in the workplace by supplying accurate, impartial information to employers and employees. It provides an information service to the workforce of Canada, publishes a newsletter and documents on health and safety and produces several CD-ROM databases and on-line databases.

13.4.2 Health and Safety Executive (HSE)

This is the regulatory body concerned with health and safety issues in the UK. It produces a wide range of publications, such as consultative documents, Approved Codes of Practice, an annual report, plan of work and leaflets. The information in the leaflets is very general and written in layman's terms, but some leaflets provide references for further reading or points of contact for advice. Some leaflets are free of charge and can be obtained from HSE Books in Sudbury. There is a catalogue of free HSE publications and a catalogue of current priced HSE publications; both are available from HSE Books.

13.4.3 International Agency for Research on Cancer (IARC)

IARC was established in 1965 by the World Health Assembly, within the framework of the World Health Organization (WHO). IARC carries out research programmes into the epidemiology of cancer and the study of potential carcinogens in its own laboratory in Lyon, and also with other international research organisations. The findings are published as IARC Monographs on the Evaluation of Carcinogenic Risks to Humans, IARC Scientific Publications or IARC Technical Reports.

13.4.4 International Commission on Occupational Health (ICOH)

This is a professional organisation whose aim is to produce knowledge and development of all matters concerning occupational health and safety. There are 27 scientific committees who organise meetings, seminars and publish various publications including a 'Code of Ethics'. An international congress is held every 3 years.

13.4.5 International Labour Organization (ILO)

The ILO was created in 1919, the initial aim being to safeguard the health of the international workforce. Its first annual International Labour Conference in 1919 adopted six ILO Conventions, which dealt with hours of work in industry, unemployment, maternity protection, night work for women and minimum age and night work for young people in industry. To date, 180 Conventions and 187 Recommendations have been made by the ILO. In 1959, the ILO established the International Occupational Safety and Health Information Centre (CIS). The aim was to collect all relevant information published on occupational health and safety world-wide. In 1973, this information was computerised, and is still available as the database 'CISDOC' today. CIS is a world-wide service; there are 120 national and collaborating centres.

13.4.6 National Institute for Occupational Safety and Health (NIOSH)

This is a US federal agency established by the Occupational Safety and Health Act of 1970. It is part of the Centers for Disease Control and Prevention (CDC), and undertakes research and makes recommendations for the prevention of illnesses and injuries in the workplace. It produces a directory, publishes numerous publications on occupational and related topics and organises conferences and seminars.

13.4.7 Occupational Safety and Health Group (OSHIG)

This has been in existence since 1990, and is a network of specialists in the health, safety, fire, environment and chemical areas. Members range from health and safety practitioners, information specialists, government and institutional members to chemists and software specialists. The aims and objectives of OSHIG are to promote awareness of the latest information in their members' subject areas, to provide a forum for sharing experiences, views and information and to disseminate information primarily to its members, but also to other relevant bodies through conferences, exhibitions and its quarterly newsletters.

13.4.8 World Health Organization (WHO)

This organisation was established in 1948. The head office is in Geneva and there are six regional offices. The aim of WHO is to ensure that people throughout the world attain the highest possible level of health as defined in its constitution. It has a wide range of duties, including the promotion of environmental hygiene and the coordination of biomedical and health services research. It also proposes conventions and regulations on causes of death and public health practices.

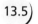

13.5 Further reading

This is not a comprehensive list and is only intended as a guide.

13.5.1 Epidemiology

Hernberg, S. *Introduction to Occupational Epidemiology*. Chelsea, MI, Lewis Publishers, 1992.

Lilienfeld, D.E. and Stolley, P.D. *Foundations of Epidemiology*, 3rd edn. Oxford, Oxford University Press, 1994.

McDonald, J.C. *Epidemiology of Work Related Diseases*. London, BMJ Books, 1995.

Monson, R.R. *Occupational Epidemiology*, 2nd edn. Boca Raton, FL, CRC Press, 1990.

Olsen, J., Merletti, F., Snashall, D. and Voylsteek, K. *Searching for Causes of Work-related Diseases*. Oxford, Oxford Medical Publications, 1991.

Steenland, K. (ed). *Case Studies in Occupational Epidemiology*. Oxford, Oxford University Press, 1993.

13.5.2 Occupational and environmental cancer/carcinogens

IARC Monographs on the Evaluation of Carcinogenic Risks to Humans. Since 1969, the IARC has produced critically evaluated monographs on the carcinogenic risk to humans of individual chemicals. IARC Monographs are distributed by WHO, and are available in the UK through The Stationery Office (London Office).

13.5.3 Occupational health and safety

Croner's Health and Safety at Work. Croner Publications Ltd, Croner House, London Road, Kingston upon Thames, Surrey, KT2 6SR. (Loose-leaf publication, updated quarterly by annual subscription.)

Holt St John, A. *Principles of Health and Safety at Work*, 2nd edn. Leicester, IOSH, 1993.

Ridley, J. *Safety at Work*, 4th edn. Oxford, Butterworth–Heinemann, 1994.

Stellman, J.M. (ed). *Encyclopaedia of Occupational Health and Safety*, 4 Vols. 4th edn. Geneva, International Labour Organization, 1998.

13.5.4 Occupational health and safety law

Barrett, B. and Howells, R. *Occupational Health and Safety Law*, 3rd edn. London, Pitman, M & E Handbooks, 1997.

Croner's Health and Safety Case Law Index. Croner Publications Ltd, Croner House, London Road, Kingston upon Thames, Surrey, KT2 6SR. (Loose-leaf publication, updated quarterly by annual subscription.)

Dewis, M. *Tolley's Health and Safety at Work Handbook*, 8th edn. Croydon, Surrey, Tolley Publishing, 1996.

Health and Safety Executive. *List of Current Health and Safety Legislation*. Sudbury, Suffolk, HSE Books (annual publication).

Kloss, D.M. *Occupational Health Law*, 2nd edn. Oxford, Blackwell Scientific Publications, 1994.

Neal, A.C. and Wright F.B. *European Communities' Health and Safety Legislation*, Vol 1. London, Chapman and Hall, 1992.

Neal, A.C. and Wright F.B. *European Communities' Health and Safety Legislation*, Vol 2. London, Chapman and Hall, 1996.

Neal, A.C. and Wright F.B. *European Communities' Health and Safety Legislation*, Vol 3. London, Chapman and Hall, 1996.

Treitel, G.H. *The Law of Contract*, 9th edn. London, Sweet & Maxwell, 1995.

Wallington, P. (ed). *Butterworth's Employment Law Handbook*, 7th edn. London, Butterworth, 1996.

Wikeley, N. *Compensation for Industrial Disease*. Aldershot, Dartmouth, 1993.

13.5.5 Occupational hygiene

Ashton, I. and Gill, F.S. *Monitoring for Health Hazards at Work*, 2nd edn. Oxford, Blackwell Science, 1992.

Clayton, G.D. and Clayton, F.E. *Patty's Industrial Hygiene and Toxicology*, Vols 1, 2A, 2B, 2C, 3A and 3B. New York, John Wiley, 1991–1994.

Croner's Handbook of Occupational Hygiene. Croner Publications Ltd, Croner House, London Road, Kingston upon Thames, Surrey, KT2 6SR (volume loose-leaf publication, updated periodically).

Harrington, J.M. and Gardiner, K. (eds). *Occupational Hygiene*, 2nd edn. Oxford, Blackwell Science, 1995.

Roach, S. *Health Risks from Hazardous Substances at Work: Assessment, Evaluation and Control*. Oxford, Pergamon Press, 1992.

13.5.6 Occupational lung disorders

Morgan, W.K.C. and Seaton, A. (eds). *Occupational Lung Diseases*, 3rd edn. Philadelphia, PA, WB Saunders, 1995.

....

Parkes, W.R. *Occupational Lung Disorders*, 3rd edn. Oxford,
   Butterworth–Heinemann, 1994.

13.5.7 Occupational medicine

Cox, R.A.F., Edwards, F.C. and McCallum, R.I. (eds). *Fitness for Work. The Medical Aspects*, 2nd edn. Oxford, Oxford Medical Publications, 1995.

Levy, B.S. and Wegman, D.H. *Occupational Health: Recognizing and Preventing Work-related Disease*, 3rd edn. Boston, Little, Brown and Co, 1994.

Raffle, P.A.B., Adams, P.H., Baxter, P.J. and Lee, W.R. (eds). *Hunter's Diseases of Occupations*, 8th edn. London, Edward Arnold, 1994 (new edition due for publication late in 1998).

Waldron, H.A. *Lecture Notes on Occupational Medicine*, 4th edn. Oxford, Blackwell Scientific Publications, 1990.

13.5.8 Statistics

Campbell, M.J. and Machin, D. *Medical Statistics. A Commonsense Approach*, 2nd edn. New York, John Wiley, 1994.

Castle, W.M. and North, P.M. *Statistics in Small Doses*, 3rd edn. Edinburgh, Churchill Livingstone, 1995.

OPCS. *Occupational Health. Decennial Supplement. Series DS No. 10*. London, HMSO, 1995.

13.5.9 Toxicology

American Conference of Governmental Industrial Hygienists. *Documentation of the Threshold Limit Values (TLV) and Biological Exposure Indices (BEI)*, 6th edn. Cincinnati, OH, ACGIH, 1991/1992 (3 volumes). (Useful summaries of toxicological data for all substances with a TLV.)

Budavari, S. (ed). *The Merck Index*, 12th edn. Encyclopaedia of Chemicals, Drugs and Biologicals. With Cross-Index of Names, Trade Names and CAS Registry Numbers. Merck and Co, 1996.

ECETOC. Technical Reports. A series of summaries of toxicological data produced by the European Chemical Industry Ecology and Toxicology Centre (ECETOC). Brussels, ECETOC. Particularly useful is Technical Report No. 71, Inventory of Critical Reviews on Chemicals: a comprehensive listing of chemical substances with references to reviews on their toxicology.

Hathaway, G.J., Proctor, N.H. and Hughes, J.P. *Chemical Hazards in the Workplace*, 4th edn. New York, Van Nostrand Reinhold, 1996.

HSE. *Risk Assessment Documents*. Sudbury, Suffolk, HSE Books. (Replaces *HSE Toxicity Reviews* and *HSE Criteria Documents*. Available from Dillons Bookstore and The Stationery Office.)

HSE. *Occupational Exposure Limits EH40*. Sudbury, Suffolk, HSE Books. (Published and revised annually. Gives advice on UK limits for exposure to airborne substances in the workplace. Available from Dillons Bookstore and The Stationery Office.)

Klaassen, C.D. (ed). *Casarett and Doull's Toxicology: The Basic Science of Poisons*, 5th edn. New York, McGraw-Hill, 1996.

Lewis, R.J. *Hawley's Condensed Chemical Dictionary*, 12th edn. New York, Van Nostrand Reinhold, 1993.

Lewis, R.J and Sax, N.I. *Dangerous Properties of Industrial Materials*, 9th edn. New York, Van Nostrand Reinhold, 1996.

Lu, F.C. *Basic Toxicology: Fundamentals, Target Organs and Risk Assessment*, 3rd edn. London, Taylor & Francis, 1996.

Timbrell, J.A. *Introduction to Toxicology*, 2nd edn. London, Taylor & Francis, 1995.

WHO/IPCS Environmental Health Criteria Documents. Geneva, World Health Organization. The International Programme on Chemical Safety (IPCS) is a joint venture of the United Nations Environment Programme, the International Labour Office and WHO. The main function of the IPCS is to evaluate the effects of chemicals on human health and the environment. The evaluations are published by WHO as Environmental Health Criteria Documents. In the UK, WHO publications are available from The Stationery Office (London Office).

13.5.10 References

Brammer, A.J., Taylor, W. and Lundborg, C. (1987) Sensorineural stages of the hand–arm vibration syndrome. *Scandinavian Journal of Work, Environment and Health*, **13** (4), 279–283.

CIBS Guide Section C4, published by the Chartered Institute of Building Services (CIBS).

Fletcher, B. (1977) Centreline velocity characteristics of rectangular unflanged hoods and slots under suction. *Annals of Occupational Hygiene*, **20**, 141–146.

Fletcher, B. (1978) Effect of flanges on the velocity in front of exhaust ventilation hoods. *Annals of Occupational Hygiene*, **21**, 265–269.

Gemne, G., Pykko, L., Taylor, W. and Pelmear P. The Stockholm Workshop scale for the classification of cold-induced Raynaud's phenomenon in the hand–arm vibration syndrome (revision of the Taylor–Pelmear scale). *Scandinavian Journal of Work, Environment and Health*, **13** (4), 275–278.

Gill, F.S. (1980) The energy implications of ventilation systems — an introductory outline. *Annals of Occupational Hygiene*, **23**, 423–433.

Griffin, M.J. (1990) *Handbook of Human Vibration*. Academic Press, London.

Olishifski, J.B. (1988) Methods of control. In *Fundamentals of Industrial Hygiene* (ed. B.A. Plog), 3rd edn. Chicago, National Safety Council.

13.6 Useful addresses

13.6.1 Advisory and information services/information providers

AEA Technology plc, Thomson House, Risley, Warrington, Cheshire WA3 6AT
Tel: +44 (0) 1925 252000
Fax: +44 (0) 1925 254535
E-mail: enquiry@aeat.co.uk
http://www.aeat.co.uk/

ASLIB, The Association for Information Management, Information House, 20–24 Old Street, London EC1V 9AP
Tel: +44 (0) 171 253 4488
Fax: +44 (0) 171 430 0514
E-mail: aslib@aslib.co.uk
http://www.aslib.co.uk/contact.html

Barbour Index plc, New Lodge, Drift Road, Windsor, Berkshire SL4 4RQ
Tel: +44 (0) 1344 884121

Fax: +44 (0) 1344 884845
http://www.barbour.org.uk

The British Library, 25 Southampton Buildings, Chancery Lane, London WC2A
1AW
Tel: +44 (0) 171 323 7949
http://portico.bl.uk

CIS, International Occupational Safety and Health Information Centre, ILO-CIS,
CH-1211, Geneva 22, Switzerland
Tel: +41 22 799 67 40
Fax: +41 22 799 85 16
E-mail: cis@ilo.org
http://turva.me.tut.fi/cis/home.html

Croner Publications, Croner House, London Road, Kingston upon Thames, Surrey
KT2 6SR
Tel: +44 (0) 181 547 3333
Fax: +44 (0) 181 547 2637
E-mail: info@croner.co.uk
http://www.croner.co.uk/

Department of Social Security Library, The Adelphi, Room 637, 1–11 John Adam
Street, London WC2N 6HT
Tel: +44 (0) 171 712 2500
Fax: +44 (0) 171 962 8491
http://www.dss.gov.uk

HSE Books, PO Box 1999, Sudbury, Suffolk CO10 6FS
Tel: +44 (0) 1787 881165
Fax: +44 (0) 1787 313995

Health and Safety Executive, Information Centre, Health and Safety Laboratory,
Broad Lane, Sheffield S3 7HQ
Tel: +44 (0) 541 545500
http://www.open.gov.uk/hse/hsehome.htm

Institute of Occupational Health, University of Birmingham, Edgbaston,
Birmingham B15 2TT
Tel: +44 (0) 121 414 6029
Fax: +44 (0) 121 414 6217
E-mail: c.a.mcroy@bham.ac.uk
http://www.birmingham.ac.uk/IOH

OSHIG, Mrs C.A. McRoy (Secretary), c/o Institute of Occupational Health, University
of Birmingham, Edgbaston, Birmingham B15 2TT
Tel: +44 (0) 121 414 6029
Fax: +44 (0) 121 414 6217
E-mail: c.a.mcroy@bham.ac.uk
http://www.panizzi.shef.ac.uk/oshig/oshig.html/

RoSPA, Edgbaston Park, 353 Bristol Road, Birmingham B5 7ST
Tel: +44 (0) 121 248 2000
Fax: +44 (0) 121 248 2001

The Stationery Office, Publications Centre, PO Box 276, London SW78 5DT
Tel: +44 (0) 171 873 0011
Fax: +44 (0) 171 873 8200
E-mail: book.orders@theso.co.uk
http://www.the-stationery-office.co.uk/

13.6.2 Audio-visual material
The British Film Institute, 21 Stephen Street, London W1P 2LN
Tel: +44 (0) 171 255 1444
Fax: +44 (0) 171 436 7950

The British Safety Council, National Safety Centre, Chancellors Road, London
    W6 9RS
Tel: +44 (0) 181 600 5581
Fax: +44 (0) 181 741 0835
E-mail: bscl@britishsafetycouncil.co.uk
http://www.britishsafetycouncil.co.uk

CFL Vision, PO Box 35, Wetherby, West Yorkshire LS23 7EX
Tel: +44 (0) 1937 541010
Fax: +44 (0) 1937 541083

13.6.3 Database providers
Canadian Center for Occupational Health and Safety (CCOHS), 250 Main Street
    East, Hamilton, Ontario, Canada L8N 1H6
Tel: +1 905 570 8094
Fax: +1 905 572 2206
E-mail: custserv@ccohs.ca
http://www.ccohs.c.ccohs/about.html/

Chapman and Hall Electronic Publishing Division, 2–6 Boundary Row, London
    SE1 8HN
Tel: +44 (0) 171 865 0066
Fax: +44 (0) 171 522 0101
E-mail: cust.serv@chall.co.uk

IRS Dialtech, The British Library, Science Reference and Information Service, 25
    Southampton Buildings, Chancery Lane, London WC2A 1AW
Tel: +44 (0) 171 412 7951
Fax: +44 (0) 171 412 7954
E-mail: irs.dialtech@bl.uk
http://www.icarus.bl.uk/sris/irs.html

Knight Ridder Information Ltd, Haymarket House, 1 Oxenden Street, London
    SW17 4EE
Tel: +44 (0) 171 839 9336

Fax: +44 (0) 171 930 2581
http://www.rs.ch/

Silver Platter Information Ltd, 10 Barley Mow Passage, Chiswick, London W4 4PH
Tel: +44 (0) 181 995 8242
Fax: +44 (0) 181 995 5159
E-mail: uk-ireland@silverplatter.com
http://www.silverplatter.com

13.6.4 International organisations/sources

American Conference of Governmental Industrial Hygienists (ACGIH), 1330
    Kemper Meadow Drive, Cincinnati OH 45240, USA
Tel: +44 (0) 513 742 2020
Fax: +44 (0) 513 742 3355
http://www.acgih.org/

Canadian Center for Occupational Health and Safety, 250 Main Street East,
    Hamilton, Ontario, Canada L8N 1H6
Tel: +1 905 570 8094
Fax: +1 905 572 2206
E-mail: custserv@ccohs.ca
http://www.ccohs.ca/

European Foundation for the Improvement of Living and Working Conditions
    (EFILWC), Wyatville Road, Loughlinstown, Co Dublin, Ireland
Tel: +00 353 1 204 3100
Fax: +00 353 1 282 6456
E-mail: postmaster@eurofound.ie
http://europa.eu.int/agencies/efilwc/index.htm

European Chemical Industry Ecology and Toxicology Centre (ECETOC), Avenue
    Louise 250, B. 63, B-1050, Brussels, Belgium
Tel: +02 649 9480
Fax: +02 649 2724

IARC, 150 cours Albert-Thomas, 69372 Lyon Cedex 08, France
Tel: 00 33 7273 8485
Fax: 00 33 7273 8575
http:// /www.iarc.fr/

ICOH, Department of Community, Occupational and Family Medicine, National
    University Hospital, Lower Kent Ridge Road, S(0511), Republic of Singapore
Tel: 00 65 774 9300
Fax: 00 65 779 1489

ILO (London Office), Millbank Tower, 21–24 Millbank, London SW1P 4QP
Tel: +44 (0) 171 828 6401
Fax: +44 (0) 171 233 5925

National Institute for Occupational Safety and Health (NIOSH), 4676 Columbia
    Parkway, Cincinnati OH 45226, USA

....

Fax: 00 1 513 533 8588
http://www.cdc.gov/niosh/homepage.html

OSHA, US Department of Labor, 200 Constitution Avenue, Washington DC 20210,
    USA
http://www.osha.gov

World Health Organization (WHO), 20 avenue Appia, CH-1211, Geneva 27,
    Switzerland
Tel: +41 22 791 2111
Fax: +41 22 791 0746
E-mail: postmaster@who.ch
http://www.who.ch:80/

13.6.5 Journals — publishers

AIHA Journal, PO Box 27632, Richmond, VA 23261–7632, USA
E-mail: infonet@aiha-org

American Journal of Industrial Medicine, John Wiley and Sons, Subscription
    Department, 9th Floor, 605 Third Avenue, New York, NY 10158–0012, USA
Tel: 212 850 6645

Annals of Occupational Hygiene, Elsevier Science Customer Service Department,
    PO Box 211, 1001 AE Amsterdam, The Netherlands
Tel: 31 20 485 3757
Fax: 31 20 485 3432
E-mail: nlinfo-f@elsvier.nl

Applied Occupational and Environmental Hygiene, Elsevier Science Customer
    Service Department, PO Box 211, 1001 AE Amsterdam, The Netherlands
Tel: 31 20 485 3757
Fax: 31 20 485 3432
E-mail: nlinfo-f@elsvier.nl

Journal of Occupational and Environmental Medicine, Williams and Wilkins, 351
    West Camden Street, Baltimore MD 21201–2436, USA
E-mail: custserv@wwilkins.com
http://www.wwilkins.com

Occupational and Environmental Medicine, BMJ Publishing Group, Journals
    Marketing Department, PO Box 299, London WC1H 9JP
Tel: +44 (0) 171 383 6415
Fax: +44 (0) 171 383 66661
E-mail: bmjsubs@dial.pipex.com

Occupational Health, Reed Business Information Ltd, Haywards Heath, West Sussex
    RH16 3BR
Tel: +44 (0) 1444 445566
Fax: +44 (0) 1444 445599

....

Occupational Health Review, Industrial Relations Services, 18–20 Highbury Place,
    London N5 1QP
Tel: +44 (0) 171 354 5858
Fax: +44 (0) 171 226 8618

Occupational Medicine, International Thomson Publishing Services (ITPS), Cheriton
    House, Northway, Andover, Hampshire, SP10 5BE
Tel: +44 (0) 1264 342713
Fax: +44 (0) 1264 342807
E-mail: christine.allingham.@itps.co.uk

Scandinavian Journal of Work, Environment and Health, Topeliuksenkatu 41 aA,
    FIN - 00250, Helsinki, Finland
Tel: 00 358 0 9 47 471
Fax: 00 358 0 9 878 3326
E-mail: maj-britt.vaariskoski@occuphealth.fi
http://paja.occcuphealth.fi/sjweh

13.6.6 Professional organisations

British Medical Association, BMA House, Tavistock Square, London WC1H 9JP
Tel: +44 (0) 171 387 4499
Fax: +44 (0) 171 388 2544
http:/www.bma.org.uk/

British Occupational Hygiene Society (BOHS) and the British Institute of
    Occupational Hygienists, Suite 2, Georgian House, Great Northern Road, Derby
    D21 1LT
Tel: +44 (0) 1332 298101
Fax: +44 (0) 1332 298099
E-mail: 100705.3356@compuserve.com
http://www.ed.ac.uk/~robin/bohs.html

Faculty of Occupational Medicine, Royal College of Physicians, 6 St Andrews Place,
    Regents Park, London NW1 4LB
Tel: +44 (0) 171 487 3414
Fax: +44 (0) 171 935 2259

Royal College of Nursing, 20 Cavendish Square, London W1M 0AB
Tel: +44 (0) 171 409 3333

13.6.7 Standards

AFNOR, Tour Europe, 92049 Paris la Défénse Cedex, France
Tel: +33 1 4291 5555
Fax: +33 1 4291 5656
E-mail: info@bsi.org.uk
http://www.afnor.fr/english/welcome.htm

ANSI, 11 West 42nd Street, New York, NY 10036, USA
Tel: 212 642 4900
Fax: 212 398 0023
http://www.ansi.org/ansi_top.html

BSI, British Standards House, 389 Chiswick High Road, London W4 4AL
Tel: +44 (0) 181 996 9000
Fax: +44 (0) 181 996 7400
E-mail: info@bsi.org.uk

CEN, Comité Européen de Normalisation, rue de Stassart 36, B-1050 Brussels, Belgium

DIN, Burggafenstrasse 6, D-10787 Berlin, Germany
Tel: +49 30 26010
Fax: +49 30 26011231
E-mail: postmaster@din.de
http://www.din.de
ISO, 1 rue de Varembé, Case postale 56, CH 1211, Geneva 20, Switzerland
Tel: +41 22 7490111
Fax: +41 22 7333430
E-mail: central@iso.ch
http://www.iso.ch/

13.6.8 Statistics

Bureau of Labor Statistics, Division of Safety and Health Statistics, Office of Safety, Health and Working Conditions, US Department of Labor, 2 Massachusetts Avenue NE, Washington DC 20212, USA
Tel: 202 606 6179
Fax: 203 606 6196
E-mail: oshstaff@bls.gov
http://stats.bls.gov/oshhome.htm
Eurostat, 2 rue mercier, L 2985, Luxembourg
Tel: +35 2 29291
E-mail: info.desk@eurostat.cec.be
http://europa.eu.int/en/communication/eurostat/

Health and Safety Executive, Epidemiology and Medical Statistics Unit, Room 244, Magdalen House, Stanley Precinct, Bootle, Merseyside L20 3QZ
Tel: +44 (0) 151 951 4540
http://www.open.gov.uk/hse/gap.htm

Health and Safety Executive (Injuries Occurring in the Workplace), Operations Unit, Room 512, Daniel House, Bootle, Merseyside L20 3QZ
Tel: +44 (0) 151 951 4604
http://www.open.gov.uk/hse/gap.htm

Index

Index

....